The Physiological Basis of
Veterinary Clinical Pharmacology

The Physiological Basis of Veterinary Clinical Pharmacology

J. Desmond Baggot, MVM, PhD, DSc, FRCVS

Formerly Professor of Preclinical Veterinary Studies, Faculty of
Veterinary Science, University of Zimbabwe, Harare and Professor of
Clinical Pharmacology, School of Veterinary Medicine, University of
California, Davis.

**Blackwell
Science**

© 2001 by
Blackwell Science Ltd
Editorial Offices:
Osney Mead, Oxford OX2 0EL
25 John Street, London WC1N 2BS
23 Ainslie Place, Edinburgh EH3 6AJ
350 Main Street, Malden
  MA 02148 5018, USA
54 University Street, Carlton
  Victoria 3053, Australia
10, rue Casimir Delavigne
  75006 Paris, France

Other Editorial Offices:

Blackwell Wissenschafts-Verlag GmbH
Kurfürstendamm 57
10707 Berlin, Germany

Blackwell Science KK
MG Kodenmacho Building
7–10 Kodenmacho Nihombashi
Chuo-ku, Tokyo 104, Japan

Iowa State University Press
A Blackwell Science Company
2121 S. State Avenue
Ames, Iowa 50014-8300, USA

First published 2001

Set in 10/12.5 pt Palatino
by DP Photosetting, Aylesbury, Bucks
Printed and bound in Great Britain by
MPG Books Ltd, Bodmin, Cornwall

DISTRIBUTORS

Marston Book Services Ltd
PO Box 269
Abingdon
Oxon OX14 4YN
(*Orders:* Tel: 01235 465500
        Fax: 01235 465555)

USA and Canada
  Iowa State University Press
  A Blackwell Science Company
  2121 S. State Avenue
  Ames, Iowa 50014-8300
  (*Orders:* Tel: 800-862-6657
        Fax: 515-292-3348
        Web www.isupress.com
        email: orders@isupress.com

Australia
  Blackwell Science Pty Ltd
  54 University Street
  Carlton, Victoria 3053
  (*Orders:* Tel: 03 9347 0300
        Fax: 03 9347 5001)

A catalogue record for this title
is available from the British Library

ISBN 0-632-05744-0

Library of Congress
Cataloging-in-Publication Data
is available

For further information on
Blackwell Science, visit our website:
www.blackwell-science.com

Contents

Preface   vii

Acknowledgements   ix

Terms and Abbreviations   x

Author's Note   xii

1   The Pharmacokinetic Basis of Species Variations in Drug
    Disposition   1

2   The Concept of Bioavailability and Applications to Veterinary
    Dosage Forms   55

3   Interpretation of Changes in Drug Disposition and Interspecies
    Scaling   92

4   Some Aspects of Dosage, Clinical Selectivity and Stereoisomerism   136

5   Drug Permeation Through the Skin and Topical Preparations   178

6   Antimicrobial Disposition, Selection, Administration and Dosage   210

7   The Bioavailability and Disposition of Antimicrobial Agents in
    Neonatal Animals   252

Appendices
    Pharmacokinetic Terms: Symbols and Units   267

Index   271

Preface

Material for this monograph has been collected over the past 25 years. The book is, in some respects, an update of *Principles of Drug Disposition in Domestic Animals* which was published in 1977, but it is more broad in scope. References to selected pre-1975 papers are included because of their inherent value.

The diversity of species in which drugs are used for clinical purposes together with the emphasis placed on the various classes of drugs distinguishes veterinary from human pharmacology. Physiological characteristics of different species essentially reflect adaptations that evolved over centuries to promote survival of the existing species. Even though each species is unique, the pattern of most physiological processes in the species within a taxonomical class can be described in mathematical terms. Species differences in the response to fixed doses or dosage regimens of drugs generally have a physiological or biochemical basis. An uncharacteristic response to dosage of a drug in animals of a particular species often warrants investigative research on the underlying mechanism to which the observed effect could be attributed.

Pharmacokinetic parameters are most useful for quantifying species differences in the bioavailability and disposition of drugs, and for calculating therapeutic dosage regimens. An assumption made in dosage calculations, which appears to be generally valid, is that the same range of therapeutic plasma concentrations is applicable to eutherian mammalian species. Disease states and pharmacokinetic-based drug interactions can alter the disposition of a drug to an extent that modification of usual dosage is required for safety and efficacy of the drug. The formulation of dosage forms determines not only the route of administration but also the clinical efficacy of a drug. Because residues of drugs and drug metabolites in the tissues and edible products of food-producing animals are unacceptable, drugs should be formulated as preparations that will be efficacious and will not prolong the persistence of residues. In formulating veterinary dosage forms, meagre consideration has been given to differences in the pharmacodynamic activity and to species variations in the bioavailability and disposition of the enantiomers of chiral drugs. Application of interspecies allometric scaling of major pharmacokinetic parameters is useful at the pre-clinical stage of drug development and may identify non-conforming species with regard to the disposition of commercially available drugs. It is well established that drug dosage cannot be extrapolated between different classes of animals (mammals, birds, fishes, reptiles). At the present time there is insufficient information available on the pharmacodynamic activity and pharmacokinetic behaviour of drugs in marsupial species to comment on the feasibility of extrapolating dosage from eutherian to marsupial mammals. The conservation of exotic animals requires protection of their natural habitats from human intrusion as the various adaptations that characterize different species have evolved in concert with their habitats.

Veterinary clinical pharmacology is an integrative discipline with the general objective of providing the requisite information for judicious selection of drug preparations for use in animals at dosages that will alleviate discomfort and pain, avoid undesirable drug interactions and effectively treat animal diseases. The specific aim of drug therapy is to readjust disease-altered physiological and/or biochemical processes to the state that is normal for the animal species. The author hopes that this book will promote postgraduate research that will both contribute to advancement of veterinary clinical pharmacology and further the well-being of animals.

J. Desmond Baggot
Ballsbridge, Dublin

Acknowledgements

To Colette for her encouragement, support and deep understanding of my academic interest and to our loving daughters Siobhán and Jen who continually enrich our lives and adapted so well to the way of life in different countries.

Terms and Abbreviations

ACE	angiotensin-converting enzyme
AChE	acetylcholinesterase
AUC_{0-24}	area under the concentration-time curve measured from $t=0$ to $t=24\,h$
AUIC	area under the inhibitory plasma concentration – time curve (with reference to antimicrobial agents)
AUMC	area under the first moment of the plasma concentration – time curve, i.e. the area under the curve of the product of time and plasma concentration over the time-span zero to infinity
b.d.	twice daily
BSP	bromosulphalein
BUN	blood urea nitrogen
C_{max}	maximum concentration of a drug
CK	creatine kinase
Cl	clearance (L/h or mL/min)
D	dose (mg)
DDT	dichlorodiphenyl-trichloroethane
DEET	diethyltoluamide
E	extraction ratio
E_H	hepatic extraction ratio
ED_{50}	median effective dose (mg/kg)
F	systemic availability (extent of absorption)
f_b	fraction of bound drug
f_u	fraction of unbound drug
FMO	flavin-containing mono-oxygenase
GABA	γ-aminobutyric acid
GFR	glomerular filtration rate
HPLC	high performance liquid chromatography
IBR	infectious bovine rhinotracheitis
ICG	indocyanine green
i.m.	intramuscular
i.o.	intraosseous
i.p.	intraperitoneal
i.v.	intravenous
k_a	absorption rate constant

k_d	disposition rate constant
K_M	Michaelis constant
LD_{50}	median lethal dose (mg/kg)
LOQ	limit of quantification
M	molar
MAT	mean absorption time
MIC_{90}	minimum inhibitory concentration required to prevent visible growth of 90% of a bacterial species *in vitro*
MLP	maximum life-span potential
MRT	mean residence time
n	number
NS	not significant
NSAIDs	non-steroidal anti-inflammatory drugs
OTC	oxytetracycline
OTC-C	conventional oxytetracycline
OTC-LA	long-acting oxytetracycline
P	probability
P_{Cr}	creatinine concentration in plasma
PASME	post-antibiotic sub-minimum inhibitory concentration effect
PCB	polychlorinated biphenyl
PCV	packed cell volume
pH	negative logarithm of the hydrogen ion concentration
pK_a	negative logarithm of the acidic ionization/dissociation constant
p.o.	*per os* (by mouth)
p.r.	*per rectum* (rectal administration)
Q	blood flow (L/h)
R_0	infusion rate required to produce steady-state plasma concentration
s.c.	subcutaneous
SD	standard deviation
SEM	standard error of the mean
t	time
$t_{\frac{1}{2}}$	half-life (i.v. administration of a drug)
U_{Cr}	creatinine concentration in urine
V	total volume of urine formed during collection period
$V_{d(area)}$	volume of distribution (L)
$V_{d(ass)}$	volume of distribution at steady-state (L)
V_{max}	maximum reaction velocity
α	absorption-rate constant
β	elimination-rate constant
β-agonists	
β-antagonists	

Author's Note

The values of pharmacokinetic terms for drugs mentioned in this monograph are average values in the various animal species, while drug doses and dosage regimens are based on average values and agree reasonably well with those usually recommended. Some emphasis is placed on veterinary dosage forms since they influence the clinical efficacy of drugs to a greater degree than is generally appreciated. Advancement of veterinary clinical pharmacology rests both on elucidating the physiological and/or biochemical basis of species variations in response to dosage of drugs and on the development of dosage forms that will most effectively deliver the drugs to their sites of action without producing adverse effects. Keen observation and attention to detail are requirements of animal management in general and of veterinary clinical pharmacology in particular.

Chapter 1
The Pharmacokinetic Basis of Species Variations in Drug Disposition

Introduction

The diversity of species in which drugs are used and studied distinguishes veterinary from human pharmacology. Another difference, which relates to clinical indications, is the emphasis placed on the various classes of drugs.

An understanding of the complex relationship between the dose of a drug and the clinically observed pharmacological effect can generally be obtained by linking the pharmacokinetic (PK) behaviour with information on pharmacodynamic (PD) activity (Fig. 1.1) (Holford & Sheiner, 1981).

Dose $\xrightarrow[\text{behaviour}]{\text{PK}}$ Plasma drug concentration $\xrightarrow[\text{activity}]{\text{PD}}$ Pharmacological effect (s)

Fig. 1.1 Schematic representation of the dose–effect relationship.

The plasma drug concentration profile occupies a central role between the dose administered and the characteristic pharmacological effect(s) produced by the drug. An inherent assumption is that the drug concentration in plasma is related to the concentration at the site of action, which can rarely be measured *in vivo*. The requirement for species differences in the dose (mg/kg) or dosage rate (dose/dosage interval) of a pharmacological agent may be attributed to variation between species in pharmacokinetic behaviour or pharmacodynamic activity, or both, of the drug. Whether a systemically acting drug produces a therapeutic or toxic effect is mainly determined by size of the dose when a single dose is administered or the dosage rate when multiple doses are administered at a constant dosage interval.

Drugs (pharmacological agents) act by modifying pre-existent physiological or biochemical processes in the body. The mechanisms of action of drugs appear to be the same in mammalian species. The clinical utility of pharmacokinetics relies on the premise that a range of therapeutic plasma concentrations can be defined for each pharmacological agent; some examples are given in Table 1.1. The pharmacodynamic properties (affinity and efficacy) of a drug are embodied in the therapeutic concentration range. There is substantial evidence to support the hypothesis that the therapeutic concentration range is the same for human beings and domestic animals. The calculation of a dosage regimen (dose and dosage interval) for a drug preparation is based upon a knowledge of the therapeutic concentration range and the pharmacokinetic parameters that describe bioavailability and disposition of the drug. Species differences in the dosage regimen for a drug preparation can generally, but not always, be attributed to variation between species in pharmacokinetic behaviour of the drug.

Table 1.1 Principal pharmacological effect and range of therapeutic plasma concentrations of some drugs.

Drug	Pharmacological effect	Therapeutic concentrations
Quinidine	Anti-arrythmic	2–6 µg/mL
Procainamide	Anti-arrythmic	6–14 µg/mL
Lignocaine (lidocaine)	Anti-arrythmic	1.5–5 µg/mL
Propranolol	Anti-hypertensive	20–80 ng/mL
Verapamil	Anti-arrythmic	80–320 ng/mL
Digoxin	Positive inotropic	0.6–2.4 ng/mL
Phenobarbitone	Anticonvulsant	10–25 µg/mL
Pethidine (meperidine)	Analgesic	0.4–0.7 µg/mL
Theophylline	Bronchodilator	6–16 µg/mL

Plasma concentration profile

Following the administration of a single dose of a drug preparation (dosage form), the factors that influence the plasma drug concentration profile include: the size of the dose (mg/kg), the formulation and route of administration of the drug preparation, the extent of both plasma protein binding and extravascular (tissue) distribution, and the rate of elimination (which refers to bio-transformation and excretion) of the drug. The significant variable associated with oral, intramuscular or subcutaneous administration, namely bioavail-ability (i.e. the rate and extent of drug absorption into the systemic circulation), can be discounted by administering the drug intravenously as a parenteral solution (if available). It is only when a drug is administered intravenously that complete systemic availability (100% absorption of the dose) can be assumed.

Some intravenous anaesthetic agents

Pharmacokinetic studies of intravenous anaesthetic agents provide useful information for comparative purposes. Following the intravenous injection of a single dose (25 mg/kg) of pentobarbital sodium to goats and dogs, the plasma concentration–time curves (plotted on arithmetic coordinates, Fig. 1.2) show that the various reflexes return and the animals of both species awaken from anaesthesia at the same plasma pentobarbitone concentrations, but at widely different times after drug administration (Davis *et al.*, 1973). The difference in the duration of anaesthetic effect is related to species variation in the rate of biotransformation (hepatic microsomal oxidation) of pentobarbitone.

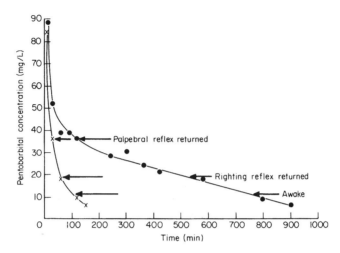

Fig. 1.2 Curves showing the decline in plasma concentrations of pentobarbital in goats (x—x) and dogs (●—●) following the intravenous injection of a single dose (25 mg/kg) of pentobarbital sodium. Arrows indicate the plasma pentobarbital concentrations (and related times) at which the various reflexes return and the animals of both species awaken from anaesthesia. (Reproduced with permission from Davis *et al.* (1973).)

The systemic clearance and the half-life of thiopentone, administered as an intravenous bolus dose, significantly differ between sheep and dogs. However, both species, as well as cats and human beings, awaken from anaesthesia at the same plasma thiopentone concentration (20 μg/mL). It is mainly redistribution of thiopentone from the highly perfused tissues (including the central nervous system (CNS)) to less well perfused tissues (such as skeletal muscle) and ultimately body fat, rather than elimination by hepatic biotransformation, that determines the duration of anaesthetic effect (Fig. 1.3) (Brodie *et al.*, 1952). Compared with mixed-breed dogs, Greyhounds and probably other lean breeds of hound (such as Whippet, Saluki and Afghan) recover more slowly from thiobarbiturate (thiopental and thiamylal) induced anaesthesia and show intermittent struggling and relapses into sleep during the recovery period. The slower and less smooth recovery of Greyhounds may be largely attributed to the lower body fat content, as a percentage of body weight, and partly to slower dose-dependent hepatic biotransformation of thiobarbiturates. Between 2 and 8 h after intravenous administration, the plasma concentrations of thiopental

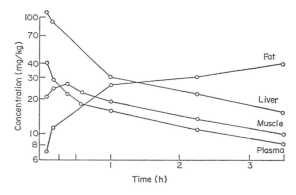

Fig. 1.3 Concentrations of thiopentone in various tissues and plasma of a dog after the intravenous administration of 25 mg/kg. (Reproduced with permission from Brodie *et al.* (1952).)

and thiamylal are significantly higher in Greyhounds than in mixed-breed dogs (Fig. 1.4) (Sams *et al.*, 1985). Premedication with acepromazine (0.25 mg/kg, i.m.) generally delays the time of awakening from thiopentone anaesthesia, although there is wide individual variation (Baggot *et al.*, 1984). The delayed awakening may have a pharmacodynamic rather than pharmacokinetic basis, or could be due to the sedative effect of the acepromazine.

Propofol, a highly lipophilic intravenous anaesthetic, rapidly induces anaesthesia of ultra-short duration in goats, dogs and human beings. Both redistribution and biotransformation of the drug contribute to the brief duration of anaesthetic effect. Even though the disposition kinetics of propofol differ among species and between mixed-breed dogs and Greyhounds (Zoran *et al.*, 1993), the blood propofol concentration at which dogs and seemingly goats return to the sternal position and human beings regain consciousness appears to be the same (1 μg/mL). The systemic clearance, expressed as mL/min·kg, of propofol exceeds hepatic blood flow in all species, particularly in goats (*vide infra*, Table 1.14). It can be concluded that another organ (the lungs) or extra-hepatic tissue contributes to the metabolism, which takes place by conjugation reactions (glucuronide and sulphate synthesis), of propofol.

Ketamine, a dissociative anaesthetic, is administered as a racemic mixture (present in the parenteral preparation) and is initially metabolized by the liver to N-desmethylketamine (metabolite I), which in part is converted by oxidation to the cyclohexene (metabolite II) (Fig. 1.5). The major metabolites found in urine are glucuronide conjugates that are formed subsequent to hydroxylation of the cyclohexanone ring. As the enantiomers differ in anaesthetic potency and the enantioselectively formed (metabolite I has approximately 10% activity of the parent drug) interpretation of the relationship between the anaesthetic effect and disposition of ketamine is complicated. On a pharmacodynamic basis, the S(+) enantiomer is three times as potent as the R(−) enantiomer (Marietta *et al.*, 1977; Deleforge *et al.*, 1991), while the enantiomer that undergoes N-demethylation (hepatic microsomal reaction) differs between species (Delatour *et al.*, 1991). Based on the observed minimum anaesthetic

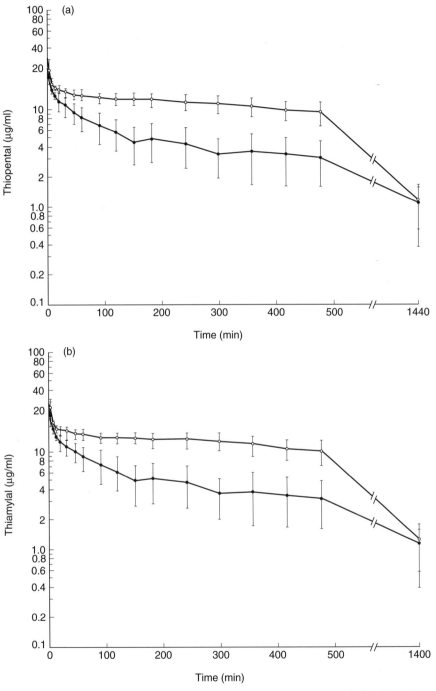

Fig. 1.4 Comparison of plasma thiobarbiturate concentration–time curves in Greyhounds and mixed-breed dogs following the intravenous administration of single doses (15 mg/kg) of thiopental and thiamylal (a) —Plasma thiopental concentrations in Greyhound (o—o) and mixed-breed dogs (●—●) after being given 15 mg of thiopental/kg, iv; mean ± SD. (b) —Plasma thiamylal concentrations in Greyhound (o—o) and mixed-breed dogs (●—●) after being given 15 mg of thiamylal/kg, iv; mean ± SD. (Reproduced with permission from Sams *et al.*, (1985).)

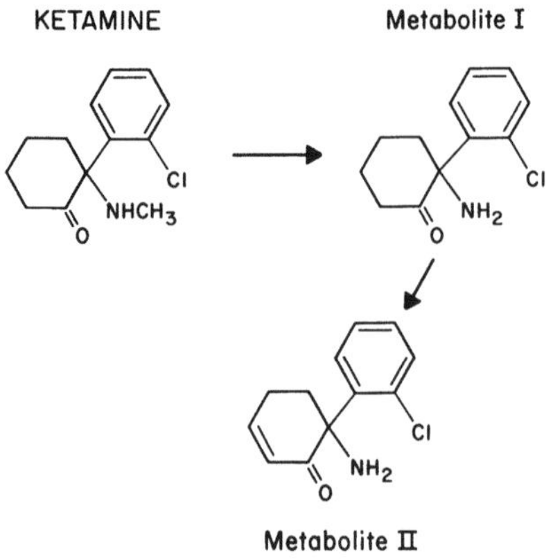

KETAMINE   Metabolite I

Metabolite II

Fig. 1.5 Initial biotransformation (oxidative reactions) of ketamine. Both the parent drug and, to a lesser extent (10%), metabolite I are pharmacologically active.

concentration of ketamine in plasma (2 µg/mL), the duration of anaesthesia produced by a single intravenous dose relates mainly to distribution and partly, depending on the size of the dose, to biotransformation of the drug. The half-life of ketamine is shorter in domestic animals (sheep, 0.5 h; horses, 0.7 h; cattle, 0.9 h; dogs, 1 h; cats, 1.1 h), apart from pigs (2.3 h), than in human beings (2.5 h).

Species variations in dosage

Low dose requirements (relative to dogs) of xylazine (α_2-adrenoceptor agonist) for cattle and morphine (mainly µ-opioid agonist) for cats may be attributed to higher sensitivity of receptor sites in the central nervous system of the susceptible species to these drugs (Table 1.2). Brahman cattle appear to be even more sensitive than other breeds of cattle to xylazine, while the sedative dose for Isle of Rhum red deer (off the west coast of Scotland), although similar to that for cattle (0.1–0.2 mg/kg, i.m.), is one-tenth of the sedative dose required for mainland red deer (Fletcher, 1974). In giraffes, xylazine should not be used alone but it could be used in conjunction with etorphine; whenever the use of etorphine is intended, the narcotic antagonist diprenorphine should be available for administration. Certain breeds of dog (notably, the Basset Hound, Great Dane and Irish Setter) appear to be susceptible to bloat, probably due to aerophagia, some hours after xylazine administration.

The idiosyncratic toxicity, manifested by neurological effects, shown by a subpopulation of (rough-haired) Collies to ivermectin ($\geqslant 100$ µg/kg, p.o.) may be attributed to a breed-related compromised blood–brain barrier (Tranquilli *et al.*, 1989), since γ-aminobutyric acid receptors that mediate neurotransmission are confined to the CNS in mammalian species. The pharmacokinetic behaviour of ivermectin does not differ between 'ivermectin-sensitive' and

Table 1.2 Species variations in drug dosage.

Drug (route of administration)	Animal species	Dose (mg/kg)	Dosage interval (h)
Single dose			
Xylazine hydrochloride (i.v.)	Dog	1.0	
	Cat	1.0	
	Horse	0.75	
	Cattle	0.075	
Morphine sulphate (i.m.)	Dog	1.0	
	Cat	0.1	
Succinylcholine chloride (i.v.)	Dog	0.3	
	Cat	1.0	
	Horse	0.1	
	Cattle	0.02	
Multiple doses			
Aspirin tablet(s) (p.o.)	Dog	10	12
	Cat	10	48
	Cow	100	12
Conventional aminophylline tablets	Dog	10	8
	Horse	5	12
Sustained-release anhydrous theophylline tablets (p.o.)	Dog	20	12
	Horse	15	24

normal Collies. A similar adverse effect has been observed in Murray Gray cattle, an Australian breed. The use of ivermectin is contra-indicated in Chelonians (tortoises, terrapins and turtles) and crocodiles.

The wide variation among species in the intravenous dose of succinylcholine (suxamethonium) required to produce a similar degree of neuromuscular blockade (depolarizing type) may be attributed to differences in the activity of pseudocholinerase, the enzyme that hydrolyses the drug. In ruminant species, at least 80% of whole blood cholinesterase activity is associated with the erythrocytes, which may account for the lower dose requirement for cattle (0.02 mg/kg) than for horses (0.1 mg/kg) and cats (1 mg/kg). Blood cholinesterase activity resides mainly in the plasma (pseudocholinesterase) of cats and horses. The eightfold longer duration of the neuromuscular blocking effect produced by succinylcholine in the rat compared with the cat was attributed to defective hydrolysis of the drug by plasma cholinesterase in the former species (Derkx *et al.*, 1971). Because succinylcholine does not produce analgesia, this drug should only be used in conjunction with an anaesthetic agent whenever a surgical procedure is to be performed.

Species differences in pharmacokinetic behaviour are far more common than in pharmacodynamic activity of drugs, but often only become evident following the administration of multiple doses at a fixed dosage interval. The long dosage interval for aspirin (acetylsalicylic acid) in cats compared with dogs is related to the slow rate of synthesis of the glucuronide conjugate, due to the relative deficiency in cats of hepatic microsomal glucuronyl transferase activity. Glucuronide synthesis is the principal metabolic pathway for salicylate elimination; following the intravenous administration of sodium salicylate, the half-life of salicylate is 25–35 h in cats (and is dose-dependent) compared with 8.6 h in dogs and 1 h in horses. Low activity of glucuronyl transferase appears to be characteristic of Felidae, as it applies not only to the domestic cat (*Felis catus*) but also to the lion (*Panthera leo*), African civet (*Viverra civetta*) and forest genet (*Genetta pardina*) (French *et al.*, 1974). Taxonomically the civet and genet belong to the Viverridae family. The combination of slow formation of the glucuronide conjugate and the accumulation of a reactive metabolite, formed by an alternative metabolic pathway, to a level that exceeds the capacity of hepatic glutathione conjugation accounts for the toxicity of paracetamol (acetaminophen) in cats. Because feline haemoglobin is particularly susceptible to oxidative damage, methaemoglobinaemia consistently occurs in paracetamol toxicity. Parenteral preparations containing benzyl alcohol (as a preservative) should not be administered to cats; benzyl benzoate lotion should not be applied to cats. The relatively long dosage interval (12 h) for aspirin (100 mg/kg, p.o.) in cows is related to slow absorption of salicylate from the reticulo-rumen rather than hepatic metabolism, which takes place rapidly in cattle.

Therapeutic (i.e. safe and clinically effective) dosage regimens for conventional (immediate-release) aminophylline tablets are 10 mg/kg at 8-h intervals for dogs and 5 mg/kg at 12-h intervals for horses. These oral dosage regimens will maintain plasma theophylline concentrations within the therapeutic range (6–16 µg/mL) and produce the desired pharmacological effect (bronchodilation). The systemic availability of theophylline, administered as conventional aminophylline tablets, exceeds 90% in both species. Dosage intervals can be extended to 12 h for dogs and 24 h for horses by administering appropriate doses of sustained-release anhydrous theophylline tablets. A longer dosage interval for the horse than for the dog is unusual for a lipid-soluble drug, since most lipid-soluble drugs are more rapidly metabolized by the liver of horses than of dogs. Even though the optimum oral dosage regimen for metronidazole, which is indicated for the treatment of anaerobic infections (e.g. pleuropneumonia, liver abscesses, peritonitis), is the same (15–20 mg/kg administered at 8 h dosage intervals) for dogs and horses, it is usual to use a 12 h dosage interval for horses based on economic considerations and convenience of drug administration.

A dosage interval of 12 h appears to be appropriate to use in dogs for oral sustained-release anhydrous theophylline tablets (Koritz *et al.*, 1986) and oral sustained-release morphine sulphate tablets (Dohoo *et al.*, 1994). Following oral administration of these sustained-release dosage forms, the average systemic availability of theophylline is 76% and of morphine is 21%. Gastrointestinal transit time in monogastric species makes it unlikely that oral sustained-release dosage forms would provide drug for absorption for longer than 24 h. Controlled-release ruminal boluses for use in cattle, due to their retention in the reticulo-rumen, either continuously release drug (generally an anthelmintic) into ruminal fluid over a prolonged period (e.g. the ivermectin ruminal bolus, 135 days; fenbendazole ruminal bolus, up to 140 days; moranel tartrate ruminal bolus, at least 90 days) or intermittently release pulse doses at a regular (approximately 3-week) interval (e.g. oxfendazole ruminal bolus for cattle). The higher dosage requirement of some anthelmintics (e.g. benzimidazole carbamates, clorsulon) for cattle and goats than for sheep, although based solely on clinical efficacy, is probably related to more rapid hepatic metabolism of these drugs in cattle and goats. Because of the more rapid elimination of closantel in goats than in sheep, a suggested interval for repeated doses of the anthelmintic to prevent reinfection with benzimidazole-resistant *Haemonchus contortus* is 30 days for goats and 50 days for sheep (Hennessy *et al.*, 1993).

Species variations in drug disposition

Disposition is the term used to describe the simultaneous effects of distribution and elimination, that is, the processes that occur subsequent to the absorption of a drug. The factors that influence drug disposition include: the chemical nature and physicochemical properties of the drug, the extent and avidity of binding to plasma proteins and extravascular macromolecules (tissue components), the extent of extravascular distribution and, in ruminant animals, operation of the ion-trapping effect in ruminal fluid, blood flow to the organs of elimination (usually the liver and kidneys), the activity of drug-metabolizing enzymes (particularly those associated with hepatic microsomal-mediated metabolic pathways), and the efficiency of excretion (mainly renal) mechanisms. The most important pharmacokinetic parameters describing the disposition of a drug are the systemic (body) clearance (Cl_B), which measures the ability of the body to eliminate the drug, and the volume of distribution (V_d), which denotes the 'apparent' space in the body available to contain the drug. The half-life ($t_{1/2}$) expresses the overall rate of drug elimination, while the mean residence time (*MRT*), which is the statistical moment analogy to half-life, represents the average time the number of drug molecules introduced reside in the body.

Species variations in the disposition of a drug may be due to differences in the apparent volume of distribution or the rate of elimination of the drug. The apparent volume of distribution of most lipophilic organic bases (e.g. ketamine, ivermectin, macrolide antibiotics) is larger in ruminant than in monogastric species. However, differences in the rate of elimination, particularly of drugs that undergo extensive hepatic biotransformation, generally account for species variations in drug disposition.

Drug elimination processes

There are two distinct processes by which drugs are eliminated from the body: biotransformation (metabolism) and excretion; although both processes are involved in the elimination of the majority of drugs, either may predominate. Elimination is ultimately responsible for terminating the action of drugs. The mechanism(s) of elimination is determined by the molecular structure and chemical nature of the drug and by the same physicochemical properties as influence drug distribution. Biotransformation converts drugs to metabolites which are generally less active than the parent drug or inactive, more polar, less lipid-soluble and suitable for rapid removal from the body by renal excretion and, to some extent, biliary excretion.

Biotransformation

Biotransformation is the principal mechanism of elimination for lipid-soluble drugs and other foreign chemical substances (xenobiotics). Because of its high content of drug-metabolizing enzymes and rich blood supply (26–29% of cardiac output), the liver is the principal organ of drug biotransformation. The hepatic microsomal enzymes, which are associated with the smooth-surfaced (devoid of ribosomes) endoplasmic reticulum, mediate a variety of oxidative reactions and glucuronide conjugation (synthesis). Some of the enzyme-catalysed reactions involved with the biotransformation of drugs are utilized in the formation and subsequent metabolism (to facilitate excretion) of certain endogenous substances, such as steroid hormones, fatty acids, prostaglandins, leukotrienes, bile acids and bilirubin. Sites of drug biotransformation, in addition to the liver, include the lungs, kidneys, blood plasma, forestomach (in ruminant species), intestinal microorganisms, intestinal mucosa (orally administered drugs) and epidermis (topically applied drugs). The most likely major metabolic pathway for a drug can often be predicted, based on a knowledge of the functional group(s) in the molecule (Table 1.3). The general pattern of drug biotransformation is usually biphasic. The first phase comprises oxidative, reductive and hydrolytic reactions, while the second phase consists of the conjugation or synthetic reactions (Fig. 1.6) (Williams, 1967). The enzyme systems involved in phase I reactions are located primarily in the endoplasmic reticulum, while the enzymes involved in conjugation reactions (referred to as transferring enzymes) are mainly cytosolic.

Microsomal oxidative reactions constitute the most prominent phase I biotransformation pathway for a wide variety of structurally unrelated drugs (Table 1.4). Some drugs (e.g. amphetamine, diazepam, propranolol, lignocaine) simultaneously undergo more than one type of microsomal-mediated oxidative reaction. Microsomal enzymes are located primarily in liver cells, where they are associated with the smooth-surface (without ribosomes) endoplasmic reticulum (Fouts, 1961). Lipid solubility is a prerequisite for drug access to the

Table 1.3 Probable biotransformation pathways for drugs.

Functional group	Biotransformation pathways
Aromatic ring	Hydroxylation
Hydroxyl	
Aliphatic	Chain oxidation; glucuronic acid conjugation; sulphate conjugation (to a lesser extent)
Aromatic	Glucuronic acid conjugation; sulphate conjugation; methylation; ring hydroxylation
Carboxyl	
Aliphatic	Glucuronic acid conjugation
Aromatic	Ring hydroxylation; glucuronic acid conjugation; glycine conjugation
Primary amines	
Aliphatic	Deamination
Aromatic	Acetylation; glucuronic acid conjugation; methylation; sulphate conjugation; ring hydroxylation
Sulphydryl	Glucuronic acid conjugation; methylation; oxidation
Ester linkage	Hydrolysis
Amide bond	Hydrolysis

Source: Baggot (1977).

site where microsomal oxidation takes place. Microsomal drug oxidations require cytochrome P450 enzymes (haemoproteins that are localized in the smooth endoplasmic reticulum and exist in several forms), the closely associated NADPH–cytochrome P450 reductase, NADPH (reduced nicotinamide adenine dinucleotide phosphate) and molecular oxygen. The ability of the microsomal drug-metabolizing enzymes (mixed function oxidase, or cytochrome P450 mono-oxygenase, system) to catalyse various oxidative reactions may be ascribed to a common mechanism, hydroxylation (Brodie *et al.*, 1958; Gillette, 1963, 1966). The steps involved in microsomal oxidation are shown schematically (Fig. 1.7). The drug (or xenobiotic) substance reacts with the oxidized (Fe^{3+}) form of cytochrome P450 to form an enzyme–substrate complex (step 1). NADPH donates an electron to the flavoprotein (NADPH–cytochrome

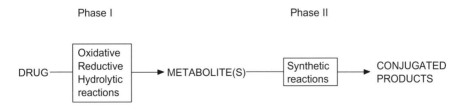

Fig. 1.6 General pattern of drug metabolism.

Table 1.4   Oxidative reactions catalysed by microsomal enzyme systems.

Oxidative reaction	Drug substrate
Aromatic hydroxylation	Amphetamine
	Phenobarbitone
	Phenytoin
	Phenylbutazone
	Propranolol
Side chain (aliphatic)	Ibuprofen
oxidation	Meprobamate
	Pentobarbitone
	Phenylbutazone
Oxidative dealkylation	
O-dealkylation	Codeine
	Griseofulvin
N-dealkylation	Diazepam
	Lignocaine
	Morphine
	Caffeine
	Theophylline
Oxidative deamination	Amphetamine
	Diazepam
Desulphuration	Parathion
(replacement of S by O)	Thiopentone
Sulphoxidation	Chlorpromazine
(S-oxidation)	Cimetidine

P450) reductase which, in turn, reduces the oxidized cytochrome P450–drug complex (step 2). A second electron is introduced from NADPH via the same flavoprotein reductase which serves to reduce molecular oxygen (O_2) and to form an 'activated oxygen'–cytochrome P450–drug intermediate (step 3). One atom of oxygen is transferred to the drug substrate to form the oxidized drug (hydroxylated product) and the second oxygen atom is released as water (step 4). Upon release of the oxidized drug, the oxidized form of cytochrome P450 is regenerated. The substrate specificity of this enzymatic reaction (cycle) is very low. High solubility in lipid is the only property that the wide variety of structurally unrelated drugs that serve as substrates for microsomal oxidation have in common.

The many isoenzymes of cytochrome P450 that exist are classified into gene families on the basis of their amino acid sequence. Of the twelve families that have been identified in mammalian species, three families (CYP1, CYP2 and CYP3) encode the enzymes involved in the majority of drug biotransformations, while the other families are involved in the metabolism of endogenous

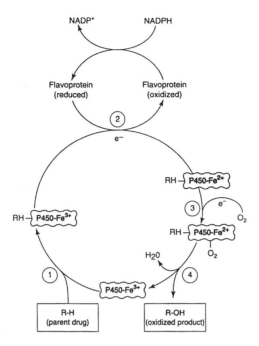

Fig. 1.7 Cytochrome P450 cycle in drug oxidations: RH, parent drug; ROH, oxidized metabolite; e⁻, electron. (Reproduced with permission from Correia (1992).)

substances. The major subfamily of cytochrome P450 isoenzymes involved in biotransformation of drugs is CYP3A (the terminal capital letter denotes the subfamily) and is expressed at significant levels extrahepatically. The subfamily CYP1A is expressed at low levels in the skin but, in common with CYP3A, the activity of the isoenzymes can be induced (or inhibited) by a variety of drugs and xenobiotics.

Based on *in vitro* studies of hepatic microsomal-catalysed oxidative reactions, using liver specimens from a variety of animal species including man, and marker substrates for the various reactions, it can be concluded that neither the measured levels of cytochrome P450 and cytochrome b_5 nor the activity of NADPH–cytochrome c reductase accounts for species variations in the capacity of oxidative reactions (McManus and Ilett, 1976; Dalvi *et al.*, 1987; Souhaili-El-Amri *et al.*, 1986). However, species variations could be attributed to differences in values of the kinetic parameters (Michaelis constant, K_M, and the maximum reaction velocity, V_{max}) associated with individual reactions.

Oxidative reactions catalysed by non-microsomal enzymes are less varied than those mediated by cytochrome P450 mono-oxygenases but are important in the metabolism of some drugs (e.g. isoproterenol, methylxanthines, methimazole, ethanol, chloral hydrate), endogenous substances (adrenalin, histamine) and naturally occurring compounds (vitamin A). Theophylline and caffeine (methylxanthines) simultaneously undergo microsomal cytochrome

P450-mediated *N*-dealkylation and non-microsomal-catalysed oxidation. A flavin-containing mono-oxygenase catalyses the reversible oxidation of parent benzimidazole sulphide anthelmintics to their sulphoxide (active) metabolites, whereas cytochrome P450 mono-oxygenases catalyse oxidation of sulphoxides to the corresponding sulphone (inactive) metabolites. Whilst most reductive reactions are catalysed by non-microsomal enzymes, some are catalysed by cytochrome P450 enzymes, generally under conditions of low oxygen tension. Drugs that contain a nitro group (e.g. chloramphenicol, nitroimidazoles, nitroxynil) and azo-compounds (prontosil) are reduced to amines. Ruminal micro-organisms efficiently perform reductive reactions and are capable of inactivating orally administered drugs containing a nitro group.

Hydrolysis is a phase I biotransformation reaction that is limited to drugs with an ester ($-$COO$-$) or an amide ($-$CONH$-$) linkage. Examples of drugs that are esters include acetylsalicylic acid (aspirin; non-steroidal anti-inflammatory drug), diphenoxylate (synthetic opioid antidiarrhoeal agent), succinylcholine (depolarizing neuromuscular blocking drug) and procaine (local anaesthetic). The esterases are found in the blood plasma, liver and other tissues, primarily in the non-microsomal soluble fraction. Hydrolytic conversion of aspirin to salicylic acid (which is pharmacologically active) takes place rapidly, but conjugation of salicylate with glucuronic acid (a phase II reaction) occurs very slowly in cats compared to other domestic animal species. The wide variation between species in the dose (mg/kg) of succinylcholine may be attributed to differences in the activity of plasma pseudocholinesterase, the enzyme that hydrolyses the drug.

The amidases, which hydrolyse amide linkages, are non-microsomal enzymes and are found principally in the soluble fraction of the liver. Procainamide (anti-arrythmic) is the amide analogue of procaine. Most amides are hydrolysed more slowly than the corresponding esters. In the horse, the half-life of procainamide is 3.5 h compared with 0.85 h for procaine. Because hydrolysis of the amide bond takes place relatively slowly, drugs containing this bond are likely to undergo biotransformation by simultaneously occurring alternative pathways. Procainamide is converted to *N*-acetylprocainamide (acetylation is a phase II conjugation reaction), which curiously has a longer half-life (6.3 h in the horse) than the parent drug. As acetylation of primary aromatic amino groups does not take place in dogs, over 50% of an administered dose of procainamide is excreted unchanged in the urine. Lignocaine (lidocaine), a local anaesthetic and anti-arrythmic drug, undergoes biotransformation by simultaneously occurring hepatic microsomal oxidative reactions (aromatic hydroxylation and *N*-dealkylation) and hydrolysis of the amide bond (Fig. 1.8) (Keenaghan & Boyes, 1972). A portion of the phase I metabolites formed undergo conjugation (phase II reaction) before excretion in the urine. The rates of the different biotransformation reactions pertaining to a drug determine the relative amounts (fraction of dose) of the metabolites that are formed; these may vary widely between species.

Phase I biotransformation reactions usually convert the parent drug to a

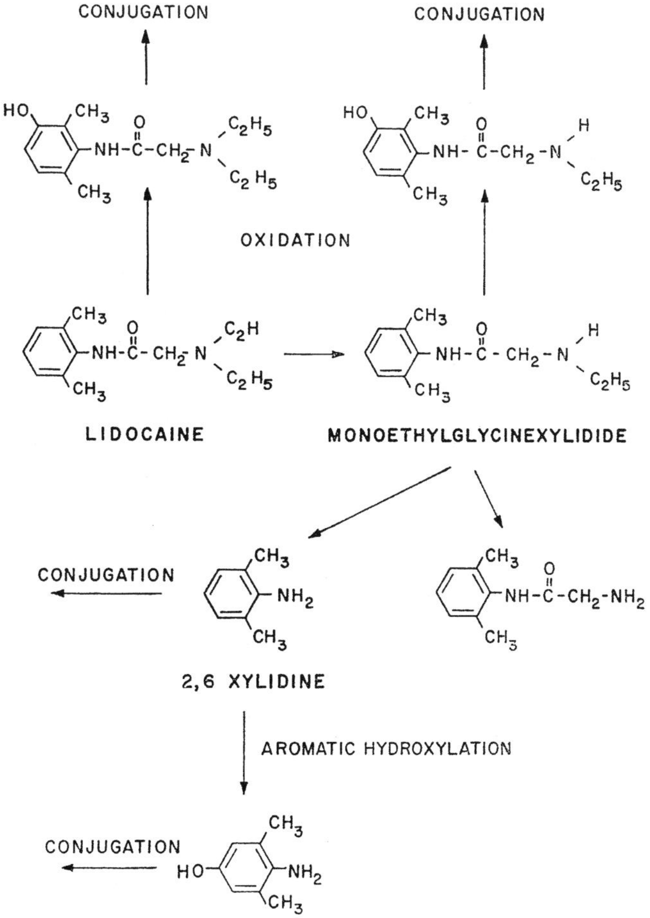

Fig. 1.8 The metabolic fate of Lidocaine (lignocaine). (Reproduced with permission from Keenaghan & Boyes (1972).)

more polar metabolite by introducing or unmasking a functional group, such as hydroxyl (−OH), carboxyl (−COOH), amino (−NH₂), or sulphydryl (−SH). If the phase I metabolites are sufficiently polar, they may be readily excreted. Otherwise, the acquired functional group enables conjugation with endogenous substances, such as glucuronic acid, acetic acid, sulphate (derived from sulphur-containing amino acids), or an amino acid (methionine, glycine), to take place. The conjugates (phase II metabolites) formed are almost invariably highly polar and rapidly excreted by the kidney (in urine) and the liver (in bile). A decrease in lipid solubility does not necessarily mean an increase in water solubility, which is the situation with some acetylated sulphonamides (e.g. sulphathiazole) particularly under acidic conditions such as occur in the urine of carnivorous species. The phase I metabolites may be either pharmacologically inactive or have modified (generally decreased) activity. Examples of

Table 1.5 Some pharmacological agents that are converted by phase I biotransformation reactions to active metabolites.

Drug	Active metabolite
Acetylsalicylic acid (aspirin)	Salicylate
Codeine	Morphine
Diazepam	Desmethyldiazepam and oxazepam
Diphenoxylate	Diphenoxin
Ketamine[a]	Norketamine (metabolite I)
Lignocaine (Lidocaine)	Desethyllignocaine
Pethidine (Meperidine)	Normeperidine
Phenylbutazone	Oxyphenbutazone
Prednisone[b]	Prednisolone
Primidone	Phenobarbital
Procaineamide	N-Acetylprocainamide[c]
Propranolol	4-Hydroxypropranolol
Sulindac[b]	Sulindac sulphide
Verapamil	Norverapamil

[a] Dissociative anaesthestic.
[b] Prednisone – prednisolone (active) and sulindac – sulindac sulphide (active) undergo interconversion.
[c] Not formed in dogs.

pharmacological agents that are converted to active metabolites are given in Table 1.5.

The principal synthetic pathways of biotransformation (phase II reactions) are glucuronide synthesis (conjugation), acetylation, sulphate conjugation, glutathione conjugation, glycine conjugation and methylation. The synthetic reactions have certain features in common (Table 1.6). They require, (i) a drug or drug metabolite (product of phase I reaction) with a suitable functional group, (ii) that energy and a conjugating agent (endogenous moiety) be supplied by the body, (iii) a transferring enzyme corresponding to the conjugating agent be present in the body, and (iv) either the conjugating agent or the drug and/or drug metabolite be in an 'activated' form, usually as a nucleotide. Apart from glutathione and certain amino acid (including glycine) conjugations, the conjugating agent becomes the 'activated' form. Because the endogenous moieties are of dietary origin, nutrition plays a key role in the regulation of synthetic reactions. The transferring enzymes (transferases) may be located in microsomes (glucuronide synthesis), the cytosol (acetylation, sulphate conjugation and methylation), or in mitochondria (glycine conjugation).

The physicochemical properties of phase II metabolites (drug conjugates) may differ significantly from those of the parent drug or phase I metabolite. In general, the phase II metabolites are pharmacologically inactive, less widely distributed and more readily excreted by both the kidneys and the liver.

Table 1.6 Synthetic (phase II) reactions.

Type of conjugation	Endogenous moiety	Transferring enzyme (location)
Glucuronide conjugation	UDP glucuronic acid	UDP-glucuronyl transferase (microsomes)
Acetylation	Acetyl CoA	N-Acetyltransferase (cytosol)
Sulphate conjugation	Phosphoadenosyl phosphosulphate	Sulphotransferase (cytosol)
Glutathione conjugation	Glutathione	GSH-S-transferase (cytosol, microsomes)
Glycine conjugation	Glycine	Acyl CoA glycine transferase (mitochondria)
Methylation	S-Adenosylmethionine	Methyltransferase (cytosol)

Species variations in conjugation reactions can depend on the occurrence of the conjugating agent (endogenous moiety), the ability to form the 'activated' nucleotide, or the amount of transferring enzyme (Williams, 1971a). While oxidative, reductive and hydrolytic reactions occur in all species, some synthetic reactions are either deficient or absent in certain species (Table 1.7). The extent to which the phase I biotransformation reactions occur varies unpredictably between species, while the phase II reactions are somewhat predictable based on the functional groups available for conjugation and the animal species.

Glucuronide synthesis (conjugation) is the most frequently occurring synthetic reaction for drugs and phase I drug metabolites. Some endogenous substances (e.g. bilirubin, thyroxine and steroids) undergo conjugation with

Table 1.7 Domestic animal species with defects in certain conjugation reactions.

Species	Conjugation reaction	Major target groups	State of synthetic reaction
Cat	Glucuronide synthesis	—OH, —COOH —NH$_2$, ＝NH, —SH	Present, slow rate
Dog	Acetylation	Ar—NH$_2$	Absent
Pig	Sulphate conjugation	Ar—OH, Ar—NH$_2$	Present, low extent

Source: Baggot (1977).

glucuronic acid before excretion. The functional group may be an amino ($-NH_2$), a carboxyl ($-COOH$), a sulphydryl ($-SH$) or a hydroxyl ($-OH$), either phenolic (attached to a ring structure) or alcoholic (attached to a straight-chain organic compound). The conjugating agent (endogenous moiety) is glucuronic acid, $C_6H_{10}O_6$, derived from glucose. The general availability of glucose in the body provides an ample supply of the conjugating agent. The process involves transfer of a glucuronyl moiety from the 'activated' form, uridine-5' diphospho-α-D-glucuronic acid (UDPGA), to the functional group on the drug and/or drug metabolite and/or endogenous substance forming the corresponding glucuronide. The transfer reaction is mediated by microsomal glucuronyl transferases located in the endoplasmic reticulum of the liver (primarily) and in other tissues (Dutton, 1966). Glucuronyl transferases are integral membrane proteins, like the cytochrome P450 mono-oxygenases. Glucuronide conjugates, being highly ionized and water-soluble, are rapidly excreted in the urine and bile. Some conjugates excreted in bile are susceptible to hydrolysis by β-glucuronidase, which is present in the intestinal bacteria. If the liberated parent drug is lipid-soluble, it will be reabsorbed and an enter-ohepatic cycle established. Enterohepatic cycling (circulation) prolongs the presence of a drug in the body and it is gradually eliminated by renal excretion. The slow rate of glucuronide synthesis in cats can be attributed to a deficiency of the transferring enzyme, microsomal glucuronyl transferase. Nonetheless, various endogenous compounds, such as bilirubin, thyroxine and steroids, form glucuronides in cats. The level of glucuronyl transferase is low in neonatal animals and newborn infants. Fish may have a low capacity to form the nucleotide UDPGA, which would limit glucuronide synthesis. In insects, glucuronide synthesis is replaced by β-glucoside conjugation (Parke, 1968).

The source of sulphate for conjugation is limited, while the enzymes responsible for sulphate activation and the transfer of sulphate to the acceptor molecule are found in the soluble fraction of the liver (Robbins & Lipmann, 1957). The relatively low capacity of the pig to synthesize ethereal sulphates is compensated for by increased glucuronide conjugation. Sulphate conjugation as well as glucuronide synthesis appear to be limited in fish (Mandel, 1971).

In domestic animal species, the endogenous moiety in amino acid conjuga-tion is often glycine, although it is the drug, or more usually the phase I metabolite of the drug, which becomes 'activated' rather than the endogenous moiety (conjugating agent). Glycine is replaced by ornithine in birds classified as anseriformes (duck, goose) and galliformes (chicken, turkey), but not in columbiformes (pigeon, dove) (Williams, 1959). Glycine conjugation takes place in both the liver and kidneys of domestic animal species other than the dog, in which it occurs only in the kidneys and may thereby be limited in extent. Conjugation with amino acids and methylation are quantitatively minor phase II reactions for drugs, but represent important reactions for endogenous compounds.

Acetylation is mainly a reaction of amino groups, of which there are different types (primary amine, amide, hydrazine and sulphonamide), and involves the transfer of the acetyl group from acetyl coenzyme A to the amino group of the drug. The transferring enzyme involved in this synthetic reaction may be specific for the amino group. The most common acetylation reaction involves primary amines and is catalysed by N-acetyltransferase. Acetylation takes place in the reticuloendothelial, rather than the parenchymal, cells of the liver, in the spleen, lungs and intestinal mucosa (Govier, 1965). Although most acetylated drugs are pharmacologically inactive, some are active (e.g. N-acetylprocainamide) or toxic (N-acetylisoniazid); the solubility of acetylsulphisoxazole is lower then that of the parent drug, particularly under acidic urinary conditions. The different types of amino group can be acetylated in all species, with the notable exceptions of the dog and fox which are unable to acetylate aromatic ($ArNH_2$) and hydrazine ($RNHNH_2$ or $ArNHNH_2$) amino groups. The inability of the dog and fox to acetylate these amino groups may be attributed to an absence of the specific transacetylases. The fractions of an oral dose of sulphadimethoxine (a slowly eliminated sulphonamide) excreted in urine over a 24-hour period as the parent (unchanged) drug, and the N^4-acetyl and N^1-glucuronide conjugates, show that acetylation of the aromatic amino groups did not occur in the dog; the glucuronide conjugate of the sulphonamide amino group was not found in urine of the cat (Table 1.8) (Williams, 1971b). The inability of the dog to acetylate certain types of amino group is compensated for by excretion of a larger fraction of the dose as parent drug or increased utilization of alternative biotransformation pathways. Although not in the case of sulphadimethoxine, the cat is generally less adept at compensating for the slow rate of glucuronide conjugation, which is a major synthetic pathway in the biotransformation of drugs and xenobiotics. Unlike its relative inability to form glucuronide conjugates, the neonate appears to have the capacity to acetylate compounds (Vest & Rossier, 1963).

Table 1.8 Excretion of sulphadimethoxine as parent drug, N^4-acetyl and N^1-glucuronide conjugates in urine of various species.

Species	Percentage of dose[a] excreted in 24 h	Percentage of 24 h excretion found as		
		Parent drug	N^4-Acetyl	N^1-glucuronide
Man	25	7	21	65
Rhesus monkey	39	6	23	66
Baboon	42	18	8	63
Squirrel monkey	9	12	37	44
Dog	26	64	0	19
Cat	34	82	18	0
Guinea pig	26	16	67	4
Hen	33	64	9	16

[a] Dose: 100 mg/kg orally except for man, when the dose was 33 mg/kg (Williams, 1971b).

Methylation, which involves the transfer of a methyl group derived from the amino acid methionine, is a relatively minor conjugation pathway for biotransformation of drugs, but plays an important role in the conversion of noradrenalin (norepinephrine) to adrenalin and the metabolism of adrenalin and histamine. Unlike other conjugation reactions, methylation does not greatly alter the physicochemical properties of the drug by increasing polarity or water solubility, and the product may therefore possess activity. Several methyltransferases exist (Axelrod, 1971) and differ from each other in the type of compound methylated which determines the reaction (O, N or S-methylation). In addition to methylation, demethylation may also occur. The sequential methylation, demethylation and remethylation of a compound could be misinterpreted as a migration of the methyl group from one position to another.

Conjugation with glutathione, a nucleophilic sulphydryl-containing tripeptide, contributes to inactivation of unstable (reactive) and potentially toxic metabolites of phase I biotransformation (specifically oxidative) reactions (Mitchell *et al.*, 1975). In this synthetic reaction, the metabolically activated drug or xenobiotic undergoes conjugation with glutathione (endogenous moiety). The enzyme glutathione-*S*-transferase, which is found in the soluble fraction (cytoplasm) of the liver and kidneys, mediates the reaction. Glutathione conjugates may subsequently be converted to *N*-acetylcysteine conjugates (mercapturic acids), mediated by a microsomal transferring enzyme (Chasseaud, 1976), which are excreted in urine and bile, depending on their molecular weight.

The synthesis of glutathione conjugates is limited by the availability of glutathione. When this is exceeded, the unstable intermediates formed may react with nucleophilic groups present on cellular macromolecules, such as protein, resulting in hepatotoxicity. Paracetamol (acetaminophen) forms predominantly glucuronide and sulphate conjugates and, to a lesser extent, enters the glutathione conjugation pathway (Fig. 1.9) (Mitchell *et al.*, 1975). Little or no hepatotoxicity occurs as long as glutathione is available for conjugation. In cats, due to slow formation of the glucuronide conjugate and limited capacity of the glutathione pathway, the reactive metabolite (*N*-acetyl-*p*-benzoquinoneimine) can accumulate. Acetylcysteine and ascorbic acid are used concurrently in the treatment of paracetamol toxicity in cats. The acetylcysteine, which is administered by intravenous injection, serves as a precursor for glutathione replenishment in the liver, while ascorbic acid (administered intravenously or orally) reduces methaemoglobin to haemoglobin. Treatment should commence immediately toxicity is suspected. Similar mechanisms may be involved in the nephrotoxicity of phenacetin, which is converted by microsomal oxidation (*O*-dealkylation) to paracetamol, and the hepatotoxicity of aflatoxin.

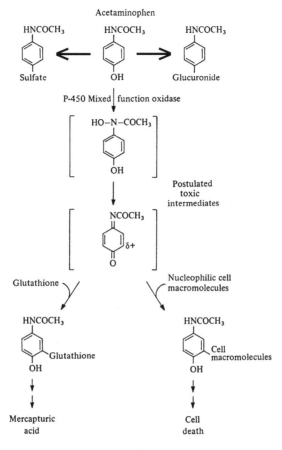

Fig. 1.9 Pathways of acetaminophen metabolism.

Metabolic activation

Prodrugs are inactive *per se,* and when formulated as oral dosage forms are intended to increase systemic availability (oral bioavailability) of the parent drug. Enalapril and pivampicillin are examples of prodrugs. Netobimin and febantel are probenzimidazole anthelmintics that, following oral administration to ruminant animals, are metabolically converted partly by ruminal microorganisms and mainly by the liver to albendazole and fenbendazole, respectively. Although triclabendazole (flukicide) is technically not a prodrug, the parent drug behaves as a prodrug. After administration of triclabendazole oral suspension to ruminant animals and horses, the parent drug is almost completely converted by hepatic first-pass metabolism (sulphoxidation) to triclabendazole suphoxide, the active metabolite. Ceftiofur, which is formulated as a parenteral dosage form, has antimicrobial activity but is very rapidly converted to the active metabolite desfuroylceftiofur which has a half-life in various animal species of 5–12 h. Ceftiofur, like triclabendazole, is technically not a prodrug.

Phase I metabolites of some drugs have activity exceeding or at least equal to that of the parent drug. Examples include phenobarbital (from primidone), ciprofloxacin (from enrofloxacin), desfuroylceftiofur (from ceftiofur) and possibly benzimidazole sulphoxides (from the corresponding sulphides).

Biotransformation, especially phase I metabolic reactions, cannot be assumed to be synonymous with detoxification because some drugs (although a minority) and xenobiotics are converted to potentially toxic metabolites (e.g. parathion, fluorine-containing volatile anaesthetics) or chemically reactive intermediates that produce toxicity (e.g. paracetamol in cats). The term 'lethal synthesis' refers to the biochemical process whereby a 'non-toxic' substance is metabolically converted to a toxic form. The poisonous plant *Dichapetalum cymosum* contains monofluoroacetate which, following gastrointestinal absorption, enters the tricarboxylic acid (Krebs) cycle in which it becomes converted to monofluorocitrate. The latter compound causes toxicity in animals due to irreversible inhibition of the enzyme aconitase. The selective toxicity of flucytosine for susceptible yeasts (*Cryptococcus neoformans*, *Candida* spp.) is attributable to its conversion (deamination) to 5-fluorouracil, which is incorporated into messenger RNA.

Changes in the rate of biotransformation

The rate of drug biotransformation is determined by drug access to and activity of drug-metabolizing enzymes. The major biotransformation pathways for lipid-soluble drugs are those mediated by cytochrome P450 enzymes associated with hepatic microsomes. Drug access to heaptic microsomal enzymes is influenced by lipid solubility of the drug, extent of binding to plasma proteins and liver blood flow, while activity of the drug-metabolizing enzymes is an inherent property of the enzyme system that can be altered, either induced (stimulated) or inhibited.

A wide variety of drugs (e.g. phenobarbital, carbamazepine, phenytoin, phenylbutazone, dexamethasone and rifampin), the chlorinated hydrocarbon insecticides (such as dichlorodiphenyl-trichloroethane (DDT), dieldrin) and environmental pollutants (notably the polychlorinated biphenyls (PCBs)) are capable of inducing hepatic microsomal enzymes. The physicochemical property that these structurally unrelated substances have in common is that of lipid solubility. The enhanced metabolizing capacity represents an increase in the concentration of enzyme protein (due to increased synthesis) rather than increased activity *per se* (Conney & Burns, 1972). Induction results in an increase in the rate of biotransformation and usually a decrease in the duration of action of the inducing substance (when administered repeatedly) and concurrently administered drugs. However, in the case of drugs that are metabolically transformed to reactive intermediates, enzyme induction may exacerbate drug-mediated tissue toxicity. Inducing substances generally increase the metabolizing capacity of cytochrome P450 isoenzymes within a subfamily, although individual isoenzymes may be separately induced. Exposure to polycyclic aromatic hydrocarbons results in dramatic induction of CYP1A subfamily both in the liver and extrahepatically. The repeated use of anticonvulsants (phenobarbital, carbamazepine, phenytoin), glucocorticoids or rifampin induces cytochrome P450 isoenzymes in the subfamily CYP3A. Topically applied dexamethasone is capable of inducing several isoenzymes of cytochrome P450 located in the epidermis. Microsomal-associated transferring enzymes that are involved in phase II biotransformation reactions, specifically glucuronide and glutathione conjugations, are inducible.

Inhibition of drug-metabolizing enzymes decreases the rate of bio-transformation reactions and prolongs the duration of action of drugs that undergo metabolism by the inhibited pathways. Imidazole-containing drugs, such as cimetidine (H_2-receptor antagonist) and ketoconazole (antifungal agent) bind tightly to the haeme iron of cytochrome P450 and competitively inhibit the metabolism of endogenous substances and concurrently adminis-tered drugs. Macrolide antibiotics, such as erythromycin, are metabolized apparently by cytochrome P450 3A (CYP3A) to metabolites that complex the haeme iron of the cytochrome and thereby render it inactive; macrolides appear to have the dual ability to induce and inhibit cytochrome P450 isoenzymes of the subfamily CYP3A (Babany *et al.*, 1988; Ortiz-de-Montellano, 1988). Certain substances, e.g. chloramphenicol, inhibit the activity of cytochrome P450 enzymes through covalent interaction with a reactive intermediate to which the substance is metabolically converted by the enzymes. At least some non-microsomal enzymes can be inhibited. Allopurinol inhibits xanthine oxidase, the enzyme that catalyses the oxidation of hypoxanthine to xanthine and uric acid. Metronidazole and disulfiram inhibit acetaldehyde dehydrogenase, which metabolizes ethanol to acetic acid.

The pharmacological action of some therapeutic agents can be attributed to inhibition of a specific enzyme which constitutes the drug receptor. Examples include the non-steroidal anti-inflammatory drugs (inhibit cyclo-oxygenases), theophylline (inhibits phosphodiesterase) and acetazolamide (inhibits carbonic anhydrase). Physostigmine and neostigmine are reversible inhibitors of cholinesterase, whereas the organophosphorus compounds 'irreversibly' inhibit cholinesterase. In the presence of organophosphate toxicity, the repe-ated administration of high doses of atropine (muscarinic receptor antagonist) can offset the muscarinic effects of the accumulated acetylcholine, but recovery is governed by the synthesis of new enzyme (acetylcholinesterase, AChE) protein. To hasten the otherwise slow recovery, repeated doses of an oxime (pralidoxime or obidoxime), which reactivates 'unaged' AChE, can be administered. The bispyridinium oxime HI-6 is a powerful reactivator of unaged AChE inhibited by the highly toxic organophorus compounds soman, sarin and tabun (nerve gases).

Disease states may alter the rate of drug metabolism directly by affecting organs and tissues involved in biotransformation reactions and indirectly by affecting hepatic blood flow, protein binding, cofactor availability and renal clearance. Extensive liver damage impairs the activities of the microsomal mixed-function oxidase system and the conjugation reactions in which the transferring enzymes are associated with hepatic microsomes (e.g. glucuronide and glutathione conjugations). Cardiac disease, by reducing blood flow to the liver, may decrease the rate of elimination (biotransformation) of high extracted (hepatic extraction ratio >0.6) drugs (e.g. pethidine, morphine, lignocaine and propranolol), as the hepatic clearance of these drugs is blood-flow limited.

Metabolic transformation mediated by intestinal micro organisms

Intestinal microorganisms are capable of metabolizing drugs and other foreign chemical substances by a variety of biotransformation reactions (Scheline, 1968). Of these, reductive and hydrolytic reactions are quantitatively of greatest importance (Williams, 1972). Metabolic transformation mediated by intestinal microorganisms may activate prodrugs, or partly inactivate drugs administered orally. In addition, hydrolysis of glucuronide conjugates of drugs excreted in the bile liberates the parent drug or phase I metabolite, which could be reabsorbed depending on lipid solubility. The cycle comprising biliary excretion, reabsorption from the intestine and return to the liver via the hepatic portal vein is referred to as the enterohepatic circulation (Fig. 1.10). When a significant fraction of the dose undergoes this cycling process, the duration of drug action will be prolonged in accordance with the decreased rate of elimination.

   An orally administered drug can be metabolized by intestinal microorganisms (e.g. sulphasalazine), by enzymes located in the intestinal mucosa and/or in the liver before entering the systemic circulation (first-pass effect). Biotransformation at these sites decreases the systemic availability of an orally administered drug, i.e. the fraction of the dose that enters the systemic circulation unchanged. In ruminant species, the ruminal microorganisms are capable of at least partially inactivating some orally administered drugs (chloramphenicol, trimethoprim, nitroxynil, digoxin) by hydrolytic and reductive reactions. The susceptibility of ruminant species to toxicity caused by ingestion of plants containing cyanogenetic glycosides (e.g. *Prunus* spp. *Acacia* spp., *Eucalyptus cladocalyx*) is due to hydrolytic release of hydrogen cyanide (prussic acid) in the rumen. The principal site of microbial biotransformation in horses is the large intestine (caecum and colon). Because of its posterior location, drugs or drug metabolites excreted in bile may undergo microbial biotransformation in the horse. Moreover drugs administered, particularly in solid/powder or semisolid/paste dosage form, in the feed or close to the time of feeding, may be conveyed by the ingesta to the large intestine. Upon release from the feed by microbial digestion, microbial biotransformation may occur. In herbivorous species, microbial biotransformation of drugs is quantitatively of much greater importance than in non-herbivorous species, while destruction

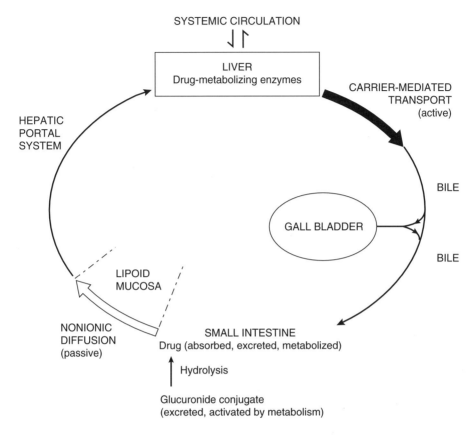

SYSTEMIC CIRCULATION

LIVER
Drug-metabolizing enzymes

CARRIER-MEDIATED
TRANSPORT
(active)

HEPATIC
PORTAL
SYSTEM

BILE

GALL BLADDER

BILE

LIPOID
MUCOSA

NONIONIC
DIFFUSION
(passive)

SMALL INTESTINE
Drug (absorbed, excreted, metabolized)

Hydrolysis

Glucuronide conjugate
(excreted, activated by metabolism)

Fig. 1.10 The enterohepatic circulation. Some drugs or their glucuronida conjugates and certain endogenous substances enter this cycle of events. The enterohepatic circulation of a drug may contribute to its duration of action. The horse, unlike other domestic animal species, does not possess a gall bladder.

of the indigenous microbial flora by antimicrobial drugs, administered orally or parenterally, can cause severe digestive disturbances, particularly in horses.

Excretion

Polar drugs and drug metabolites (particularly conjugates), due to their limited capacity to diffuse through lipid membranes, are eliminated by excretion. The kidneys are by far the most important organ of excretion, although certain compounds are excreted by the liver in the bile.

The kidneys receive the largest blood flow (22–24% of cardiac output) of any organ, relative to the percentage body weight they constitute (cattle, 0.24%; horse 0.36%; dog, 0.61%). The functional unit of the kidney is the nephron, which comprises a renal corpuscle (glomerulus and Bowman's capsule), proximal convoluted tubule, descending and ascending limbs of the loop of

Henle, distal convoluted tubule and collecting tubule. The most significant feature of the mammalian renal system is its highly developed anatomical arrangement in which renal cells are interposed between blood and tubular fluid. The hydrostatic pressure, imparted to the blood by the heartbeat, forces a 'protein-free' filtrate of plasma through the pores of the glomerular capillaries. The permeability of the glomerular capillaries is about 50 times that of the capillaries in skeletal muscle. As the glomerular filtrate passes down the renal tubules, its volume is reduced and its composition altered by the processes of tubular reabsorption and tubular secretion, resulting in the formation of urine. Many homeostatic regulatory mechanisms operate to minimize changes in the volume and composition of the internal fluid environment. Total body water comprises 60% of body weight, of which approximately one-third is extra-cellular fluid.

Renal excretion is the principal process for elimination of drugs that are predominantly ionized at physiological pH and for compounds with limited solubility in lipid (drug metabolites). Because the normal physiological processes are utilized in the excretion of drugs and drug metabolites, glomerular filtration of molecules that are not bound to plasma proteins (free drug and metabolites) invariably occurs. The glomerular filtration rate (GFR) varies among animal species. Average values of GFR, expressed in mL/min per kg body weight, for the various species are: horse, 1.65; sheep, 2.20; cattle and goats, 2.25; pig, 2.80; cat, 2.94; dog, 3.96. Endogenous creatinine clearance provides a clinically useful index of renal function (GFR).

The involvement of tubular secretion and/or reabsorption depends on the chemical nature and physicochemical properties of the compound. Tubular secretion is an active (requires the expenditure of energy), carrier-mediated, saturable process whereby certain polar organic compounds are excreted by proximal tubule cells directly into the glomerular filtrate. While plasma protein binding decreases the availability of drug molecules for glomerular filtration, it does not directly influence tubular secretion, presumably because of rapid dissociation of the drug – protein complex. Therefore, tubular secretion is generally a function of total plasma drug concentration. There are separate secretory pathways for organic anions and cations. Examples of drugs and drug conjugates that undergo tubular secretion are given in Table 1.9. As this excretion mechanism is carried-mediated, it is subject to competitive inhibition by compounds of a generally similar character that share the same pathway. A well-known example is the inhibition by probenecid of the tubular secretion of some antimicrobial agents and drugs that are weak organic acids. The ability of probenecid to inhibit tubular secretion has been used to decrease the rate of elimination of benzylpenicillin (penicillin G) and thus increase the duration of action of the penicillin as a consequence of the longer half-life. Competitive inhibition provides the only conclusive evidence that a transport process is carrier-mediated.

While a drug may enter tubular fluid both by glomerular filtration and proximal tubular secretion, its renal clearance may, nonetheless, be low due to

Table 1.9 Examples of drugs and drug conjugates that are actively secreted by proximal renal tubule cells into tubular fluid.

Acids	Bases
Penicillins[a]	Amiloride
Cephalosporins[a]	Triamterene
Furosemide	Procainamide
Benzothiadiazides (thiazide diuretics)	Quaternary ammonium compounds
Methotrexate	Cimetidine
Probenecid	
p-Aminohippurate (PAH)	
Glucuronic acid conjugates	
Sulphate conjugates	
N^4 -Acetylated sulphonamides	

[a] Nafcillin, cefoperazone and ceftriaxone are β-lactam antimicrobials that are mainly excreted by the liver in bile.

substantial reabsorption of the drug in the distal nephron (refers to the distal convoluted tubule and collecting tubule). As reabsorption takes place by passive diffusion, it is influenced by the concentration of the drug and its degree of ionization in distal tubular fluid. Because of the highly efficient reabsorption of water from the glomerular filtrate in the proximal tubule, a large concentration gradient exists between drug in distal tubular fluid and free drug in the blood. The degree of ionization is determined by the pK_a of the drug and the pH of distal tubular fluid, which is similar to that of urine. The pH of urine is mainly determined by the composition of the diet. It is generally acidic (pH 5.5–7.0) in carnivorous species, alkaline in herbivorous species (pH 7.2–8.4) and can vary over a wider range (pH 4.5–8.0) in humans. Alteration of urinary pH, which can be clinically useful in the management of drug intoxication, may affect the excretion rate of weak organic electrolytes, particularly those with pK_a values within the range 4.5–8.5. The urine pH–excretion rate dependency is substantial only when a significant fraction (> 20%) of the dose is normally excreted unchanged in the urine and the non-ionized moiety in distal tubular fluid is lipid-soluble. For drugs that are eliminated both by hepatic biotransformation and renal excretion, the fraction of dose excreted unchanged in the urine varies widely between species; it is generally lower in the herbivorous species due to more rapid biotransformation of lipid-soluble drugs in these species. Urinary acidification promotes the reabsorption from the distal nephron of weak organic acids and enhances the renal excretion of weak organic bases. Because tubular reabsorption is also influenced by the rate of urine flow, the induction of alkaline diuresis will further increase the excretion rate of weak organic acids in unchanged form (parent drug).

The liver clears compounds from arterial blood, as do the kidneys, and also from portal venous blood. Hepatic elimination processes include various biotransformation reactions, mainly microsomal oxidative reactions and conjugation reactions, and biliary excretion. Some drugs (e.g. cardiac glyco-sides, erythromycin, tetracyclines) and glucuronide conjugates of a variety of compounds, which include lipophilic drugs (e.g. morphine, sulindac, indo-methacin) or their phase I metabolites and endogenous substances (bilirubin, steroid hormones), are excreted by the liver in the bile. Glutathione conjugates, including that of sulphobromophthalein (BSP), are excreted in bile. Most of the compounds excreted in bile are polar and have molecular weights exceeding 300 g/mol. Species variations in the extent of biliary excretion are likely to occur for polar compounds with molecular weights in the range 300–500 g/mol (Williams, 1971a).

Bile is an exocrine secretion of hepatic cells, mainly periportal hepatocytes. It is composed of bile salts, bile pigments (bilirubin glucuronide) and other substances dissolved in an alkaline electrolyte solution (pH 7.8–8.4). Bile is secreted continuously at the rate of 0.5–0.75 mL/h per kg body weight and is temporarily stored in the gall bladder, with the exception of the horse and certain other species (including camelids and giraffe) which do not possess a gall bladder. Upon stimulation by the hormone cholecystokinin-pancreozymin (CCK), secreted by cells of the upper small intestinal mucosa, the gall bladder contracts and releases the stored bile. Consequently the flow of bile into the duodenum is intermittent, apart from the horse in which bile flow is con-tinuous. Some of the components of bile, in particular bile salts, are reabsorbed in the intestine, conveyed back to the liver in the portal vein and re-excreted in the bile (enterohepatic circulation). Because of its anterior location, the forest-omach of ruminant species does not participate in the enterohepatic circulation of drugs. However, drugs that passively diffuse form the systemic circulation into the rumen or enter the rumen via saliva, which is alkaline (pH 8.2–8.4) and is secreted at a daily rate of 100–190 L in cattle and 6–16 L in sheep, may be slowly reabsorbed. The unbound fraction of weak organic acids in plasma is available for diffusion into saliva and the cycle of excretion in saliva and slow reabsorption form reticulo-ruminal fluid could contribute to the long half-lives of phenylbutazone (55 h) and carprofen (43 h) in cattle.

Organic anions (including glucuronic acid and glutathione conjugates) and cations are actively secreted by hepatocytes into bile by carrier-mediated transport processes which appear to have features similar to those in the proximal renal tubule. In addition, neutral organic compounds (e.g. cardiac glycosides) are actively transported into bile. The liver is proficient in removing protein-bound drugs from the blood so that extensive binding to plasma albumin does not deter biliary excretion, whereas it would delay glomerular filtration.

Glucuronide conjugates excreted in bile may be hydrolysed by β-glucuronidase, which is present in intestinal microorganisms, and the liberated drug or, to a lesser extent, phase I metabolite (which is less lipid-soluble) may be reabsorbed by passive diffusion. When a significant fraction of the dose undergoes enterohepatic circulation, elimination of the drug is slow. It is usual for these drugs to be gradually eliminated by renal excretion (e.g. most tetracycline antibiotics, cardiac glycosides). The contribution of biliary excretion as a mechanism of drug elimination lies in the hepatic clearance of organic anions and cations and of neutral organic compounds that do not undergo enterohepatic circulation.

Rate of elimination

Elimination refers to biotransformation (metabolism) and excretion. Half-life is the pharmacokinetic parameter used to measure the overall rate of drug elimination. Following the intravenous injection of a single dose, the half-life expresses the time required for the plasma concentration, as well as the amount of drug in the body, to decrease by 50% through elimination processes, that is, during the elimination phase of the disposition curve (Fig. 1.11). At therapeutic dosage, the majority of drugs are eliminated by first-order kinetics, which implies that a constant *fraction* (50%) is eliminated each clinically relevant half-life. The clinically relevant half-life is that associated with the therapeutic range of plasma concentrations of the drug and it is used in the selection of a dosage interval. Another application of this pharmacokinetic parameter is in the comparison of the rate of drug elimination in different species.

Species variations in half-life

Mammals and birds

There are wide species variations in the half-lives of most drugs that are eliminated mainly by hepatic metabolism (Table 1.10). The only property these drugs have in common is that they are relatively lipid-soluble, which is also a feature of xenobiotics (including drugs) that induce hepatic microsomal enzymes. With regard to comparison of species, the general trend is that drug half-lives are shorter in cattle and horses (herbivorous species) than in dogs and cats (carnivorous species), while the half-lives are considerably longer (i.e. drug elimination takes place more slowly) in human beings than in domestic animals. There are, however, notable exceptions to this trend, such as the methylxanthines (caffeine and theophylline) in horses and phenylbutazone in cattle, that defy explanation at the present time. Although a wide range of values exists for the half-life of phenylbutazone in cattle (42–66 h), it does not appear to be dose-dependent in this species. The average half-life of phenylbutazone in dromedaries (*Camelus dromedarius*), goats and sheep is

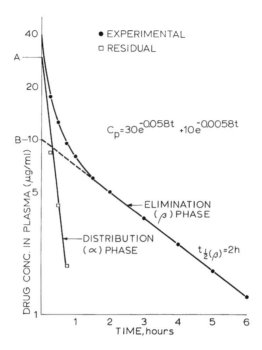

Fig. 1.11 Semilogarithmic graph showing the decline in plasma drug concentrations (with time) following the intravenous injection of a single dose (10 mg/kg). The biexponential equation of the disposition curve is shown (inset). The half-life, $t_{1/2 \, (\beta)}$, of drug is calculated from the expression $t_{1/2 \, (\beta)} = 0.693/\beta$, where β (0.0058 min^{-1}) is the negative logarithm of the slope of the linear terminal portion (elimination phase) of the disposition curve. (Reproduced with permission from Baggot, (1977).)

12.5 h, 15.9 h and 17.9 h, respectively. Because of differences in the rate of hepatic metabolism, the half-life of some drugs (e.g. sulphamethazine, trimethoprim, ceftiofur, closantel) is shorter in goats than in sheep, while the half-life of certain other drugs (e.g. phenylbutazone, norfloxacin) is shorter in donkeys than in horses.

Two drugs that have unusually long half-lives in dogs are naproxen (a non-steroidal anti-inflammatory drug) and phenobarbitone, which is used for the control of *grand mal* epilepsy. The half-life of naproxen is 74 h in mongrel dogs (35 h in Beagles), 13.9 h in humans, 8.3 h in horses and 1.9 h in Rhesus monkeys. Flunixin, ibuprofen and salicylate have half-lives in dogs of 3.7 h, 4.6 h and 8.6 h, respectively. The half-life of phenobarbitone is 64 h in mongrel dogs (32 h in Beagles), 96–120 h in humans, 24–48 h in baboons and 18 h in horses. Because of the short half-lives of phenytoin, sodium valproate, carbamazepine and clonazepam in dogs relative to humans (Table 1.11), the dosage intervals that would be required in dogs for anti-convulsant effectiveness make conventional dosage forms of these drugs impractical for therapeutic use. The half-life of diazepam *per se* in dogs is 3.2 h, while that of the combined parent drug and active metabolites (desmethyldiazepam and oxazepam) is 7.6 h, compared with

Table 1.10 Species variations in the half-lives of some drugs that are mainly eliminated by hepatic metabolism.

Drug	Cattle	Horse	Dog	Human
Pentobarbitone	0.8	1.5	4.5[c]	22.3
Thiopentone	3.3	2.5	8.3	11.5
Salicylate	0.8	1.0	8.6	12.0
Phenylbutazone	42–66	4.1–4.7[a]	2.5–6.0[a]	72.0[a]
Flunixin	6.9	1.9	3.7	–
Morphine	–	1.0	0.95	1.9
Ketamine	0.9	0.7	1.0	2.5
Caffeine	3.8	18.2	4.25	4.9
Theophylline	6.9	14.8	5.7	9.0
Norfloxacin	2.4	6.4	3.6	5.0
Enrofloxacin	1.7	5.0	3.4	–
Chloramphenicol	3.6	0.9	4.2	4.6
Metronidazole	2.8	3.9	4.5	8.5
Trimethoprim[b]	1.25	3.2	4.6	10.6
Sulphadiazine[b]	2.5	3.6	5.6	9.9
Sulphadimethoxine[b]	12.5	11.3	13.2	40

[a] Half-life is dose-dependent.
[b] Half-life may be influenced by urinary pH reaction.
[a] Half-life of pentobarbitone in mongrel dogs is 8.2 h when plasma concentration-time data are analysed according to a three-compartment pharmacokinetic model.

Table 1.11 Comparison of the average half-lives following the intravenous administration (apart from carbamazepine) of a single dose of anticonvulsant drugs in dogs and human beings.

	Half-life (h)		Therapeutic range plasma concentrations (µg/mL)
Drug	Dog	Human	
Phenobarbitone	64	96	10–25
Phenytoin	3.5–4.5[a]	15–24[a]	10–20
Sodium valproate	2	14	40–100
Carbamazepine (p.o.)	1.5	15	4–10
Clonazepam	1.5–2.5[a]	24–36[a]	0.01–0.08
Diazepam	7.6[b]	32.9[b]	>0.6

[a] Half-life is dose-dependent.
[b] Parent drug and active metabolites.

32.9 h in humans. The rapid conversion of diazepam to metabolites with lower (about one-third) anticonvulsant activity may explain the variable clinical effectiveness of the drug, which must be injected intravenously, in controlling *status epilepticus* in the dog (Frey & Loscher, 1985).

The half-life of pethidine (meperidine), which is eliminated by hydrolysis and *N*-demethylation (microsomal oxidative reaction) or conjugation with glucuronic acid is 0.7–0.9 h in goats, dogs and cats, 1.1 h in horses and pigs, 1.2 h in Rhesus monkeys and 3.2 h in human. Because it undergoes rapid biotransformation, the duration of analgesia produced by pethidine is short in domestic animals. The principal indication for use of pethidine in dogs and cats is pre-anaesthetic medication. Unlike morphine, the dose (3.3 mg/kg) of pethidine hydrochloride is the same for both species and should be administered by intramuscular injection. The preferred sites for intramuscular injection of parenteral drug preparations in dogs are the lumbar epaxial musculature and the quadriceps femoris muscle (Autefage *et al.*, 1990). Pethidine is indicated in horses for the relief of visceral pain associated with spasmodic colic; the dose (2.2 mg/kg) is administered by intramuscular injection. The prime site for intramuscular injection in the neck of horses appears to be at the level of the fifth cervical vertebra, ventral to the funicular part of the ligamentum nuchae but dorsal to the brachiocephalic muscle (Boyd, 1987). However, a higher degree of analgesia and fewer side-effects are produced by the concomitant use, at reduced dosage, of xylazine hydrochloride (0.25 mg/kg) or the more potent detomidine hydrochloride (0.025 mg/kg), administered by slow intravenous injection, and butorphanol tartrate (0.05 mg/kg) injected intravenously. The half-life of flunixin meglumine (non-steroidal anti-inflammatory drug), which binds extensively to plasma proteins and is eliminated both by hepatic metabolism and renal excretion is short in cats (1.5 h) and horses (1.9 h) compared with dogs (3.7 h) and cattle (6.9 h). In common with some other drugs that undergo partial excretion in bile, the half-life of flunixin is shorter in donkeys (0.5 h) than in horses (1.9 h). The half-lives of several extensively metabolized drugs (e.g. hexobarbitone, caffeine, theophylline, diazepam) are shorter in laboratory animal species (mice, rats, guinea pigs and rabbits) and Rhesus monkeys than in domestic animals. Consistent with this trend is that the average half-life of antipyrine, a marker substance used to indicate hepatic microsomal oxidative activity, is shorter in laboratory animals (0.2–1.4 h) and Rhesus monkeys (1.2 h) than in domestic animals (1.75–3.25 h) and human beings (10.3–12.7 h); antipyrine half-life is shorter in goats than in sheep. Pygmy (dwarf) goats metabolize at least some drugs, e.g. sulphonamides (hydroxylation) and chloramphenicol (glucuronide conjugation), more rapidly than other breeds of goat. Based on antipyrine half-life, there appears to be an approximately threefold difference in hepatic microsomal oxidative activity between Pygmy goats and other breeds.

Individual variation is generally wider in humans than in domestic or laboratory animal species. It has been hypothesized (Boxenbaum, 1982) that the lesser quantitative ability of humans to metabolize drugs, especially by hepatic

microsomal oxidative reactions, may be correlated with their enhanced longevity (maximum life-span potential).

Even though the half-lives of a variety of drugs that undergo extensive
hepatic metabolism conform to a general pattern in mammalian species, the
rates of oxidative, reductive and hydrolytic reactions (phase I metabolic
pathways) are unpredictable. There is less uncertainty associated with the
conjugation reactions (phase II metabolic pathways), because some are either
defective or absent in certain species. For example, cats slowly synthesize
glucuronide conjugates of drugs with functional groups suitable for conjugation; dogs are unable to acetylate aromatic amino groups. The amino acid used
for conjugation may differ between primate and non-primate species (Smith &
Williams, 1974) as well as between mammalian and avian species (Williams,
1967).

Like in mammals, wide variations exist between avian species in the half-
lives of drugs that are eliminated mainly by hepatic metabolism (Dorrestein &
van Miert, 1988). The apparent half-life of chloramphenicol (50 mg/kg, i.m.) in
a variety of avian species ranges from 0.5 h in Columbiformes (pigeons) to 3.5 h
in Galliformes (poultry) (Clark *et al.*, 1982), while that of ceftiofur (10 mg/kg,
i.m.) ranges from 2.5 h in cockatiels to 7.9 h in Amazon parrots (Tell *et al.*, 1998).
The half-life of enrofloxacin, which is metabolized by various oxidative reactions and formation of conjugates, is 7.0 h in chickens compared with 4.1 h in
turkeys. Following oral administration of norfloxacin (20% oral solution,
10 mg/kg), the apparent half-life of the drug is similar in chickens (11.1 h),
turkeys (9.1 h) and geese (10.65 h), but the peak plasma concentration (C_{max})
attained is significantly lower in turkeys (Laczay *et al.*, 1998). The differences
between chickens and turkeys, sheep and goats, horses and donkeys in the rate
of elimination of some lipid-soluble drugs are unpredictable, but the trend is
that such drugs are eliminated more rapidly by turkeys, goats and donkeys
than by chickens, sheep and horses, respectively.

Renal excretion is the principal elimination process for drugs that are predominantly ionized at physiological pH and for compounds with limited
solubility in lipid (polar drugs and drug metabolites). Due to their chemical
nature and physicochemical properties, these drugs are generally less widely
distributed in extravascular tissues than lipophilic drugs. There is less pronounced variation between species in the half-lives of drugs that are mainly
eliminated by renal excretion than of drugs that undergo extensive hepatic
metabolism. The clinically relevant half-life of gentamicin in domestic animal
species (dog, 1.25 h; cat, 1.36 h; cattle, sheep and goats, 1.4–1.8 h; pig, 1.9 h; horse
and donkey, 2.5 h), with the exception of the pig, reflects the relative (not
actual) rate of glomerular filtration and is independent of the urinary pH
reaction. For comparative purposes, the half-life of gentamicin, which is
eliminated solely by glomerular filtration, is 0.6 h in rats, about 1 h in guinea
pigs and rabbits, 2–3 h in humans, about 3 h in llamas and camels, 1.25–3.4 h in
various avian species, 12 h in channel catfish (*Ictalurus punctatus*) at 22°C, and
an average of 51 h in three reptilian species.

Penicillins and cephalosporins have short half-lives (0.5–1.5 h) in domestic animals because these antibiotics are secreted by the proximal renal tubules and, due to their high degree of ionization, are not reabsorbed from the distal nephron. The half-lives of lipid-soluble weak organic acids (e.g. sulphadimethoxine, sulphadiazine, phenobarbitone) and organic bases (e.g. trimethoprim, procainamide, amphetamine) of which a significant fraction (>20%) of the dose is eliminated by renal excretion may be influenced by the urinary pH reaction. Under acidic urinary conditions, which are normally present in carnivorous species, weak acids are reabsorbed from the distal renal tubules, whereas the excretion of weak bases is enhanced.

The tetracyclines, apart from doxycycline and minocycline, are slowly eliminated by renal excretion (glomerular filtration). Their slow elimination can be attributed to enterohepatic circulation whereby drug excreted by the liver in bile is reabsorbed from the intestine. The half-life of oxytetracycline differs widely between animal species; goat (3.4 h), cattle (4.0 h), sheep (5.2 h), dog (6.0 h), pig (6.0 h), donkey (6.5 h), horse (9.6 h), and red-necked wallaby (*Macropus rufogriseus*) (11.4 h). Doxycycline, unlike other tetracyclines, is eliminated by biliary excretion and diffusion into the intestine. The half-life of doxycycline is relatively short in dogs (7.0 h) and cats (4.6 h) compared with human beings (16 h). The half-life of doxycycline in chickens (4.8 h) is shorter than in turkeys (10 h) (Santos *et al.*, 1996). Minocycline is mainly eliminated by hepatic metabolism.

The basis of the species variation in the half-life of digoxin is difficult to explain, as this drug is primarily eliminated by renal excretion. The average half-life of digoxin is 7.8 h in cattle, 11.7 h in ferrets 7.2 h in sheep, 23 h in horses, 28 h in dogs, 35 h in cats and 39 ± 13 h in human beings. Variation in the half-life could be attributed to the extremely wide extravascular distribution, the tissue binding of the drug, the very low and narrow range of therapeutic plasma concentrations (0.6–2.4 ng/mL) and the contribution of enterohepatic circulation to prolongation of the rate of elimination. Because plasma protein binding of digoxin in the various species is low (18–36%), protein binding would not be a contributing factor.

The half-lives of a small number of drugs are dose-dependent, i.e. their elimination obeys zero-order kinetics, in certain species. In order to ascertain whether the elimination of a drug obeys linear (first-order) or non-linear (zero-order) kinetics, the drug should be administered intravenously at three, or more, dose levels (mg/kg); usually the just-effective dose, double and four times the just-effective dose. Dose-dependent elimination can generally be attributed to saturation of a major metabolic pathway for a drug, even when administered at therapeutic dosage. Examples include phenylbutazone in horses and dogs, rifampin in horses, salicylate in cats, phenytoin, salicylate and ethanol in humans. When sulphonamides are administered at high dosage (≥100 mg/kg), hydroxylation (a major metabolic pathway for these drugs in herbivorous species and in dogs) is capacity-limited (Vree *et al.*, 1985). When the plasma concentration falls below the saturation level of the capacity-limited metabolic pathway, the elimination of the drug changes from zero-order (constant rate) to first-order (exponential) kinetics.

Fish

Compared to those of mammalian and avian species, the half-lives of antimicrobial agents in poikilothermic species (fish and reptiles) are prolonged, which is consistent with their much lower metabolic turnover rate (Calder, 1984), and are influenced by ambient (in the case of fish, water) temperature (Table 1.12). The average half-life of trimethoprim, administered intravenously as trimethoprim–sulphadiazine combination, in carp (*Cyprinus carpio* L.) is 40.7 h at 10°C and 20 h at 24°C (Nouws *et al.*, 1993) compared with 1.25 h in cattle, 3.2 h in horses, 4.6 h in dogs and 10.6 h in human beings. Sulphadiazine half-life similarly differs widely between species: carp (47 h at 10°C; 33 h at 24°C), cattle (2.5 h), horses (3.6 h), dogs (5.6 h) and human beings (9.9 h). The prolonged half-lives of lipid-soluble antimicrobial agents in fish, although mainly due to much slower hepatic metabolism, could be partly attributed to lower renal function and a greater degree of enterohepatic circulation. Glomerular filtration and passive diffusion across the gill membranes may contribute to the excretion of lipophilic drugs in fish (Brodie & Maickel, 1962). Oxytetracycline is slowly eliminated by glomerular filtration because the drug

Table 1.12   Half-lives of some antimicrobial agents in various species of fish.

Antimicrobial agent	Fish species	Acclimatization temperature (°C)	Half-life (h)
Trimethoprim	Carp (*Cyprinus carpio*)	10	40.7
		24	20.0
Sulphadiazine	Carp (*Cyprinus carpio*)	10	47.0
		24	33.0
Sulphadimidine	Carp (*Cyprinus carpio*)	10	50.3
	Rainbow trout (*Oncorhynchus gairdneri*)	20	25.6
		10	20.6
		20	14.7
Ciprofloxacin	Rainbow trout (*Oncorhynchus gairdneri*)	12	11.2
	Carp ((*Cyprinus carpio*)	20	14.5
	African catfish (*Clarias gariepinus*)	25	14.2
Florfenicol	Atlantic salmon (*Salmo salar*)	10.8 ± 1.5[a]	12.2
Oxytetracycline	Rainbow trout (*Oncorhynchus gairdneri*)	12	89.5
	African catfish (*Clarias gariepinus*)	25	80.3
Gentamicin	Channel catfish (*Ictalurus punctatus*)	22	12.0

[a] Sea water.

undergoes enterohepatic circulation. The half-life of oxytetracycline is 80.3 h in African catfish (*Clarias gariepinus*) at 25°C and 89.5 h in rainbow trout (*Salmo gairdneri*) at 12°C (Grondel *et al.*, 1989), compared with half-lives in the range 3.4–9.6 h in domestic animals. In poikilothermic species, the elimination of antimicrobial agents increases (i.e. half-life decreases) with increase in ambient temperature. Florfenicol may be indicated in controlling outbreaks of furunculosis (caused by *Aeromonas salmonicida*) in salmon in a salt water environment. The half-life of florfenicol in Atlantic salmon (*Salmo salar*), held in tanks of running sea water at 10.8 ± 1.5°C, is 12.2 h (Varma *et al.*, 1994) which is approximately four times the half-life of the drug in cattle. The antibacterial activity of florfenicol is not affected by acetyl transferase, the bacterial enzyme responsible for the majority of the plasmid-mediated resistance to chloramphenicol and thiamphenicol (Syriopoulou *et al.*, 1981).

The half-life of enrofloxacin in fingerling rainbow trout (*Oncorhynchus mykiss*) at 15°C is 27.4 h (Bowser *et al.*, 1992), which is several times the half-life of the drug in mammalian species: cattle (1.7 h), dogs (3.4 h), llamas (3.4 h), camels (3.6 h), sheep (3.7 h), horses (5 h), pigs (5.5 h) and cats (6.7 h). Enrofloxacin is converted by *N*-deethylation (a hepatic microsomal-mediated reaction) to ciprofloxacin, an antimicrobial agent in its own right. Although enrofloxacin and ciprofloxacin have a similar spectrum of antibacterial activity, they differ in the degree of activity (quantitative susceptibility) in that ciprofloxacin is generally the more active (lower MIC_{90}). (The MIC_{90} is the minimum inhibitory concentration of an antimicrobial agent that, after 18–24 h of incubation, prevents the visible growth of 90% of a certain bacterial species isolated from a species of animal.) The half-life of ciprofloxacin in rainbow trout (*Oncorhynchus gairdneri*) acclimatized at 12°C is 11.2 h, in carp (*Cyprinus carpio*) at 20°C is 14.5 h and in African catfish (*Clarias gariepinus*) at 25°C is 14.2 h (Nouws *et al.*, 1988), compared with half-lives in domestic animals that range from 1.25 h in sheep to 4.7 h in horses. Following the intramuscular administration of enrofloxacin (5 mg/kg) to red pacu (*Colossoma brachypomum*) acclimatized at 25°C, the peak plasma concentration (C_{max}) of enrofloxacin was 1.6 µg/mL and the apparent elimination half-life was 28.9 h; the C_{max} of ciprofloxacin was 0.05 µg/mL and the apparent $t_{1/2}$ was 53 h (Lewbart *et al.*, 1997). Enrofloxacin administered intramuscularly at the same dose to gopher tortoises (*Gopherus polyphemus*) produced a C_{max} of 2.4 µg/mL and the apparent $t_{1/2}$ was 23.1 h (Prezant *et al.*, 1994). Ciprofloxacin is eliminated far more slowly than enrofloxacin in red pacu, whereas both the parent drug and active metabolite are eliminated at approximately the same rate, based on their apparent half-life values, in cattle, horses and dogs. This difference could be largely due to the slower metabolic conversion of enrofloxacin to ciprofloxacin.

Applications of half-life

Useful applications of half-life include selection of the dosage interval associated with a dosage regimen, prediction of the time required to attain a steady-state (plateau) concentration during constant intravenous infusion, and species comparison of the overall rate of elimination of a drug (or marker substance for an elimination process). Because of the availability in research papers of half-life values for drugs and the hybrid nature of half-life, this parameter is generally used for interspecies allometric scaling of drug elimination. Although useful under certain circumstances, the predictive value of this application of half-life depends upon knowledge of the elimination process for the drug and the judicious selection of the species to be included in the scaling technique.

It should be appreciated that half-life is a composite (hybrid) pharmacokinetic parameter which expresses the relationship between the volume of distribution (area method) and the systemic (body) clearance of the drug.

$$t_{1/2} = \frac{0.693 \cdot V_{d(area)}}{Cl_B}$$

The disposition curve for the majority of drugs can be readily separated into distribution and elimination phases. It is on the elimination phase that the half-life is based. Drugs that selectively bind to tissue components (e.g. aminoglycoside antibiotics) have a prolonged terminal elimination phase that is often associated with subtherapeutic plasma concentrations (Fig. 1.12) (Riviere, 1988). For example, the half-life of gentamicin (10 mg/kg, i.v.) in sheep based on the clinically relevant elimination phase is 1.75 h, while that based on the prolonged terminal phase is 88.9 h (Brown *et al.*, 1986). Whenever a semilogarithmic plot of the plasma concentration–time data shows deviation of the elimination phase from linearity, the existence of a 'deep' peripheral compartment can be suspected. For drugs that show linear pharmacokinetic behaviour, dissimilar values of clearance based on single-dose studies and average steady-state plasma concentrations (multiple-dose study) provide definitive evidence of the presence of a 'deep' peripheral compartment (Browne *et al.*, 1990). Requirements of the study design are that the duration of blood sampling be prolonged and the analytical method employed be sufficiently sensitive to detect and precisely measure the drug substance of interest at low concentrations. The relevance of a particular half-life depends upon the intended application, whether it be selection of the dosage interval or tentative prediction of the withdrawal period. The disposition of a drug should be determined at both ends of the recommended dose range. A disproportionate increase in plasma concentration of the drug with increase in dose is evidence of non-linear pharmacokinetic behaviour.

When a conventional (immediate-release) dosage form of a drug is administered orally or by other than intravenous (for example, i.m. or s.c.) injection, the half-life based on the decline phase of the plasma concentration–time curve is an apparent, rather than the true, half-life of the drug. This is because absorption continues after the time (t_{max}) of the observed peak plasma concentration (C_{max}). The apparent half-life varies not only with the route (and site) of administration but also with the formulation of the dosage form of the drug (Baggot & Brown, 1998).

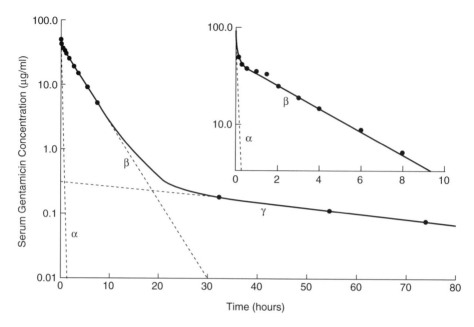

Fig. 1.12   Serum concentration–time profile of gentamicin in an animal after intravenous administration, illustrating three phases of disposition. Alpha and beta phases, relevant for therapeutic monitoring, are the only phases evident when drug concentrations are monitored over a short time after dosing (inset). When a sensitive assay is employed to monitor drug concentrations for prolonged periods, the third (gamma) phase becomes evident. It is this last phase that is responsible for predicting tissue withdrawal times. (Reproduced with permission from Riviere (1988).)

Extent of distribution

After entering the systemic circulation, irrespective of the route of adminis-tration, drugs are conveyed throughout the body in the circulating blood for distribution to tissues and for elimination (biotransformation and excretion). It is only the free (unbound) fraction of drug in the systemic circulation that is available for extravascular distribution; the fraction bound to plasma proteins becomes available as the concentration of drug in the plasma declines. The rate at which a drug distributes extravascularly can be limited either by perfusion (lipophilic drugs) or by diffusion (ionized and polar drugs). The extent of distribution is determined by the chemical nature and related physicochemical properties of the drug (in particular lipid solubility and, in the case of weak organic acids and bases, degree of ionization), extent of binding to plasma proteins and to extravascular tissue components, and by the body composition of the animal species. The most notable differences have been found between ruminant and monogastric species, mainly for lipid-soluble organic bases. Following parenteral administration, these drugs passively diffuse from the systemic circulation into ruminal fluid (pH 5.5–6.5), where they become 'trapped' by ionization. Because of the large capacity of the reticulo-rumen (100–225 L in cattle and 10–25 L in sheep and goats), a significant fraction of the amount of drug in the body may temporarily accumulate in the forestomach. The more widely a drug is distributed, the lower the concentration and fraction in the plasma of the amount of drug in the body. Digoxin and lipophilic weak bases (e.g., diazepam, xylazine) distribute widely in extravascular tissues, whereas the distribution of weak organic acids (e.g. furosemide, phenylbuta-zone) is largely limited to the extracellular fluid. An analogous situation applies to antimicrobial agents.

The pharmacokinetic term that is used to estimate the extent of distribution of a drug is the volume of distribution (V_d). This parameter indicates the *apparent* space (L/kg) in the body available to contain the drug. Volume of distribution relates the amount of drug in the body to the concentration in the plasma or blood, depending upon the fluid measured, at any time after pseudo-distribution equilibrium has been attained. Based on this parameter, the extent of distribution of drugs can be categorized as wide ($>0.7 \text{L/kg}$), moderate ($0.3–0.7 \text{L/kg}$) or limited ($<0.3 \text{L/kg}$). Application to antimicrobial agents pla-ces macrolides, lincosamides, fluoroquinolones and trimethoprim in the widely distributed category; metronidazole, rifampin and sulphonamides are moderately well distributed, while β-lactam antibiotics and aminoglycosides are in the limited distribution category. Even though tetracyclines distribute widely, extravascular distribution of doxycycline (a highly lipid-soluble member of this class) is limited by extensive binding to plasma proteins. Differences in clinical efficacy of individual tetracyclines are attributable to their pharmacokinetic properties (absorption, distribution and excretion) rather than to quantitative differences in the susceptibility of microorganisms. Volume of distribution does not reveal the pattern of distribution of a drug, which can be determined only by measuring the level (amount) of drug in the various organs and tissues of the body.

The volume of distribution (area method) can be calculated from the equation

$$V_{d(area)} = \frac{\text{Dose}}{\text{AUC} \cdot \beta}$$

where AUC is the total area under the plasma concentration–time curve and β is the overall elimination rate constant of the drug, obtained from the linear terminal (elimination) phase of the semilogarithmic disposition curve follow-ing drug administration as an intravenous bolus dose. The AUC can be estimated by the trapezoidal rule, from the time of drug administration to the last measured plasma concentration, with extrapolation to infinite time. Alternatively, the AUC can be obtained from the experimental constants that define the equation describing the biexponential disposition curve:

$$\text{AUC}_{i.v.} = \frac{A}{\alpha} + \frac{B}{\beta}$$

When the drug is administered by an extravascular route, correction for dose must be made in the systemic availability (F) and the apparent first-order elimination rate constant, obtained from the late decline phase of the curve, should be substituted for β in the area method equation.

Because of differences in the body composition of various animal species, the extent of binding to plasma proteins and the rate of elimination of a drug, the volume of distribution may differ between species (Table 1.13). Apart from the extent of distribution of a drug being wide, moderate or limited in the different species, there is no obvious pattern in this parameter. This may be due partly to differences in the analytical methodology employed, because the majority of pharmacokinetic studies of a drug are performed on a single species at any one laboratory. Xylazine is an exception in that the disposition of the drug was studied in sheep, horses and dogs at the same laboratory and coincidentally there was remarkably little variation in the apparent volume of distribution between the species (Garcia-Villar *et al.*, 1981). The volume of distribution of anitimicrobial agents in fish may be categorized similarly to that in mammals, varies between different species of fish, and may be influenced by the temperature of the water in which the fish are acclimatized.

Because the volume of distribution, serving as a proportional factor, relates the plasma concentration to the amount of drug in the body, this term is applied in calculating the size of the dose (mg/kg) required to achieve a desired plasma concentration:

$$\text{Dose}_{i.v.} = C_{p(ther)} \cdot V_{d(area)}$$

Table 1.13   Volume of distribution of some drugs in different species.

Drug	$V_{d(area)}$ (L/kg)		
	Sheep (S)/goat (G)	Horse	Dog
Phenylbutazone	0.10 (S)	0.19	0.20
Furosemide	–	0.24	0.25
Thiopentone	1.00 (S)	0.74	0.85
Theophylline	0.65 (S)	1.02	0.82
Diazepam	–	0.63	0.56
Xylazine	2.74 (S)	2.46	2.52
Gentamicin	0.24 (G)	0.25	0.33
Ampicillin	0.50 (S)	0.30	0.27
Sulphadiazine	0.39 (S)	0.46	0.42
Trimethoprim	1.20 (G)	1.38	1.85
Enrofloxacin	2.52 (S)	2.49	2.45
Thiamphenicol	1.06 (S)	–	0.76
Metronidazole	–	0.66	0.98
Ivermectin	5.30 (S)	–	2.40

where $C_{p(ther)}$ is a plasma concentration within the therapeutic range for a pharmacological agent or a multiple of the minimum inhibitory concentration (MIC) for an antimicrobial agent. When the volume of distribution of a drug varies widely between species, the dosage requirement will differ for the various species. It is only when a drug is administered by intravenous injection that a desired plasma concentration will reliably be produced. Drug administration by an extravascular route may require upward adjustment of the dose to compensate for incomplete systemic availability of the drug. Allowance cannot be made in the size of dose for variation in the rate of drug absorption either between different formulations of the drug administered to a single species or the same formulation administered to different animal species.

When the dose of a drug is administered as an intravenous bolus, the volume of distribution at steady-state ($V_{d(ss)}$) can be calculated. This parameter represents the volume in which a drug would appear to be distributed during steady-state if the drug existed throughout that volume at the same concentration as in the measured fluid (plasma or blood). The volume of distribution at steady-state is generally calculated by a non-compartmental method, which is based on the use of areas (Benet & Galeazzi, 1979) and does not require the application of a compartmental pharmacokinetic model or mathematical description of the disposition curve:

$$V_{d(ss)} = \frac{\text{Dose}_{IV} \cdot \text{AUMC}}{(\text{AUC})^2}$$

where AUC is the total area under the curve (zero moment) and AUMC is the area under the first moment of the plasma concentration–time curve, that is, the area under the curve of the product of time and plasma concentration over the time-span zero to infinity. The value obtained for $V_{d(ss)}$ is generally smaller than that of $V_{d(area)}$; as the elimination rate constant for a drug decreases, $V_{d(area)}$ approaches the value of $V_{d(ss)}$.

The volume of distribution at steady-state is useful for determining the significance of changes in the extent of distribution of a drug in the presence of disease states and for comparing volumes of distribution of the enantiomers of a chiral drug or differences between neonatal and adult animals of the same species. The $V_{d(ss)}$ values of flunixin, ketoprofen and phenylbutazone (non-steroidal anti-inflammatory drugs) are larger in newborn foals than in adult horses because of the larger extracellular fluid volume in the newborn foal. It is unlikely that lower binding of these drugs to plasma proteins contributes significantly to the larger volume of distribution, because the relative hypoalbuminaemia in newborn foals, unlike in piglets, is not pronounced. In dosage calculations, $V_{d(area)}$ rather than $V_{d(ss)}$ should be used.

Clearance

The systemic (body) clearance of a drug represents the *sum* of the clearances by the various organs that contribute to elimination of the drug. It can be calculated by dividing the systemically available dose by the *total* area under the plasma concentration–time curve (from zero time to infinity):

$$Cl_B = \frac{F \cdot \text{Dose}}{\text{AUC}}$$

It is only when the drug is administered intravenously that complete systemic availability ($F = 100\%$, or unity) of the dose can be assumed. Following the administration of a single dose by any route, the total area under the curve can be estimated by the linear trapezoidal rule, from zero time to the last measured plasma drug concentration, with extrapolation to infinite time, assuming log–linear decline:

$$AUC_{(\text{any route})} = \sum_{i=O}^{n-1} \frac{t_{i+1} - t_i}{2}(C_i + C_{i+1}) + \frac{C_{p(\text{last})}}{\beta \text{ or } k_d}$$

where $C_{p(\text{last})}$ is the last measured plasma concentration and β or k_d is the apparent first-order rate constant associated with the elimination or late decline phase of plasma concentration following intravenous or extravascular administration, respectively, of the drug. The accuracy of this method for estimating the total area under the curve (AUC) depends on the number of plasma concentration–time points from the time of drug administration to the last measured plasma concentration, the precision and sensitivity of the analytical method used to quantify plasma concentrations of the drug, and the relative area under the extrapolated portion of the curve, which should be less than 10% of the total area. When the decline of drug concentration is exponential and there are long intervals between the plasma concentration–time points, an improved estimate of AUC may be obtained by using a combination of the linear trapezoidal rule and, during the decline phase, the log trapezoidal method (Gibaldi & Perrier, 1982). If the drug is administered by an extravascular (includes oral) route and the systemic availability (F) is not known, the term Cl_B/F should be reported. This situation arises whenever an intravenous dosage form of the drug is not available.

By definition, the systemic clearance of a drug is the product of the apparent volume of distribution, calculated by the area method, and the overall elimination rate constant:

$$Cl_B = V_{d(\text{area})} \cdot \beta$$

The concept of clearance is extremely useful in clinical pharmacokinetics because the systemic clearance of a drug is usually constant over the range of plasma concentrations of clinical interest. This is because the elimination of most drugs obeys first-order (linear) kinetics whereby a constant *fraction* is eliminated per unit of time. For drugs that exhibit dose-dependent elimination, clearance will vary with the plasma concentrations attained. Elimination of these drugs obeys zero-order (non-linear) kinetics, which implies that a constant *amount* of drug is eliminated per unit of time. Examples of drugs that are eliminated by zero-order kinetics when administered at therapeutic dosage include phenylbutazone in dogs (Dayton *et al.*, 1967) and horses (Piperno *et al.*, 1968), salicylate in cats (Yeary & Swanson, 1973), and phenytoin in human beings (Houghton & Richens, 1974).

Clearance may be regarded as the volume of blood or plasma (depending on the fluid used for drug assay) from which a drug would appear to be removed per unit time to account for its elimination (i.e. biotransformation and excretion). For comparative purposes, clearance is expressed in units of mL/min·kg. Although drug concentrations are usually measured in plasma, clearance based on plasma drug concentrations can have values that are not 'physiological'. Blood clearance may be determined from plasma clearance provided the drug rapidly equilibrates between erythrocytes and plasma and the blood-to-plasma distribution ratio or the erythrocyte-to-plasma concentration ratio at equilibrium is determined (Benet, 1984); knowledge of the haematocrit is required for the conversion.

The systemic clearance, based on measurement of plasma concentrations, of a variety of drugs shows wide species variations (Table 1.14). For drugs that undergo extensive hepatic biotransformation, systemic clearance mainly reflects the capacity of the liver to metabolize these drugs. The systemic clearance of ketamine, based on plasma concentrations in sheep (67 mL/min·kg) is over twice that in horses (28 mL/min·kg) and dogs (29 mL/min·kg) and over four times that in pigs (12 mL/min·kg), cats (13 mL/min·kg) and human beings (15 mL/min·kg). Both distribution and hepatic biotransformation contribute to the duration of ketamine anaesthesia by influencing the time required for the plasma concentration to decline to the minimum effective concentration (2 μg/mL). As the clearance of propofol is based on blood propofol concentrations, the value obtained can be interpreted physiologically. The clearance of propofol exceeds hepatic blood flow, which indicates that the drug is simultaneously metabolized by the liver and at extrahepatic sites (e.g. the lungs). The high value of clearance, particularly in goats (275 mL/min·kg), accounts for the short half-life of propofol (15 min in goats compared with 91 min in dogs). Systemic clearance is additive; in the case of propofol, systemic clearance is the sum of clearances by the liver and extrahepatic tissues.

Enrofloxacin is mainly eliminated by hepatic metabolism, and systemic clearance of the drug varies between species. In sheep, horses, dogs and pigs the average clearance of enrofloxacin is in the range 5.75–8.56 mL/min·kg, while enrofloxacin clearance (mL/min·kg) differs more widely between other species: rabbits (17.9), llamas (12.0), chickens (3.3), turkeys (8.9), houbara bustard (5.7) and fingerling rainbow trout (*Oncorhynchus mykiss*) at 15°C (1.25). Systemic clearance of enrofloxacin represents mainly hepatic clearance composed of a variety of metabolic pathways, which include *N*-deethylation to ciprofloxacin.

The systemic clearance of ciprofloxacin in sheep, horses, dogs and pigs is in

Table 1.14 Systemic clearance of some drugs in different species.

Drug	Process of elimination[a]	Cl_B (mL/min·kg) Sheep (S)/ goat (G)	Horse	Dog	Pig	Human
Flunixin	M	0.65 (S)	1.10	0.86	–	–
Furosemide	E	–	12.9	7.25	–	2.1
Thiopentone	M	3.75 (S)	3.43	1.96	–	3.9
Theophylline	M	1.10 (G)	0.67	1.67	0.63	0.65
Metoclopramide	M + E	59.0 (G)	–	25.3	–	6.2
Ketamine	M	67 (S)	28	29	12	15
Propofol[b]	M	275 (G)	–	59	–	31
Gentamicin	E	1.68 (G)	1.20	3.10	1.66	0.82
Ampicillin	E	5.15 (S)	2.89	3.90	4.50	1.7
Ceftriaxone	E	3.70 (S)	5.22	3.26	–	0.24
Sulphadoxine	M(+E)	0.70 (G)	0.32	–	0.48	–
Sulphadiazine	M(+E)	0.63 (S)	1.45	0.92	–	0.55
Trimethoprim	M(+E)	20.7 (G)	5.03	4.77	5.18	2.2
Enrofloxacin	M	7.80 (S)	5.75	8.56	7.00	–
Ciprofloxacin	M + E	18 (S)	9.7	13	17	7.0
Metronidazole	M(+E)	–	1.97	2.50	–	1.3
Oxytetracycline	E	3.40 (G)/2.25 (S)	1.25	4.03	2.88	–

[a] M, metabolism; E, excretion.
[b] Clearance of propofol is based on concentrations in blood.

the range 10–18 mL/min·kg, while in carp (*Cyprinus carpio*) acclimatized at 20°C, African catfish (*Clarias gariepinus*) at 25°C and rainbow trout (*Oncorhynchus gairdneri*) at 12°C ciprofloxacin clearance (mL/min·kg) is 2.5, 4.5 and 4.8, respectively (Nouws *et al.*, 1988).

Trimethoprim, a lipophilic organic base, is mainly eliminated by hepatic metabolism and to a variable extent, depending on the species, by renal excretion. The systemic clearance of trimethoprim in goats (20.7 mL/min·kg), which predominantly represents hepatic clearance, is four times higher than in horses, dogs and pigs (4.8–5.2 mL/min·kg) and several times higher than in carp (*Cyprinus carpio*), 0.78 mL/min·kg and 2.35 mL/min·kg at 10°C and 24°C, respectively. The systemic clearance of sulphadiazine (and other sulphonamides) does not vary so widely between mammalian species (0.5–1.5 mL/min·kg), but is significantly lower in fish (e.g. in carp it is 0.13 mL/min·kg and 0.20 mL/min·kg at 10°C and 24°C, respectively). The clearance of sulphadimidine in carp (*Cyprinus carpio*) varies with temperature of the water: it is 0.27 mL/min·kg at 10°C and 0.41 mL/min·kg at 20°C.

Because the extravascular distribution of gentamicin (and other aminoglycoside antibiotics) is limited (average $V_{d(area)}$) is about 250 mL/kg in mammalian and avian species), and the drug binds to a low extent to plasma proteins and is eliminated solely by glomerular filtration, the systemic clearance of gentamicin would be expected to reflect the glomerular filtration rate (GFR) in the various species (Table 1.15). This relationship holds true for the majority of species, apart from cats (and human beings) in which gentamicin clearance relative to GFR is somewhat lower than would be expected. Systemic clearance of gentamicin represents renal clearance of the drug and is lower than the GFR because some proximal tubular reabsorption occurs. The clearance of gentamicin in domestic animal species (1.2–3.1 mL/min·kg) is lower than in rabbits and guinea pigs (3.4 mL/min·kg and 4.0 mL/min·kg, respectively) and higher than in chickens and turkeys (0.78 mL/min·kg and 0.83 mL/min·kg, respectively). In llamas (*Lama glama*), gentamicin clearance is 0.51–1.05 mL/min·kg (Dowling *et al.*, 1996; Lackey *et al.*, 1996) and probably varies with the state of hydration. In channel catfish (*Ictalurus punctatus*) acclimatized at 22°C, the systemic clearance of gentamicin is 0.13 mL/min·kg (Setzer, 1985). The efficiency of renal excretion, like the capacity of hepatic metabolism, in eliminating drugs is significantly lower in piscine than in mammalian species.

Table 1.15   The relationship between glomerular filtration rate (GFR) and systemic clearance of gentamicin in various species.

Species	GFR (mL/min·kg)	Gentamicin clearance (mL/min·kg)
Dog	3.96	3.10
Cat	2.94	1.61
Pig	2.80	1.66
Goat	2.26	1.68
Cattle	2.25	1.32
Sheep	2.20	1.56
Human	1.84	0.82
Horse	1.65	1.20
Donkey	–	1.25
Turkey	1.32	0.83
Chicken	1.23	0.78

Based on the relationship between plasma and/or serum concentrations and clinical effectiveness of gentamicin, with due consideration of safety, the recommended dosage regimens are 2–4 mg/kg administered intramuscularly at 8–12 h intervals for horses, donkeys and llamas, and 3–5 mg/kg administered intramuscularly or subcutaneously at 8–12 h intervals for dogs and at 12–24 h intervals for cats. The average systemic clearance (mL/min·kg) of gentamicin is 0.80, 1.20, 1.25, 3.10 and 1.61 in llamas, horses, donkeys, dogs and cats, respectively. An empirical dosage regimen for gentamicin in gopher snakes (*Pituophis melanoleucus catenifer*) is 2.5 mg/kg administered intramuscularly in the anterior half of the body, to avoid the renal first-pass effect, at a 72-h dosage interval (Bush *et al.*, 1978).

Oxytetracycline distributes widely in the body, undergoes enterohepatic circulation and, in most species, is eliminated relatively slowly by renal excretion (glomerular filtration). Species differences in both volume of distribution and systemic clearance contribute to the wide variation between species in the half-life of oxytetracycline. The clearances of oxytetracycline in rainbow trout (*Oncorhynchus gairdneri*) and African catfish (*Clarias gariepinus*) are 0.27 mL/min·kg and 0.19 mL/min·kg, respectively. These clearance values are much lower than in domestic animals (1.25–4.04 mL/min·kg) and, although determined at different acclimatization temperatures, indicate a difference in clearance of the drug between fish species (Grondel *et al.*, 1989). Further support for species variation is provided by the difference in systemic clearance of sulphadimidine between rainbow trout (*Oncorhynchus gairdneri*) (0.685 mL/min·kg) and carp (*Cyprinus carpio*) (0.269 mL/min·kg) acclimatized at the same water temperature (10°C) (van Ginneken *et al.*, 1991) and in ciprofloxacin clearance, which in rainbow trout at 12°C is 4.77 mL/min·kg and in carp at 20°C is 2.47 mL/min·kg (Nouws *et al.*, 1988).

Dosage rate

Dosage rate is defined as the systemically available dose divided by the dosage interval. When designing dosage regimens with the objective of maintaining plasma concentrations within the therapeutic range for a drug, systemic clearance is probably the most important pharmacokinetic parameter. Under multiple dosage conditions (i.e. the repeated administration of a fixed dose at a constant dosage interval), the dosage rate required to provide a desired average steady-state concentration, $C_{p(avg)}$, of the drug is

$$\text{Dosage rate} = \frac{F \cdot \text{Dose}}{\text{Dosage interval}} = C_{p(avg)} \cdot Cl_B$$

Assuming knowledge of the average steady-state concentration desirable for a drug, the dosage rate is dependent on the systemic clearance of the drug. For example, knowledge of the therapeutic range of plasma concentrations for theophylline (6–16 µg/mL) and of the systemic availability (90–100%) and clearance of the drug provides the basis for calculating oral dosage regimens for conventional aminophylline tablets. The dosage rates that would provide an average steady-state plasma theophylline concentration of 10 µg/mL and produce a sustained bronchodilator effect are 10 mg/kg administered at 8-h intervals to dogs and 5 mg/kg administered at 12-h intervals to horses or cats. The systemic clearance of theophylline in the horse and cat is 40 mL/h·kg, which is similar to clearance of the drug in human beings. Systemic clearance of theophylline in dogs is much higher (100 mL/h·kg) than in horses, cats and humans.

The average steady-state plasma concentration of a drug is neither the arithmetic nor the geometric mean of the maximum desirable and minimum effective concentrations. Rather, it is a plasma concentration within the therapeutic range which, when multiplied by the dosage interval, corresponds to the total area under the curve following the administration of a single intravenous dose, or the area under the curve during a dosage interval at steady-state.

$$C_{p(avg)} = \frac{AUC}{Dosage\ interval}$$

For example, the total area under the curve following a single 400 mg oral dose of metronidazole to human beings is 80.0 μg·h/mL and the area under the curve during a 12-h dosage interval at steady-state is 82.3 μg·h/mL. Oral systemic availability of the drug is complete (98.9%). The average observed steady-state plasma metronidazole concentration (6.9 ± 1 μg/mL; mean ± SE) closely agrees with the average predicted steady-state concentration (6.3 ± 0.5 μg/mL) (Jensen & Gugler, 1983).

When a drug is administered by continuous intravenous infusion, the infusion rate (R_0) required to provide a desired steady-state plasma concentration is

$$R_0 = C_{p(ss)} \cdot Cl_B$$

Based on this equation, it follows that the concentration at steady-state is directly proportional to the rate of infusion and inversely proportional to the systemic clearance of the drug. While the rate of infusion determines the steady-state concentration that will be attained, the time required to reach steady-state is determined *solely* by the rate of elimination (half-life) of the drug. For practical purposes it can be assumed that a plasma concentration within 90% of the desired steady-state (plateau) concentration will be achieved after continuously infusing the drug solution at a constant rate for a period corresponding to four times the half-life of the drug. It follows that the time required to achieve steady-state is appreciable for drugs with long half-lives. This disadvantage can be overcome by simultaneously administering a loading dose and starting the infusion of the drug. An alternative to slowly administering the loading dose as a single entity is to administer it in increments at short intervals, (e.g. dysrhythmic drugs). Intravenous infusion is the only mode of drug administration that allows precise control over the entry of a drug into the systemic circulation and avoids fluctuations in plasma concentration which is a feature of dosage regimens.

Mean residence time

The mean residence time (MRT) represents the average time the molecules of a drug reside in the body following the administration of a single dose. Calculation of MRT is based on total areas under the plasma concentration–

time curves, which are estimated by numerical integration using the trapezoidal rule (from time zero to the last measured plasma concentration) with extrapolation to infinite time.

$$MRT = \frac{AUMC}{AUC}$$

where AUC is the total area under the curve (zero moment) and AUMC is the area under the (first) moment curve obtained from the product of plasma concentration and time vs. time from time zero to infinity. The areas under the extrapolated portion of the curves are estimated by

$$\frac{C_{p(last)}}{\beta} \quad \text{for AUC}$$

and

$$\frac{t^* \cdot C_{p(last)}}{\beta} + \frac{C_{p(last)}}{\beta^2} \quad \text{for AUMC}$$

where β is the overall elimination rate constant of the drug and t^* is the time of the last measured plasma drug concentration ($C_{p(last)}$). It is desirable that the areas under the extrapolated portion of the curves be less than 10% of the total AUC and less than 20% of the total AUMC.

When the drug is administered as an intravenous bolus dose, the total areas under the curves can be calculated from the coefficients and exponents of the equation describing the disposition curve and obtained by compartmental pharmacokinetic analysis of the plasma concentration–time data.

$$AUC_{i.v.} = \frac{A}{\alpha} + \frac{B}{\beta}$$

$$AUMC_{i.v} = \frac{A}{\alpha^2} + \frac{B}{\beta^2}$$

Regardless of whether the data are analysed by a compartmental or non-compartmental method, the duration of blood sampling and the limit of quantification of the analytical method used to measure the drug concentration are important features of the pharmacokinetic study. The MRT, after an intravenous bolus dose of a drug can be estimated from either plasma drug concentration or urinary excretion data (Rowland & Tozer, 1989).

The advantages of using non-compartmental methods for calculating pharmacokinetic parameters, such as systemic clearance (Cl_B), volume of distribution ($V_{d(area)}$), systemic availability (F) and mean residence time (MRT), are that they can be applied to any route of administration and do not entail the selection of a compartmental pharmacokinetic model. The important assumption made, however, is that the absorption and disposition processes for the drug being studied obey first-order (linear) pharmacokinetic behaviour. The first-order elimination rate constant (and half-life) of the drug can be calculated by regression analysis of the terminal four to six measured plasma concentration–time data points. When the drug is administered as an intravenous bolus dose, the volume of distribution at steady-state ($V_{d(ss)}$) can be calculated.

$$V_{d(ss)} = \frac{\text{Dose}_{i.v.} \cdot \text{AUMC}}{(\text{AUC})^2} = \text{MRT}_{i.v} \cdot Cl_B$$

Disease-induced change in the volume of distribution at steady-state can be due to a change in either the mean residence time or systemic clearance, or both, of the drug.

It may be appropriate in most instances to consider the product of 0.693 and $\text{MRT}_{i.v.}$ as the 'effective' half-life of a drug requiring a multi-compartment model for analysis of the disposition curve (Gibaldi & Perrier, 1982). The effective half-life ($t_{1/2(eff)}$) is best obtained following both single and multiple (steady-state) dosing. Under these conditions, it is a direct and accurate parameter reflecting accumulation from the administered dosage form of the drug and the dosage regimen applied (Boxenbaum & Battle, 1995).

References

Autefage, A., Fayolle, P. & Toutain, P.-L. (1990) Distribution of material injected intramuscularly in dogs. *American Journal of Veterinary Research*, **51**, 901–904.

Axelrod, J. (1971) Methyltransferase enzymes in the metabolism of physiologically active compounds and drugs. In: *Concepts in Biochemical Pharmacology*, (eds B.B. Brodie & J.R. Gillette), Part 2, pp. 609–619. Springer–Verlag, Berlin.

Babany, G. Larrey, D. & Pessayre, D. (1988) Macrolide antibiotics as inducers and inhibitors of cytochrome P-450 in experimental animals and man. In: *Progress in Drug Metabolism*, (ed. G.G. Gibson), pp. 61–98. Taylor and Francis, London.

Baggot, J.D. (1977) *Principles of Drug Disposition in Domestic Animals: The Basis of Veterinary Clinical Pharmacology*: W.B. Saunders, Philadelphia.

Baggot, J.D. & Brown, S.A. (1998) Basis for selection of the dosage form. In: *Development and Formulation of Veterinary Dosage Forms*, (eds G.E. Hardee & J.D. Baggot), 2nd edn., pp. 7–143. Marcel Dekker, New York.

Baggot, J.D., Toutain, P.L., Brandon, R.A. & Alvinerie, M. (1984) Effect of premedication with acetylpromazine on the disposition kinetics of thiopental. *Journal of Veterinary Pharmacology and Therapeutics*, **7**, 197–202.

Benet, L.Z. (1984) Pharmacokinetic parameters: which are necessary to define a drug substance? *European Journal of Respiratory Diseases*, **65** (Suppl. 134), 45–61.

Benet, L.Z. & Galeazzi, R.L. (1979) Noncompartmental determination of the steady-state volume of distribution. *Journal of Pharmaceutical Sciences*, **68**, 1071–1074.

Bowser, P.R., Wooster, G.A., St Leger, J. & Babish, J.G. (1992) Pharmacokinetics of enrofloxacin in fingerling rainbow trout (*Oncorhynchus mykiss*). *Journal of Veterinary Pharmacology and Therapeutics*, **15**, 62–71.

Boxenbaum, H. (1982) Interspecies scaling, allometry, physiological time, and the ground plan of pharmacokinetics. *Journal of Pharmacokinetics and Biopharmaceutics*, **10**, 201–227.

Boxenbaum, H. & Battle, M. (1995) Effective half-life in clinical pharmacology. *Journal of Clinical Pharmacology*, **35**, 763–766.

Boyd, J.S. (1987) Selection of sites for intramuscular injections in the neck of the horse. *Veterinary Record*, **121**, 197–200.

Brodie, B.B. & Maickel, R.P. (1962) Comparative biochemistry of drug metabolism. In: *Metabolic Factors Controlling Duration of Drug Action*. Proceedings of the First International Pharmacological Meeting, Vol. 6, (eds B.B. Brodie & E.G. Erdos), pp. 299–324. Macmillan, New York.

Brodie, B.B., Bernstein, E. & Mark, L.C. (1952) The role of body fat in limiting the duration of action of thiopental. *Journal of Pharmacology and Experimental Therapeutics*, **105**, 421–426.

Brodie, B.B., Gillette, J.R. & LaDu, B.N. (1958) Enzymatic metabolism of drugs and other foreign compounds. *Annual Review of Biochemistry*, **27**, 427–454.

Brown, S.A., Coppoc, G.L., Riviere, J.E. & Anderson, V.L. (1986) Dose-dependent pharmacokinetics of gentamicin in sheep. *American Journal of Veterinary Research*, **47**, 789–794.

Browne, T.R., Greenblatt, D.J., Schumacher, G.E. *et al.* (1990) New pharmacokinetic methods III: Two simple tests for 'deep pool effect'. *Journal of Clinical Pharmacology*, **30**, 680–685.

Bush, M., Smeller, J.M., Charache, P. & Arthur, R. (1978) Biological half-life of gentamicin in gopher snakes. *American Journal of Veterinary Research*, **39**, 171–173.

Calder III, W.A. (1984) *Size, Function and Life History*. Harvard University Press, Cambridge, Mass.

Chasseaud, L.F. (1976) Conjugation with glutathione and mercapturic acid excretion. In: *Gutathione: Metabolism and Function*, (eds I.M. Arias & W.B. Jacoby), pp. 77–114. Raven Press, New York.

Clark, C.H., Thomas, J.E., Milton, J.L. & Goolsby, W.D. (1982) Plasma concentrations of chloramphenicol in birds. *American Journal of Veterinary Research*, **43**, 1249–1253.

Conney, A.H. & Burns, J.J. (1972) Metabolic interactions among environmental chemicals and drugs. *Science*, **178**, 576–586.

Correia, M.A. (1992) Drug biotransformation. In: *Basic and Clinical Pharmacology*, (ed. B.G. Katzung), 5th edn. pp. 49–59. Appleton & Lange, Norwalk, Conn.

Dalvi, R.R., Nunn, V.A. & Juskevich, J. (1987) Hepatic cytochrome P-450 dependent drug metabolizing activity in rats, rabbits and several food-producing species. *Journal of Veterinary Pharmacology and Therapeutics*, **10**, 164–168.

Davis, L.E., Neff-Davis, C.A. & Baggot, J.D. (1973) Comparative pharmacokinetics in domesticated animals. In: *Research Animals in Medicine*, (ed. L.T. Harmison), pp. 715–732. Publication No. (NIH) 72–333, United States Department of Health, Education and Welfare, Washington D.C.

Dayton, P.G., Cucinell, S.A., Weiss, M. & Perel, J.M. (1967) Dose dependence of drug plasma level decline in dogs. *Journal of Pharmacology and Experimental Therapeutics*, **158**, 305–316.

Delatour, P., Jaussaud, P., Courtot, D. & Fau, D. (1991) Enantioselective N-demethylation of ketamine in the horse. *Journal of Veterinary Pharmacology and Therapeutics*, **14**, 209–212.

Deleforge, J., Davot, J.L., Boisrame, B. & Delatour, P. (1991) Enantioselectivity in the anaesthetic effect of ketamine in dogs. *Journal of Veterinary Pharmacology and Therapeutics*, **14**, 418–420.

Derkx, F.H.M., Bonta, I.L. & Lagendijk, A. (1971) Species-dependent effect of neuromuscular blocking agents. *European Journal of Pharmacology*, **16**, 105–108.

Dohoo, S., Tasker, R.A.R. & Donald, A. (1994) Pharmacokinetics of parenteral and oral sustained-release morphine sulphate in dogs. *Journal of Veterinary Pharmacology and Therapeutics*, **17**, 426–433.

Dorrestein, G.M. & van Miert, A.S.J.P.A.M. (1988) Pharmacotherapeutic aspects of medication of birds. *Journal of Veterinary Pharmacology and Therapeutics*, **11**, 33–44.

Dowling, P.M., Ferguson, J.G. & Gibney, R.F. (1996) Pharmacokinetics of gentamicin in llamas. *Journal of Veterinary Pharmacology and Therapeutics*, **19**, 161–163.

Dutton, G.J. (1966) The biosynthesis of glucuronides. In: *Glucuronic Acid, Free and Combined Chemistry, Biochemistry, Pharmacology and Medicine*, (ed. G.J. Dutton), pp. 185–299. Academic Press, New York.

Fletcher, J. (1974) Hypersensitivity of an isolated population of red deer (*Cervus elaphus*) to xylazine. *Veterinary Record*, **94**, 85–86.

Fouts, J.R. (1961). The metabolism of drugs by subfractions of hepatic microsomes. *Biochemical and Biophysical Research Communications*, **6**, 373–378.

French, M.R., Bababunmi, E.A., Golding, R.R. *et al.* (1974) The conjugation of phenol, benzoic acid, 1-naphthylacetic acid and sulphadimethoxine in the lion, civet and genet. *FEBS Letters*, **46**, 134–137.

Frey, H.-H. & Loscher, W. (1985) Pharmacokinetics of anti-epileptic drugs in the dog: a review. *Journal of Veterinary Pharmacology and Therapeutics*, **8**, 219–233.

Garcia-Villar, R., Toutain, P.L., Alvinerie, M. & Ruckebusch, Y. (1981) The pharmacokinetics of xylazine hydrochloride: an interspecific study. *Journal of Veterinary Pharmacology and Therapeutics*, **4**, 87–92.

Gibaldi, M. & Perrier, D. (1982) *Pharmacokinetics, 2nd* edn. pp. 409–417, 445–449. Marcel Dekker, New York.

Gillette, J.R. (1963) Metabolism of drugs and other foreign compounds by enzymatic mechanisms. *Recent Progress in Drug Research*, **6**, 13–73.

Gillette, J.R. (1966) Biochemistry of drug oxidation and reduction by enzymes in hepatic endoplasmic reticulum. *Advances in Pharmacology*, **4**, 219–261.

van Ginneken, V.J.Th., Nouws, J.F.M., Grondel, J.L., Driessens, F. & Degen, M. (1991) Pharmacokinetics of sulphadimidine in carp (*Cyprinus carpio* L.) and rainbow trout (*Salmo gairdneri* Richardson) acclimated at two different temperature levels. *Veterinary Quarterly*, **13**, 88–96.

Govier, W.C. (1965) Reticuloendothelial cells as the site of sulfanilamide acetylation in the rabbit. *Journal of Pharmacology and Experimental Therapeutics*, **150**, 305–308.

Grondel, J.L., Nouws, J.F.M., Schutte, A.R. & Driessens, F. (1989) Comparative pharmacokinetics of oxytetracycline in rainbow trout (*Salmo gairdneri*) and African catfish (*Clarias gariepinus*). *Journal of Veterinary Pharmacology and Therapeutics*, **12**, 157–162.

Hennessy, D.R., Sangster, N.C., Steel, J.W. & Collins, G.H. (1993) Comparative pharmacokinetic disposition of closantel in sheep and goats. *Journal of Veterinary Pharmacology and Therapeutics*, **16**, 254–260.

Holford, N.H.G. & Sheiner, L.B. (1982) Understanding the dose-effect relationship:

clinical application of pharmacokinetic–pharmacodynamic models. *Clinical Pharmacokinetics*, **6**, 429–453.

Houghton, G.W. & Richens, A. (1974) Rate of elimination of tracer doses of phenytoin at different steady-state serum phenytoin concentrations in epileptic patients. *British Journal of Clinical Pharmacology*, **1**, 155–161.

Jensen, J.C. & Gugler, R. (1983) Single- and multiple-dose metronidazole kinetics. *Clinical Pharmacology and Therapeutics*, **34**, 481–487.

Keenaghan, J.B. & Boyes, R.N. (1972) The tissue distribution, metabolism and excretion of lidocaine in rats, guinea pigs, dogs and man. *Journal of Pharmacology and Experimental Therapeutics*, **180**, 454–463.

Koritz, G.D., McKiernan, B.C., Neff-Davis, C.A. & Munsiff, I.J. (1986) Bioavailability of four slow-release theophylline formulations in the Beagle dog. *Journal of Veterinary Pharmacology and Therapeutics*, **9**, 293–302.

Lackey, M.N., Belknap, E.B., Greco, D.S. & Fettman, M.J. (1996) Single intravenous and multiple dose pharmacokinetics of gentamicin in healthy llamas. *American Journal of Veterinary Research*, **57**, 1193–1199.

Laczay, P., Semjen, G., Nagy, G. & Lehel, J. (1998) Comparative studies on the pharmacokinetics of norfloxacin in chickens, turkeys and geese after a single oral administration. *Journal of Veterinary Pharmacology and Therapeutics*, **21**, 161–164.

Lewbart, G., Vaden, S., Deen, J. *et al.* (1997) Pharmacokinetics of enrofloxacin in the red pacu (*Colossoma brachypomum*) after intramuscular, oral and bath administration. *Journal of Veterinary Pharmacology and Therapeutics*, **20**, 124–128.

McManus, M.E. & Ilett, K.F. (1976) Mixed function oxidase activity in a marsupial, the quokka (*Setonix brachyurus*). *Drug Metabolism and Disposition*, **4**, 199–202.

Mandel, H.G. (1971) Pathways of drug biotransformation: biochemical conjugations. In: *Fundamentals of Drug Metabolism and Drug Disposition*, (eds B.N. LaDu, H.G. Mandel & E.L. Way), pp. 149–186. Williams and Wilkins, Baltimore, Md.

Marietta, M.P., Way, W.L., Castagnoli, N. & Trevor, A.J. (1977) On the pharmacology of the ketamine enantiomorphs in the rat. *Journal of Pharmacology and Experimental Therapeutics*, **202**, 157–165.

Mitchell, J.R., Potter, W.Z., Hinson, J.A., Snodgrass, W.R., Timbrell, J.A. & Gillette, J.R. (1975) Toxic drug reactions. In: *Concepts in Biochemical Pharmacology*, (eds J.R. Gillette & J.R. Mitchell), Part 3, pp. 383–419. Springer–Verlag, Berlin.

Nouws, J.F.M., Grondel, J.L., Schutte, A.R. & Laurensen, J. (1988) Pharmacokinetics of ciprofloxacin in carp, African catfish and rainbow trout. *Veterinary Quarterly*, **10**, 211–216.

Nouws, J.F.M., van Ginneken, V.J.T., Grondel, J.L. & Degen, M. (1993) Pharmacokinetics of sulphadiazine and trimethoprim in carp (*Cyprinus carpio* L.) acclimated at two different temperatures. *Journal of Veterinary Pharmacology and Therapeutics*, **16**, 110–113.

Ortiz de Montellano, P.R. (1988) Suicide substrates for drug metabolizing enzymes: mechanisms and biological consequences. In: *Progress in Drug Metabolism*, (ed. G.G. Gibson), pp. 99–148. Taylor and Francis, London.

Parke, D.V. (1968) *The Biochemistry of Foreign Compounds*, pp. 117–136. Pergamon Press, Oxford.

Piperno, E., Ellis, D.J., Getty, S.M. & Brody, T.J. (1968) Plasma and urine levels of phenylbutazone in the horse. *Journal of the American Veterinary Medical Association*, **153**, 195–198.

Prezant, R.M., Isaza, R. & Jacobson, E.R. (1994) Plasma concentrations and disposition kinetics of enrofloxacin in gopher tortoises (*Gopherus polyphemus*). *Journal of Zoo and Wildlife Medicine*, **25**, 82–87.

Riviere, J.E. (1988) Veterinary clinical pharmacokinetics. Part 1: Fundamental concepts. *Compendium on Continuing Education for the Practicing Veterinarian*, **10**, 24–30.

Robbins, P.W. & Lipmann, F. (1957) Isolation and identification of active sulfate. *Journal of Biological Chemistry*, **229**, 837–851.

Rowland, M. & Tozer, T.N. (1989) *Clinical Pharmacokinetics: Concepts and Applications*, 2nd edn. pp. 479–485. Lea and Febiger, Philadelphia.

Sams, R.A., Muir, W.W., Detra, R.L. & Robinson, E.P. (1985) Comparative pharmaco-kinetics and anesthetic effects of methohexital, pentobarbital, thiamylal, and thio-pental in Greyhound dogs and non-Greyhound, mixed-breed dogs. *American Journal of Veterinary Research*, **46**, 1677–1683.

Santos, M.D.F., Vermeersch, H., Remon, J.P. *et al.* (1996) Pharmacokinetics and bioa-vailability of doxycycline in turkeys. *Journal of Veterinary Pharmacology and Ther-apeutics*, **19**, 274–280.

Scheline, R.R. (1968) Drug metabolism by intestinal microorganisms. *Journal of Phar-maceutical Sciences*, **57**, 2021–2037.

Setzer, M.D. (1985) Pharmacokinetics of gentamicin in channel catfish (*Ictalurus punc-tatus*). *American Journal of Veterinary Research*, **46**, 2558–2561.

Smith, R.L. & Williams, R.T. (1974) Comparative metabolism of drugs in man and monkeys. *Journal of Medical Primatology*, **3**, 138–152.

Souhaili-El Amri, H. Batt, A.M. & Siest, G. (1986) Comparison of cytochrome P-450 content and activities in liver microsomes of seven animal species, including man. *Xenobiotica*, **16**, 351–358.

Syriopoulou, V.P., Harding, A.L., Goldman, D.A. & Smith, A.L. (1981) *In vitro* anti-bacterial activity of fluorinated analogs of chloramphenicol and thiamphenicol. *Antimicrobial Agents and Chemotherapy*, **19**, 294–297.

Tell, L., Harrenstien, L., Wetzlich, S. *et al.* (1998) Pharmacokinetics of ceftiofur sodium in exotic and domestic avian species. *Journal of Veterinary Pharmacology and Therapeutics*, **21**, 85–91.

Tranquilli, W.J., Paul, A.J. & Seward, R.L. (1989) Ivermectin plasma concentrations in Collies sensitive to ivermectin-induced toxicosis. *American Journal of Veterinary Research*, **50**, 769–770.

Varma, K.J., Sutherland, I., Horsberg, T.E. *et al.* (1994) Florfenicol: pharmacokinetics and efficacy in Atlantic salmon. In: *Proceedings of the Sixth International Congress of EAVPT* (Edinburgh), (ed. P. Less), pp. 220–221. Blackwell, Oxford.

Vest, M.F. & Rossier, R. (1963) Detoxification in the newborn: the ability of the newborn infant to form conjugates with glucuronic acid, glycine, acetate and glutathione. *Annals of the New York Academy of Sciences*, **111**, 183–197.

Vree, T.B., Hekster, Y.A., Nouws, J.F.M. & Dorrestein, G.M. (1985) Pharmacoki-netics of sulfonamides in animals. In: *Pharmacokinetics of Sulfonamides Revisited*, (eds T.B. Vree & Y.A. Hekster), *Antibiotics and Chemotherapy*, Vol. 34, pp. 130–170. Karger, Basel.

Williams, R.T. (1959) *Detoxification Mechanisms, 2nd* edn. pp. 732–740. Chapman and Hall, London.

Williams, R.T. (1967) Comparative patterns of drug metabolism. *Federation Proceedings,* **26**, 1029–1039.

Williams, R.T. (1971a) Species variations in drug biotransformations. In: *Fundamentals of Drug Metabolism and Drug Disposition,* (eds B.N. LaDu, H.G. Mandel & E.L. Way), pp. 187–205. Williams and Wilkins, Baltimore, Md.

Williams, R.T. (1971b). The metabolism of certain drugs and food chemicals in man. *Annals of the New York Academy of Sciences,* **179**, 141–154.

Williams, R.T. (1972) Toxicologic implications of biotransformation by intestinal microflora. *Toxicology and Applied Pharmacology,* **23**, 769–781.

Yeary, R.A. & Swanson, W. (1973) Aspirin dosages for the cat. *Journal of the American Veterinary Medical Association,* **163**, 1177–1178.

Zoran, D.L., Riedesel, D.H. & Dyer, D.C. (1993) Pharmacokinetics of propofol in mixed-breed dogs and Greyhounds. *American Journal of Veterinary Research,* **54**, 755–760.

Chapter 2
The Concept of Bioavailability and Applications to Veterinary Dosage Forms

Introduction

Bioavailability is defined as the rate and extent to which a drug, administered by any route, enters the systemic circulation unchanged. In addition to the chemical nature and related physicochemical properties of the drug substance, the formulation of the dosage form and the route of administration affect the bioavailability of the drug and may thereby influence the intensity and duration of the pharmacological effects produced (Fig. 2.1). It is only when a drug is injected intravenously that the onset of action is immediate and complete systemic availability ($F = 100\%$) can be assumed. When a drug is administered orally or by an extravascular parenteral route (e.g. intramuscular or subcutaneous injection), knowledge of the systemic availability (extent of

FACTORS AFFECTING THE CONCENTRATION OF A DRUG AT ITS SITE OF ACTION

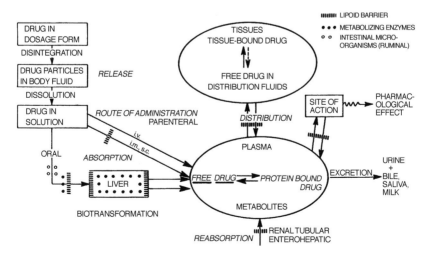

Fig. 2.1 Factors affecting the bioavailability and concentration of a drug at its site of action. (Reproduced with permission from Baggot (1977).)

absorption) is required for calculating clearance and dosage of the drug. Because the absorption process affects the rate of elimination to a variable degree, the value obtained for half-life is 'apparent' rather than 'true', which is based on the overall rate of elimination following intravenous injection of a single dose, while the mean residence time should be qualified by the route of drug administration (e.g., $MRT_{p.o.}$). The variety of veterinary dosage forms that are available for drug administration to animals, e.g. solutions, suspensions, oral pastes, tablets (conventional and sustained-release), long-acting parenteral preparations, modified-release ruminal boluses and formulated products for rectal administration, increases the need for an understanding of bioavailability.

Estimation of bioavailability

An indication of the rate of drug absorption can be obtained from the peak (maximum) plasma concentration (C_{max}) and the time taken to reach the peak concentration (t_{max}), based on the measured plasma concentration–time data. However, the blood sampling times determine how well the peak is defined and, in particular, t_{max}. Both C_{max} and t_{max} may be influenced by the rate of drug elimination, while C_{max} is also affected by the extent of absorption. The term C_{max}/AUC, where AUC is area under the curve from time zero to infinity or to the limit of quantification (LOQ) of the analytical method, provides additional information on the rate of absorption. This term, which is expressed in units of reciprocal time (h^{-1}), can easily be calculated. In spite of the imprecision of the estimation provided by C_{max}, it generally suffices for clinical purposes.

Even though the absorption rate constant (k_a) defines the rate of absorption, its accurate determination is largely dependent on the adequacy of the plasma concentration–time data associated with the absorption phase of the drug. When a drug is administered orally, as a conventional (immediate-release) dosage form, or injected intramuscularly as an aqueous parenteral solution, the absorption and disposition kinetics can often be analysed in terms of a one-compartment pharmacokinetic model with apparent first-order absorption. The plasma concentration–time curve is described by the equation

$$C_p = \frac{F \cdot Dose \cdot k_a}{V_d(k_a - k_d)}(e^{-k_d t} - e^{-k_a t})$$

where k_a and k_d are the apparent first-order absorption and disposition (composite of distribution and elimination) rate constants, respectively, and the coefficient represents the zero-time intercept (in units of concentration) of the back-extrapolated disposition (linear terminal) phase, which corresponds to the zero-time intercept of the absorption phase obtained graphically by the method of residuals (Fig. 2.2) (Gibaldi & Perrier, 1982). When there is a delay in

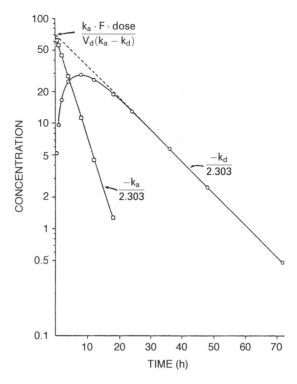

Fig. 2.2 Semilogarithmic graph of plasma drug concentration (○) after oral administration of a dose. The absorption phase is obtained by the method of residuals following back-extrapolation of the linear terminal (disposition) phase. Residual values are denoted by the dashed line. The zero-time intercept (in units of concentration) is log [F·Dose·k_a/V_d (k_a–k_d)]. (Reproduced with permission from Gibaldi & Perrier (1982).)

absorption, the time at which the back-extrapolated (disposition phase) and residual (absorption phase) lines intersect indicates the lag time, i.e. the time between drug administration and the beginning of absorption. The lag time can vary from a few minutes to some hours depending on dissolution of the dosage form, gastric emptying time or binding of the drug by feed constituents. Too few data points during the absorption phase, which is a common shortcoming of the design of many studies, detract from accurate estimation of the absorption rate constant. However, the pharmacokinetic approach generally indicates whether absorption is a first-order process. Alternatively, the absorption rate constant can be indirectly obtained by non-compartmental analysis of the plasma concentration–time data and calculation of the mean absorption time (MAT), based on the difference between the mean residence times following extravascular (MRT$_{n.i.}$, non-instantaneous) and intravenous administration (MRT$_{i.v.}$) of the drug:

$$MAT = MRT_{n.i.} - MRT_{i.v}$$

Assuming that absorption approximates a first-order process, which is generally valid for conventional dosage forms, $MAT = 1/k_a$. Knowledge of k_a allows calculation of the absorption half-life:

$$t_{1/2}(a) = \frac{0.693}{k_a} = 0.693 \cdot MAT$$

When absorption takes place rapidly, which is usual for conventional dosage forms, $k_a > k_d$, but when absorption takes place slowly and $k_a < k_d$ the 'flip-flop' phenomenon occurs, whereby the rate of absorption controls the rate of elimination of the drug. This situation applies not only to sustained-release oral dosage forms administered to dogs, but also to phenylbutazone and meclofenamic acid in horses, salicylate administered as an aspirin bolus to cattle and oral suspensions of benzimidazole anthelmintics in ruminant species.

The variety of methods that may be used to estimate the rate of drug absorption shows the uncertainty associated with determining this component of bioavailability. Fortunately, the extent of absorption (systemic availability), in conjunction with the peak plasma concentration and apparent half-life, is of greater interest in designing drug dosage regimens.

The usual method for estimating systemic availability (F) of a drug after extravascular (p.o., i.m.) administration of the dose employs the method of corresponding areas:

$$F = \frac{AUC_{p.o./i.m.}}{AUC_{i.v.}}$$

where AUC is the *total* area under the plasma concentration–time curve relating to the route of drug administration. The total area under the curve can be estimated by the linear trapezoidal rule, from zero time to the last measured plasma drug concentration, with extrapolation to infinite time, assuming log–linear decline:

$$AUC_{(\text{any route})} = \sum_{i=0}^{n-1} \frac{t_{i+1} - t_i}{2}(C_i + C_{i+1}) + \frac{C_{p(last)}}{\beta \text{ or } k_d}$$

where $C_{p(last)}$ is the last measured plasma concentration and β or k_d is the apparent first-order rate constant associated with the elimination or late decline phase of plasma concentration following intravenous or extravascular administration, respectively, of the drug (Fig. 2.3) (Baggot, 1977). The accuracy of this method depends upon the completeness with which the plasma concentration–time data define the curve; the relative area under the extrapolated portion should be less than 10% of the total area under the curve. Correction should be made for the size (mg/kg) of the extravascularly administered dose when it differs from that given by intravenous injection. The application of this method for estimating systemic availability involves the assumption that clearance of the drug is not changed by the route of administration. A crossover design, with an appropriate washout period between the phases of the bioavailability study, should be used whenever feasible.

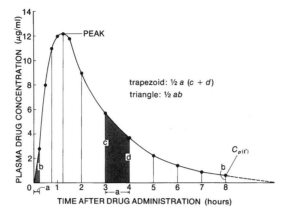

Fig. 2.3 Application of the trapezoidal rule for estimating area under the curve (AUC). The observed (measured) plasma drug concentration–time data are plotted on arithmetic coordinates. Total area under the curve is obtained by adding together areas of the trapezoids, the triangle from time zero to the first measured datum point and the calculated area under the extrapolated (terminal) portion of the curve, $C_{p(t^*)}/k_d$, where $C_{p(t^*)}$ is the last measured datum point and k_d is the apparent first-order disposition rate constant. The sample collection times and duration of sampling determine how well and/or completely the curve is defined.

When the AUC for an oral dosage form is compared with AUC following intravenous injection of a parenteral dosage form (suitable for intravenous administration), the absolute bioavailability (systemic availability) is obtained, whereas comparison of the AUCs for two oral dosage forms (test and reference) estimates the relative bioavailability of the test product. A similar situation applies to the comparison between two parenteral preparations administered by intramuscular injection, for example, the comparison in cattle or pigs of a long-acting oxytetracycline product with the conventional (immediate-release) dosage form of oxytetracycline.

The systemic availability of a drug can be estimated by comparing the cumulative urinary excretion of the unchanged (parent) drug after extra-vascular administration with the amount excreted unchanged after intravenous injection of the drug. Using this approach, the systemic availability of oxytetracycline was determined in pigs following the intramuscular injection (*m. biceps femoris*) of single doses (20 mg/kg) of a conventional (OTC-C) and a long-acting (OTC-LA) preparation and a single intravenous dose (20 mg/kg) of the conventional preparation (Fig. 2.4) (Xia *et al.*, 1983). Both the conventional and the long-acting product provided over 95% systemic availability (absolute bioavailability) of oxytetracycline. This method is an alternative to comparing area under the plasma concentration–time curves (AUCs), but it is cumbersome to apply because the total volume of urine voided during the excretion period for the drug (at least four half-lives) must be measured. In addition, the stability of the drug in urine during the collection period and storage of the samples must be assured. The use of cumulative urinary excretion data to compare the

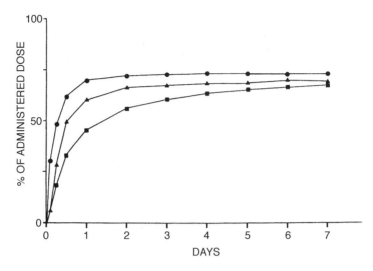

Fig. 2.4 Cumulative urinary excretion of oxtetracycline (OTC) in pigs after intravenous injection of conventional OTC preparation (●, $n=3$) and intramuscular injection of the conventional preparation (▲, $n=4$) and a long-acting OTC preparation (■, $n=6$). (Reproduced with permission from Xia *et al.* (1983).)

systemic availability of different dosage forms of a drug administered by the same extravascular route (p.o. or i.m.), i.e., relative bioavailability, assumes that the ratio of the total amount excreted unchanged to the amount absorbed remains constant. It is always preferable to base estimation of the rate of drug absorption on plasma concentrations rather than on urinary excretion data.

Factors influencing bioavailability

The aqueous solubility of a drug or dosage form determines its availability for absorption, while lipid solubility of the drug, which applies to neutral molecules and to the non-ionized form of weak organic acids and organic bases, influences the absorption process (passive diffusion). Except when administered as an oral liquid preparation (aqueous solution, elixir or syrup), the availability of a drug for absorption is mainly influenced by dissolution of the dosage form. Dissolution can be enhanced by formulating a soluble salt of the drug (e.g. phenobarbital sodium, phenytoin sodium, propranolol hydrochloride, quinidine sulphate) or a micronized form (e.g. griseofulvin, clonazepam, spironolactone). Through its influence on dissolution, the salt chosen can affect oral bioavailability; for example, oxytetracycline hydrochloride provides higher oral bioavailability of oxytetracycline than the less soluble oxytetracycline dihydrate; doxycycline is formulated as the hyclate, monohydrate and hydrochloride salts.

When a drug is administered orally to a monogastric animal, it must be relatively stable in the strongly acidic environment in the stomach (e.g. penicillin V, cephalexin monohydrate, erythromycin estolate) and be accessible to the mucosal epithelial lining, particularly of the small intestine, for absorption. Gastric emptying, the nature of the ingesta, intestinal motility and blood flow to the villi influence both the rate and extent of drug absorption. There are differences between monogastric species in the rate of gastric emptying, which is dependent on the volume of gastric contents; distension of the stomach is the primary physiological stimulus to increase gastric emptying. By promoting gastric emptying, metoclopramide can increase the rate of absorption of soluble drugs while intestinal transit rate influences the availability of drug for absorption when administered as a sustained-release dosage form. An effective pH of 5.3 in the microenvironment of the intestinal mucosal surface, rather than the reaction of intestinal contents (pH 6.6), is consistent with observations on the absorption of drugs that are weak organic acids or organic bases. Under normal conditions, weak acids with $pK_a > 3$ and bases with $pK_a < 7.8$ are well absorbed from the small intestine (Hogben *et al.*, 1959). An alteration in the pH of the stomach or small intestinal contents can markedly change the degree of ionization of drugs that are weak organic acids or bases. At pH values below the pK_a, weak acids exist mainly in the non-ionized form; the converse applies to weak bases. Lipid-soluble neutral molecules (e.g. digoxin, chloramphenicol) and fluoroquinolones (amphoteric) are well absorbed, although the systemic availability of norfloxacin is much lower than that of enrofloxacin/ciprofloxacin or marbofloxacin. Absorption of the quaternary antimuscarinic agents (propantheline and methscopolamine) is slow and incomplete, which could account for their relatively selective antispasmodic effect.

First-pass effect

Having traversed the gastrointestinal mucosal barrier, drug molecules are conveyed in the hepatic portal blood to the liver, where they are exposed to the 'first-pass' effect before entering the systemic circulation (Fig. 2.5). The oral bioavailability of fenbendazole, which is sequentially oxidized in the liver to fenbendazole sulphoxide (oxfendazole) and fenbendazole sulphone (inactive metabolite), is 27.1% in pigs weighing between 32 and 45 kg (Petersen & Friis, 2000). In Equidae (horses, ponies and donkeys) and ruminant species (cattle, sheep and goats) triclabendazole (flukicide), administered as an oral suspension, is converted by hepatic first-pass metabolism to triclabendazole sulphoxide (active), which is subsequently converted to the sulphone (inactive metabolite). Suxibuzone (6 mg/kg), administered orally to horses, is completely converted by first-pass hepatic metabolism (hydrolysis) to phenylbutazone (Delbeke *et al.*, 1993). The first-pass effect can substantially reduce the systemic availability (absolute oral bioavailability) of lipid-soluble drugs that undergo extensive biotransformation in the liver (e.g. diazepam, propranolol). The systemic availability of drugs that are highly extracted by the

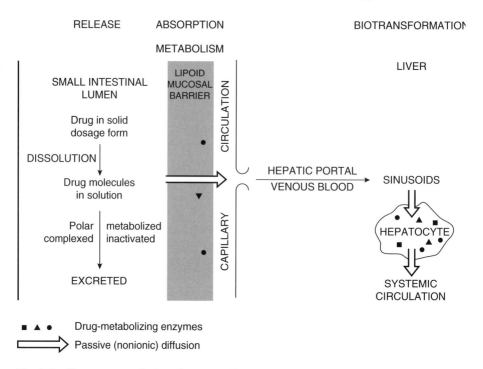

Fig. 2.5 The processes that are interposed between the oral administration of a drug as a solid dosage form and entry of the molecules into the systemic circulation.

liver (hepatic extraction ratio, $E_H > 0.6$) is sensitive to small changes in the hepatic extraction ratio (systemic clearance, i.v. divided by liver blood flow). Some drugs that show incomplete systemic availability following oral administration to dogs are presented in Table 2.1. While presystemic metabolism occurs mainly in the liver, it can also take place in the mucosa of the small intestine during the process of absorption. Metabolism in the mucosal epithelial cells can decrease the oral bioavailability of some drugs (e.g. salicylate) or can activate prodrugs (e.g. pivampicillin). As the metabolites of the majority of drugs are inactive, low systemic availability must be compensated for by increasing the size (mg/kg) of the oral relative to the intravenous dose. Some drugs, however, are converted to active metabolites with generally lower activity than the parent drug (e.g. N-desmethyldiazepam and oxazepam are rapidly formed from diazepam; oxyphenbutazone is the principal metabolite of phenylbutazone), while the metabolites of a small number of drugs have similar activity (e.g. phenobarbitone formed from primidone) or greater activity (e.g. ciprofloxacin formed from enrofloxacin) than the parent drug. Induction of hepatic microsomal drug metabolizing enzyme activity, as occurs during chronic treatment with phenobarbitone, could further reduce (generally) or increase the systemic availability (when activity of parent drug and active metabolites are combined) of extensively metabolized drugs. Because of

Table 2.1 Systemic availability of some orally administered drugs in dogs.

Drugs (dosage form)	Dose (mg/kg)	Systemic availability (%)	Site of metabolism/ other factor
Phenobarbitone (tablet)	10	86–96	Liver
Valproic acid (tablet)	40	78	Liver
Phenytoin (tablet)	15	36[a]	Liver
Salicylate (aspirin tablet)	250 mg total	45	Liver
Ibuprofen (gelatin capsule)	5	60–86	Liver
Naproxen[b] (gelatin capsule)	5	68–100	–
Theophylline (conventional aminophylline tablet)	10	91	Liver
Diazepam (tablet)	2	1–3 86[c]	Liver + (intestinal mucosa)
Lidocaine (solution)	10	15	Liver
Procainamide (tablet)	25	85[a,f]	–
Propranolol (conventional tablet)	80 mg total	2–17	Liver
Verapamil (conventional tablet)	0.5	15	Liver
Digoxin (Lanoxin tablet)	1 mg total	80	Dissolution
Cephalexin monohydrate (capsule)	20	57	Dissolution
Norfloxacin (tablet)	5	35[a]	Dissolution + liver
Enrofloxacin (tablet)	5	100[d]	–
Allopurinol (tablet)	15	70[e]	Intestine + liver (xanthine oxidase)

[a] Average oral bioavailability; wide individual dog variation.
[b] Naproxen has an unusually long half-life in dogs.
[c] Total active benzodiazepine.
[d] Total antimicrobial active fluoroquinolone.
[e] Average oral bioavailability is 14% in the horse.
[f] Dogs do not form *N*-acetylprocainamide (active metabolite).

wide variation in dissolution between different brands of digoxin tablets (De Rick *et al.*, 1979) and the narrow range of therapeutic plasma concentrations (0.6–2.4 ng/ml), digoxin tablets with the same formulation, or which have been shown to be bioequivalent, should be used in an animal on maintenance therapy. The use of a differently formulated tablet, or either an elixir or encapsulated hydroalcoholic solution (which provide higher systemic availability of digoxin, $F \geq 95\%$ than tablets) would, in effect, be changing the therapeutic dose. The altered clinical effect would only become fully evident after 6–8 days when a new steady-state plasma concentration has been attained. To avoid hepatic first-pass metabolism, glyceryl trinitrate (nitroglycerin) is formulated as a variety of dosage forms, which include parenteral solution, tablet or spray for sublingual application and transdermal therapeutic system, for use in humans, and as an ointment (2%) for topical application to dogs (cardiogenic pulmonary oedema) or horses (acute laminitis).

Antimicrobial agents most likely to be affected by the first-pass effect include trimethoprim, sulphonamides, fluoroquinolones, chloramphenicol, metronidazole and rifampin. The metabolites of trimethoprim, sulphonamides, most fluoroquinolones and chloramphenicol are inactive, while ciprofloxacin and sarafloxacin formed by *N*-dealkylation of enrofloxacin and difloxacin, respectively, and desacetylrifampin have antimicrobial activity similar to or greater than (ciprofloxacin) the parent drug. Certain antimicrobial agents (chloramphenicol and erythromycin) inhibit hepatic microsomal enzyme activity, whereas rifampin is a potent inducer of hepatic microsomal enzymes.

Effect of food

When an antimicrobial agent is administered to dogs either in conjunction with food or shortly after feeding, the oral bioavailability may be either increased or decreased depending on the drug preparation, although the systemic availability of amoxycillin, ampicillin prodrugs, fluoroquinolones, clarithromycin and enteric-coated formulations of erythromycin is not affected by the time of feeding relative to oral dosing. Ampicillin prodrugs (hetacillin, pivampicillin and bacampicillin) are hydrolysed in the intestinal mucosa during the absorption process to liberate ampicillin which enters the systemic circulation after passing unaffected through the liver. The presence of food in the stomach decreases the systemic availability of most penicillins, oral cephalosporins (cephalexin, cefadroxil, cefuroxime, cefixime), trimethoprim–sulphonamide combinations (in particular trimethoprim) and tetracyclines (except doxycycline). Feeding shortly before dosing increases the systemic availability of doxycycline, erythromycin estolate, nitrofurantoin, ketoconazole and griseofulvin (micronized).

The systemic availability of oral penicillins and cephalosporins is much lower in horses, apart from foals, than in dogs, and there exists the potential to seriously disturb the balance of commensal microorganisms in the colon. The systemic availability of amoxicillin (5% oral suspension of the trihydrate) is 30–50% in 5- to 10-day-old Thoroughbred foals compared with 5–15% in adult horses (Baggot *et al.*, 1988a), and of cefadroxil (5% oral suspension) is 68% in 1-month-old foals and decreases to 14.5% in foals 5 months of age (Duffee *et al.*, 1997). Pivampicillin (acidified aqueous suspension) provides systemic availability (ampicillin) of 40–53% in foals between 11 days and 4 months of age and decreases to 31–36% in adult horses (Ensink *et al.*, 1994). Penicillin V, the phenoxymethyl analogue of penicillin G, cannot be recommended (due to low systemic availability (less than 5% in adult horses) and the digestive disturbances caused) for the treatment of bacterial infections in horses (Baggot *et al.*, 1990).

Foals treated orally with erythromycin and rifampin for *Rhodococcus equi* infection (pneumonia) could serve as a potential reservoir of *Clostridium difficile* and excrete the microorganism, resistant to both antimicrobial agents, in the faeces. It would appear that erythromycin is the offending drug; it may promote the growth of *C. difficile* in the intestine of the foal and a variable fraction of the oral dose, seemingly irrespective of the dosage form, is excreted in the faeces (Baverud *et al.*, 1998). Coprophagic behaviour of mares housed with erythromycin-treated foals would lead to ingestion of the resistant microorganism and the antibiotic, which would severely disrupt the commensal bacterial flora of the large intestine resulting in acute colitis in the mares. The available evidence suggests that acute colitis associated with *C. difficile* in adult horses is a nosocomial infection (Baverud *et al.*, 1997). The stomach of the horse has a small capacity (8.5% of the gastrointestinal tract) compared to the pig (29%) and the dog (62%) and, unlike other monogastric species, a major part of the stomach is lined with stratified squamous epithelium. Expressed on the basis of volume capacity, the stomach of the horse, pig and dog can hold 7–14 L, 5.5–7 L and 3–8 L, respectively. Although the average pH of gastric contents is 4.5–6.0, the pH reaction can vary over a remarkably wide range of acidity (pH 1.13–6.8) (Schwarz *et al.*, 1926), which is influenced both by the nature of the feed and the pattern of feeding. In horses fasted for 12 h, gastric pH is relatively low (pH 2.1–2.4) (Sangiah *et al.*, 1988).

As the systemic availability of most antimicrobial agents administered orally (pastes) or by nasogastric tube (aqueous suspensions) to horses is significantly decreased by feeding shortly before dosing, food should be withheld for up to 2 h after administration of an antimicrobial agent. The systemic availability of rifampin (5 mg/kg) in adult horses is 68% when the drug is administered 1 h before feeding and significantly lower (26%) when administered 1 h after feeding (Table 2.2). In horses fasted overnight and for 3 h after dosing, the bioavailability of metronidazole, administered via nasogastric tube as an aqueous suspension, is 75% (Baggot *et al.*, 1988b), and of trimethoprim and sulphadiazine, combined in a commercially available oral paste formulation, is 67% and 58%, respectively (van Duijkeren *et al.*, 1994). The oral bioavailability of pyrimethamine, suspended in corn syrup, is 56% (Clarke *et al.*, 1992). Feeding

Table 2.2 Oral bioavailability in horses of rifampin (5 mg/kg; aqueous suspension), metronidazole (20 mg/kg; aqueous suspension), pyrimethamine (1 mg/kg; suspended in corn syrup), trimethoprim (5 mg/kg) and sulphadiazine (25 mg/kg; oral paste combination preparation).

Pharmacokinetic parameter	Rifampin		Metronidazole 3 h before feeding	Pyrimethamine suspended in corn syrup	Trimethoprim–sulphadiazine oral paste 3 h before feeding	
	1 h before feeding	1 h after feeding			Trimethoprim	Sulphadiazine
Lag time (h)	0.28	0.27	0.30			
C_{max} (µg/mL)	3.30 ± 1.42	1.21 ± 1.10	21.2 ± 3.1	0.18 ± 0.03	1.72 ± 0.36	12.1 ± 4.5
t_{max} (h)	1.5	2.25	1.5	2.89 ± 2.09	1.2 ± 0.32	2.6 ± 0.48
MAT (h)	2.80 ± 1.47	2.48 ± 1.19	3.38 ± 4.09	—	—	—
$t_{1/2 \,(d)}$ (h)	7.26 ± 1.78	6.91 ± 0.90	6.0 ± 2.94	9.86 ± 5.74	2.58 ± 0.61	8.15 ± 5.63
$MRT_{p.o.}$ (h)	9.32 ± 1.96	9.00 ± 0.68	9.41 ± 4.32	—	—	—
F (%)	67.6 ± 25.8	25.6 ± 17.2	74.5 ± 13.0	56 ± 14	67.0 ± 20.3	57.6 ± 14.8

horses close to the time of administering phenylbutazone in various oral dosage forms changes the pattern without altering the extent of absorption (oral bioavailability) of the drug. The availability of a drug for absorption from the small intestine of the horse, particularly when administered in conjunction with or shortly after feeding, may be limited by adsorption to the ingested feed, especially hay. Under these circumstances absorption may occur in two phases, initially (1–2 h after drug administration) from the small intestine and several (8–10) hours later from the large intestine (major site) following microbial digestion of the fibrous material (Maitho *et al.*, 1986; van Duijkeren *et al.*, 1995). The pH reaction of large intestinal contents in the horse is 6.6–6.8 which is conducive to the absorption of most lipid-soluble drugs, although a more acidic environment (pH 6.3 in the duodenum) would favour the absorption of weak organic acids (e.g. non-steroidal anti-inflammatory drugs, sulphonamides).

The oral bioavailability of penicillin V and tetracyclines (oxytetracycline, chlortetracycline and tetracycline) in pigs is low (<20%), whereas the systemic availability of enrofloxacin, trimethoprim and sulphadiazine is high (>80%) and not affected by feeding at the time of drug administration. The presence of food in the stomach of pigs markedly decreases the oral bioavailability of spiramycin (from 60% to 24%) and lincomycin (from 73% to 41%) (Nielsen 1997; Nielsen & Gyrd-Hansen, 1998). The oral bioavailability of amoxycillin, administered intragastrically via a tube as a solution/suspension of amoxycillin trihydrate, in fasted pigs is 33% and in fed pigs is 28% (Agerso & Friis, 1998), which shows that absorption of amoxycillin from the gastrointestinal tract of pigs, like in dogs, is not affected by food.

Rectal bioavailability

The rectal administration of immediate-release dosage forms of certain drugs could serve as an alternative to oral administration in dogs (and horses). Compared with drug absorption from intramuscular injection sites, absorption following oral administration takes place more slowly, the C_{max} is lower and the extent of absorption (systemic availability) is more variable, largely due to the first-pass effect on drugs that undergo hepatic biotransformation. There are, however, some drugs that should not be administered by intramuscular injection because of the irritation and tissue damage produced or precipitation and erratic absorption from the injection site (e.g. diazepam, phenytoin). Rectally administered lipid-soluble drugs formulated in appropriate dosage forms could provide more reliable absorption than from the stomach and small intestine, particularly if the influence of the first-pass effect is decreased. An important advantage of rectal over oral administration is *partial* avoidance of the hepatic first-pass effect. In dogs, the caudal rectal haemorrhoidal veins bypass the portal circulation and drain directly into the caudal vena cava. Avoidance of the hepatic first-pass effect in dogs may be less than in human beings. Following the rectal administration of a parenteral formulation of diazepam to dogs, the systemic availability of the parent drug is somewhat higher (2.7–7.4%) than following oral administration of diazepam in tablet form (1–3%), while the sum of diazepam and active metabolites (N-desmethyldiazepam and oxazepam), formed by hepatic microsomal oxidative reactions, estimates rectal bioavailability to be 66–80% (Papich & Alcorn, 1995) and oral bioavailability to be 74–100% (Loscher & Frey, 1981). The rectal administration of a parenteral preparation of diazepam (5 mg/mL) at a dose of 2 mg/kg provides a clinically effective plasma benzodiazepine concentration (> 150 ng/mL) and constitutes an alternative mode of diazepam administration to intravenous injection in the emergency treatment of dogs with convulsive seizures. Chronic phenobarbital therapy, by inducing hepatic microsomal oxidative activity, reduces the rectal bioavailability and total active benzodiazepine concentration in plasma, because the hepatic clearance of diazepam and active metabolites (N-desmethyldiazepam and oxazepam) is increased (Wagner *et al.*, 1998).

Three different formulations (fatty suppository, hydrophilic suppository and liquid suspension) containing racemic ketoprofen as active ingredient administered to horses after manual evacuation of the rectum provided relatively low (about 28%) systemic availability of the non-steroidal anti-inflammatory drug (Corveleyn *et al.*, 1996). The oral bioavailability of racemic ketoprofen (micronized powder in hard gelatin capsules) administered to horses with restricted access to food is 54.2% and 50.5% for S(+)- and R(–)-enantiomers, respectively (Landoni & Lees, 1995). Following oral administration of racemic ketoprofen as an oil-based paste to horses with restricted access to food, the oral bioavailability is very low (5.75% and 2.7% for S (+)- and R(–)-enantiomers, respectively). These results clearly show the profound influence that formulation (dosage form) can have on the oral bioavailability of a drug that is incompletely available systemically. At the present stage of formulation development, the oral bioavailability of racemic ketoprofen is superior to rectal bioavailability of the drug in horses. Because venous drainage of the rectum of the horse, unlike the human and the dog, appears to be substantially into the hepatic portal vein, minimal avoidance of hepatic first-pass metabolism of drugs absorbed from the rectum would be expected in horses. The rectal bioavailability of cisapride (1 mg/kg; finely ground tablets in propylene glycol) in horses is very low (1.23%), making this route of administration clinically ineffective (Cook *et al.*, 1997).

Ruminant species

The anatomical arrangement of the gastrointestinal tract and associated digestive physiology distinguish ruminant (cattle, sheep and goats) from monogastric (horses, pigs, dogs and cats) species. These distinguishing features form the basis of the marked difference between ruminant and monogastric species in the oral bioavailability of drugs, and determine the oral dosage forms that are appropriate to use.

The volume capacity of the mature reticulo-rumen is 100–225 L in cattle and 10–25 L in sheep and goats, and accounts for 60% of the total capacity of the gastrointestinal tract. The forestomach contents vary from liquid to semisolid consistency and the pH reaction is normally maintained within the range 5.5–6.5, due to the copious secretion of alkaline saliva (pH 8.2–8.4) which is particularly rich in bicarbonate and phosphate buffers, but devoid of amylase. The daily secretion of saliva is 100–190 L in cattle and 6–16 L in sheep. The turnover rate of reticulo-ruminal fluid has been estimated to be 2.0 per day for cattle and 1.1–2.2 per day for sheep (Hungate, 1966). Despite the stratified squamous nature of its epithelial lining, the rumen has considerable absorptive capacity (Phillipson & McAnally, 1942; Masson & Phillipson, 1951). Because absorption takes place by passive diffusion, lipid-soluble drugs, whether they be neutral molecules or the non-ionized form of weak organic acids or bases, may be absorbed from the rumen. Ruminal microorganisms are capable of metabolizing (or degrading) some drugs (e.g. trimethoprim, chloramphenicol, digitalis glycosides, nitroxynil) either by a hydrolytic or reductive reaction which would decrease the amount of drug (i.e. fraction of the orally administered dose) available for absorption. Intraruminal microbial biotransformation reactions make ruminant animals susceptible to toxicity caused by ingestion of plants containing cyanogenetic glycosides (cyanide poisoning) or accumulated nitrate (nitrite poisoning). Over-use of nitrogenous fertilisers contributes to the incidence of nitrite poisoning. Antidotal substances that are used, injected intravenously, to treat these toxicities are sodium nitrite followed by sodium thiosulphate for cyanide poisoning and methylthioninium chloride (methylene blue) for nitrite poisoning. In ruminant animals, where chemical compounds can be altered (activated or detoxified) by microbial action in the forestomach and where the whole physiological tempo of the body is so dependent on ruminal activity, no pharmacological or toxicological investigation can be interpreted without full consideration of the basic diet and feeding regimen (Clark & Wessels, 1952).

After comminution by rechewing and microbial digestion, the liquid component with suspended particles of reticulo-ruminal contents is 'pumped' in a two-stage process by the omasum into the abomasum (true stomach). Omasal transfer of ingesta is regulated by the volumes of fluid in the reticulo-rumen and the abomasum. The omasum facilitates the transfer of ingesta when the fluid volume in the reticulo-rumen is increased or the volume in the abomasum is decreased. During the transfer process, water and electrolytes are absorbed and the size of particulate matter in the ingesta is reduced. The abomasum, which accounts for approximately 4–5% of the capacity of the gastrointestinal tract in adult cattle and 7.5% of gastrointestinal tract capacity in sheep and goats, is the only component of the ruminant stomach that secretes digestive juices. Secretions from the fundic area contain hydrochloric acid, pepsin and, in suckling pre-ruminant animals, rennin (a milk-coagulating enzyme). The pH reaction of abomasal contents usually remains close to 3.0 (Masson & Phillipson, 1952). Lipid-soluble drug molecules that were not absorbed from reticulo-ruminal fluid may be absorbed by passive diffusion from the abomasum and small intestine. Drug molecules absorbed from the forestomach, the abomasum or small intestine must pass through the liver where they are subjected to 'first-pass' metabolism before entering the systemic circulation.

Because of the large volume of reticulo-ruminal contents, a drug can attain only a low concentration in the reticulo-rumen whether it is administered in solution or as a solid dosage form. Dissolution of solid dosage forms, dilution in the large volume of fluid and binding to particulate matter would decrease the rate, but not necessarily the extent, of drug absorption. Lipid-soluble neutral molecules and the non-ionized form of weak organic electrolytes, particularly organic acids because of the acidic reaction of ruminal fluid (pH 5.5–6.5), should normally be well absorbed from the reticulo-rumen. When aspirin in a solid dosage form (60 grain, which is equivalent to 3.9 g, oral bolus) was administered to cows, the drug was slowly absorbed and systemic availability was 50–70% (Gingerich *et al.*, 1975). The 12-h dosage interval for aspirin in adult cattle is based on the rate of absorption, rather than the half-life, of salicylate. In a study of the oral bioavailability of sulphamethazine (an organic acid, pK_a 7.4) administered to yearling cattle in different oral dosage forms, it was shown that 81% of the dose is available systemically from an oral solution, 63% from a rapid-release bolus and 32% from a slow-release bolus (Bevill *et al.*, 1977). The estimation of bioavailability of sulphamethazine was based on the cumulative urinary excretion of the drug.

Benzimidazole anthelmintics (e.g. albendazole, fenbendazole, oxfendazole, which is fenbendazole sulphoxide), probenzimidazoles (e.g. netobimin and febantel, which are metabolically converted to albendazole and fenbendazole, respectively) and various flukicides (e.g. closantel, rafoxanide, oxyclozanide, triclabendazole) are administered to ruminant animals as oral suspensions. This is because of their poor solubility in water which may be advantageous, since slow but adequate absorption increases the duration of anthelmintic activity. In sheep, reduction in the level of feed intake decreases the rate of onward passage of digesta from the rumen to the abomasum and small intestine. It has been shown (Hennessy *et al.*, 1995) that orally administered oxfendazole associated extensively with particulate digesta in the reticuloru-men. Following passage of this material into the abomasum, the drug is released and subsequently absorbed from the small intestine. When the rate of passage of digesta from the rumen was decreased by temporarily reducing feed intake, the systemic availability of oxfendazole was increased due to the extended time available for absorption of the drug to take place (Ali & Hennessy, 1995). Diet-hay and concentrate feeding, compared with grazing on pasture, was shown to affect the C_{max} and AUCs of the flukicides rafoxanide and triclabendazole sulphoxide administered as oral suspensions to 4- to 5-month-old parasite-free lambs (Taylor *et al.*, 1993); the systemic availability of both drugs was higher in the housed lambs fed hay and concentrates than in the lambs grazing on pasture due to slower passage of the digesta from the rumen to the abomasum and small intestine.

Reducing the level of feed intake (for 36 h before and 36 h after dosing) extends the residence time of ivermectin, administered as an oral solution, in the reticulo-rumen and increases the systemic availability and anthelmintic efficacy of the drug. In sheep with reduced feed intake 97% of ivermectin-resistant *Haemonchus contortus* were removed, compared with 53% in sheep maintained on a high level of feed intake (Ali & Hennessy, 1996). The systemic availability of orally administered anthelmintics is increased, with the likely exception of morantel which undergoes extensive first-pass metabolism, by extending the time for absorption to take place. Spontaneous closure of the reticular groove, which occurs reflexly in some animals, would decrease the systemic availability and clinical efficacy of anthelmintics. Reticular groove closure is more likely to occur when drugs are administered as oral solutions (e.g. levamisole, ivermectin) than as oral suspensions (e.g. benzimidazoles, probenzimidazoles and various flukicides). Should rapid absorption of a drug (e.g. a non-steroidal anti-inflammatory drug) from the gastrointestinal tract of an adult ruminant animal be desired, an oral solution of the drug could be administered immediately after inducing closure of the reticular groove. This can generally be achieved in cattle by administering orally a solution containing sodium bicarbonate and in sheep by administering orally a copper sulphate solution or injecting intravenously a dose (0.3 unit/kg) of lysine–vasopressin. Closure of the reticular groove would be unwanted in the case of an oral liquid, such as dimeticone emulsion or poloxalene, used to treat frothy bloat in cattle.

Modified-release dosage forms

Modified-release dosage forms include sustained-release tablets or capsules containing pharmacological agents for oral administration to monogastric animals (principally dogs), slow-release ruminal boluses containing trace elements for oral administration to ruminant animals, and controlled-release ruminal boluses containing anthelmintics or production enhancers (e.g. monensin) for administration to cattle or sheep within a specified range of body weight.

A sustained-release dosage form provides an initial amount of drug sufficient to produce a desired therapeutic plasma concentration, and continuously releases the drug at a constant (zero-order) rate which will maintain the therapeutic concentration for an extended period (recommended dosage interval). The margin of safety of the drug (active ingredient) is an important consideration in the selection of a candidate drug, because sustained-release products contain a large amount of the drug and the possibility of 'dose-dumping' with resultant toxicity exists.

Following the administration of a sustained-release dosage form (tablet or capsule) to dogs, the duration of drug availability for absorption is limited by the residence time of the dosage form in the stomach and small intestine. This has been estimated to be 9–12 h. By including the large intestine, the availability of a drug for absorption could be extended by a further 8–10 h in horses. In the development of a sustained-release dosage form for use in dogs, the aim is to provide effective plasma concentrations throughout the dosage interval (12 h) with an acceptable degree of fluctuation (i.e. C_{max}: C_{min} ratio) in steady-state concentrations. The latter is determined both by the half-life of the drug and the dosage interval (Theeuwes & Bayne, 1977). Suitable candidate drugs should have reasonably high oral bioavailability, which implies reliable absorption from the gastrointestinal tract and only partial inactivation by the first-pass effect unless active metabolites are formed, a half-life in the range 4–6 h, and a relatively high potency but reasonably wide range of therapeutic plasma concentrations (combined parent drug and active metabolites). Because of variation between dogs and human beings in the oral bioavailability and the rate of elimination of most lipid-soluble drugs, those that would be suitable for formulating as sustained-release dosage forms may differ between the two species.

Theophylline meets the criteria which make it a suitable candidate drug for formulating as a sustained-release oral preparation for use in dogs. Oral bioavailability of the conventional oral dosage form (aminophylline tablets) is 91%, the average half-life of theophylline in dogs is 5.8 h, and the range of therapeutic plasma concentrations is 6–16 µg/mL. Of the sustained-release oral dosage forms that are commercially available, anhydrous theophylline in tablet form (200 and 300 mg) is preferred for use in dogs. This product has an oral bioavailability (theophylline) of 76% and the dosage regimen (20 mg/kg administered at 12-h intervals) is predicted to maintain plasma concentrations within the therapeutic range with less fluctuation than other sustained-release products in peak-to-trough theophylline concentrations (Koritz *et al.*, 1986).

Other drugs of veterinary interest that have been formulated as sustained-release oral dosage forms include morphine, propranolol, quinidine, procainamide, verapamil and diltiazem. Of these, sustained-release morphine sulphate tablets (15 mg) have the greatest potential for use in dogs over 10 kg body weight. A shortcoming of the use of opioid drugs to maintain analgesia in dogs is their short duration of action. Because the oral bioavailability of morphine in dogs is low (less than 20%) and the half-life is about 1 h, it could be considered unsuitable as a candidate drug for formulating as a sustained-release oral dosage form. Nonetheless, the results obtained in a pharmacokinetic study of the commercially available sustained-release oral product indicate that this dosage form could have potential use at a dosage regimen of 1–2 mg/kg administered at 8- or 12-h intervals for the management of chronic pain in dogs (Dohoo, 1997). Phenytoin is a likely candidate drug for formulating as a sustained-release dosage form, which could enable this drug to be used in dogs for the treatment of generalized tonic-clonic seizures (*grand mal* epilepsy). The average oral bioavailability of the conventional dosage form is 36%, the half-life in dogs is 3.5–4.5 h (dose-dependent) and the therapeutic range of plasma concentrations is 10–20 µg/mL. The short half-life of valproic acid in dogs (2 h) probably makes this anticonvulsant drug less suitable than phenytoin for formulation as a sustained-release dosage form, even though the oral bioavailability of valproic acid is 78% and the range of therapeutic plasma concentrations is 40–100 µg/mL. It could be difficult to avoid a high degree of fluctuation in plasma valproate concentrations during a 12-h dosage interval.

Modified-release ruminal boluses use to advantage the anatomical arrangement of the forestomach of ruminant animals. Slow-release ruminal boluses containing trace elements (cobalt oxide; copper oxide; cobalt and copper in sodium phosphate glass matrix; selenium as sodium selenate) are commercially available for administration to cattle and sheep, and the compound bolus can be administered to adult deer. Controlled-release ruminal boluses are designed either to continuously release drug (an anthelmintic or production enhancer) at a constant rate for a prolonged specified period or to intermittently deliver pulse doses at predetermined intervals. Each delivery system is designed for use in either cattle or sheep within a specified range of body weight and, after oral administration, is retained in the reticulo-rumen at least throughout the entire period of drug release. The retention of controlled-release delivery systems in the reticulo-rumen is dependent either on density or geometry of the system (Fig. 2.6). The various types of ruminal boluses and their technological design were described by Klink *et al.* (1998).

The ivermectin (Ivomec) ruminal bolus, designed for use in cattle between 100 and 400 kg body weight, contains 1.72 g of ivermectin which is continuously released into ruminal fluid at a constant rate (12.5 mg/day) over a period of 135 days. The fenbendazole (Panacur) ruminal bolus, for use in cattle between 100 and 300 kg body weight, contains 12 g of the benzimidazole sulphide which is continuously released into ruminal fluid for up to 140 days. Withdrawal periods associated with the ivermectin and fenbendazole controlled-release systems are 180 days and 200 days, respectively, and neither system should be administered to cows producing milk for human consumption. The morantel tartrate (Paratect Flex) ruminal bolus, for use in cattle over 100 kg body weight, contains 11.8 g of morantel base which is released, at a rate of approximately 150 mg/day, into ruminal fluid over a period of at least 90 days. There is no withdrawal period associated with the morantel tartrate ruminal bolus. The Captec, also known as the Laby (1974), system is a controlled-release ruminal capsule designed for use in sheep within a specified range of body weight (35–70 kg). This system is used to continuously deliver either albendazole (32.5 mg/day) or ivermectin (1.6 mg/day) over a period of 100 days. The modified-release ruminal bolus containing oxfendazole (Autoworm), designed for use in grazing cattle between 200 and 400 kg body weight, delivers pulse doses (each 1.25 g) of fenbendazole sulphoxide (oxfendazole) at 3-week intervals over a period of 105 days (Jacobs *et al.*, 1987; Rowlands *et al.*, 1988). It is significant that the 3-week interval between release of successive doses roughly coincides with the prepatent period of the major gastrointestinal tristrongylids of cattle. The modified-release bolus containing five tablets of oxfendazole (Autoworm 5) releases the first dose 21 days after administration,

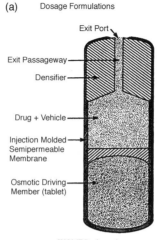

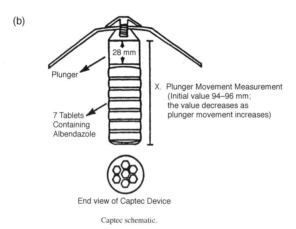

Fig. 2.6 Technological design of (a) controlled-release ruminal bolus containing ivermectin for administration to cattle and (b) controlled-release ruminal capsule containing albendazole or ivermectin for administration to sheep. (Reproduced with permission from Klink *et al.* (1998).)

while the bolus containing six tablets (Autoworm 6) releases the first dose on the day of administration. The withdrawal period associated with both intermittent-release products is 6 months.

Intramuscular injection

Drug absorption from an intramuscular injection site is mainly determined by the formulation of the parenteral preparation and is influenced by the vascularity of the injection site, the volume deposited at any one site, the concentration of drug in the preparation and by certain physicochemical properties (lipid solubility and pK_a) of the drug. The barrier to absorption is the capillary endothelium which most drugs penetrate by passive diffusion, although small molecules enter the systemic circulation by bulk flow through intercellular pores in the endothelial membrane. Absorption is generally assumed to be a first-order process but this assumption is often invalid, particularly during the initial period when the process obeys zero-order (non-linear) kinetics. Local and systemic factors that influence the rate of drug absorption seldom remain constant while absorption is taking place.

The extent of absorption (systemic availability) of a drug is estimated by the method of corresponding areas. Comparison of total AUC following the intramuscular injection of a parenteral preparation (solution or suspension) with that following the intravenous injection of a bolus dose of the drug (parenteral solution) provides an estimation of *absolute* bioavailability, while comparison of AUCs following intramuscular injection of different parenteral preparations (one of which must be a reference formulation) at the same injection site or of the same parenteral preparation at different injection sites estimates the *relative* bioavailability. A crossover design with an appropriate washout period between the phases of the bioavailability study should be used whenever feasible.

When the parenteral preparation is an aqueous non-irritating solution of the drug, absorption is generally rapid, in that the peak plasma concentration is attained within 30–60 min after giving the injection, and complete (i.e. systemic availability is 100%). Absorption does not significantly influence the rate of elimination (half-life) of the drug. The intramuscular (*m. serratus ventralis cervicis*) and subcutaneous injection of gentamicin sulphate 5% solution (50 mg gentamicin base/mL) to horses provided similar plasma concentration profiles of gentamicin (Fig. 2.7) and AUCs, which reflect the relative extent of absorption, did not significantly differ between the two routes of administration (Gilman *et al.*, 1987). Following the intravenous, intramuscular and subcutaneous administration of gentamicin (3 mg/kg) to dogs, the absolute biavailability (i.m., 95.98%, s.c. 94.30%) and peak plasma concentration (i.m., 10.7 µg/mL; s.c., 10.2 µg/mL) of the drug were similar (Wilson *et al.*, 1989). A parenteral solution of indomethacin administered to sheep (1 mg/kg) by intramuscular injection (semitendinous muscle) provides rapid absorption and almost complete systemic availability (91.0 ± 32.8%) of the drug, although there is wide interanimal variation. While the average half-life is somewhat longer following intramuscular (21.25 ± 4.4 h) than intravenous administration (17.4 ± 4.6 h) of the drug, the difference between the routes is not statistically significant (Vinagre *et al.*, 1998). The half-life of indomethacin in dogs and human beings is 7.9 h and 11.2 h, respectively. This non-steroidal anti-inflammatory drug undergoes extensive enterohepatic circulation.

Bumetanide (potent loop diuretic) administered by intramuscular injection to horses (15 µg/kg) is rapidly absorbed in that the peak plasma concentration

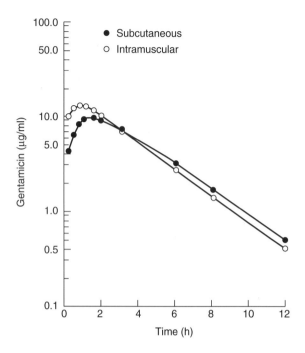

Fig. 2.7 Concentrations of gentamicin in plasma of horses (*n* = 6) after intramuscular or subcutaneous administration of gentamicin sulphate (4 mg/kg). The mean values (± SD) for AUC (subcutaneous 53.16 ± 6.52 µg·h/mL; intramuscular 60.79 ± 11.49 µg·h/mL) were not significantly different (Student's *t*-test, paired comparison, *P* > 0.05). (Reproduced with permission from Gilman *et al.* (1987).)

(34 ± 10 µg/mL) is attained within 8–10 min, the absolute bioavailability is 70–80%, and the drug is rapidly eliminated with an apparent half-life of 11–27 min (harmonic mean is 15 min) compared with 6.3 min when administered by intravenous injection (Delbeke *et al.*, 1986). Following intramuscular administration of the parenteral combination preparation containing ticarcillin disodium and clavulanate potassium (in the ratio 30:1, Timentin®, at a dose of 50 mg/kg ticarcillin and 1.68 mg/kg clavulanic acid) to dogs (gluteal muscles), both drugs are rapidly absorbed from the injection site and the absolute bioavailability of ticarcillin and clavulanic acid is 91% and 65%, respectively (Garg *et al.*, 1987). When the combination preparation was administered intramuscularly to 3-day-old foals (semimembranosus and semitendinosus muscles), the absolute bioavailability of ticarcillin was 100% and of clavulanic acid 88% (Wilson *et al.*, 1991). Even though the intramuscular route of administration provides satisfactory bioavailability and somewhat prolongs the elimination of both drugs in dogs and neonatal foals, this route cannot be recommended because of the local irritation, although short-lasting, produced at the injection site. Intravenous administration of the combination preparation may be effective for the treatment of ticarcillin-resistant Enterobacteriaceae

infections in dogs and is a useful alternative to an aminoglycoside for the treatment of various bacterial infections in neonatal foals. When cefazolin sodium (33% solution) was administered by intramuscular (gluteal muscles) and intravenous injection to horses, the absolute bioavailability of cefazolin was 78.4 ± 18.8% and the apparent half-life (i.m. injection) ranged from 49 to 99 min compared with the true half-life (i.v. injection) of 35–46 min (Sams & Ruoff, 1985). This study shows that cefazolin is well absorbed from the intramuscular injection site and absorption controls the rate of elimination of the drug, which is an example of the 'flip-flop' phenomenon. Because many parenteral solutions are well outside the physiological pH range, are hypertonic, or contain non-aqueous vehicles in their formulations, their absorption is somewhat erratic and at least some degree of tissue irritation with associated pain is produced at the site of injection. Although lipid solubility promotes diffusion of a drug through the capillary endothelium, some degree of water solubility at physiological pH is required to obviate precipitation of the drug at the injection site. Examples of drugs that are incompletely absorbed include ampicillin, dicloxacillin, cephradine, chlordiazepoxide, while some other drugs (e.g. diazepam, phenytoin, quinidine, digoxin) are unsuitable for intramuscular injection. Formulations of sparingly soluble drugs which contain a water-miscible solvent (such as propylene glycol) may cause precipitation of the drug at the intramuscular injection site so that absorption becomes limited by dissolution of the precipitated drug. This situation applies to diazepam and phenytoin and may explain the low bioavailability (46%) of a parenteral preparation of meclofenamic acid administered intramuscularly (middle gluteal muscle) to horses relative to oral bioavailability (71%) of the drug (Snow *et al.*, 1981). Although intramuscular injection is not a recommended route for administration of flunixin meglumine, the bioavailability of the drug following intramuscular injection (1.1 mg/kg in the gluteal muscles) appears to be 100% (Dyke *et al.*, 1997).

Long-acting (prolonged-release) parenteral preparations are formulated with a non-aqueous (such as oil) vehicle (solution), or a poorly soluble salt of the drug is used (usually an aqueous suspension). These preparations provide slow absorption of the drug over an extended period due to its gradual or staged availability for absorption. While the sodium salt of ceftiofur (as a reconstituted aqueous solution) is rapidly and completely absorbed (systemic availability, 100%) after intramuscular injection in various species (Brown *et al.*, 1991; Courtin *et al.*, 1997; Craigmill *et al.*, 1997), the ceftiofur cystalline-free, acid-sterile oil suspension is more slowly absorbed (S.A. Brown, unpublished data). Following intramuscular injection of ceftiofur sodium at single doses of 1.1 and 2.2 mg ceftiofur free acid equivalents per kilogram body weight to sheep, the C_{max} values of ceftiofur and metabolites (measured as desfuroylceftiofur acetamide by high performance liquid chromatography (HPLC) were 4.33 and 7.13 µg/mL, the apparent half-lives were 6.5 h and 7.65 h, respectively, and the AUC (from time zero to the limit of quantification of the assay) was proportional to the dose administered. From the time peak plasma concentration was reached (t_{max}, 0.5–1 h), the disposition curves following intravenous and intramuscular administration of ceftiofur sodium were roughly parallel (Craigmill *et al.*, 1997). Following the intramuscular injection at two sites (left and right hindquarters) of a single dose of ceftiofur sodium (2.2 mg ceftiofur free acid equivalents per kilogram body weight) to horses, the C_{max} of ceftiofur and related metabolites was 4.46 ± 0.93 μg/mL and occurred at 1.25 h after drug administration. The plasma concentration declined exponentially from the time the peak was attained to 12 h after drug administration (0.47 ± 0.15 μg/mL). The apparent half-life of ceftiofur metabolites was 3.15 h and the $MRT_{i.m.}$ was 6.10 ± 1.27 h (Jaglan *et al.*, 1994).

Avermectins and milbemycins (macrocyclic lactones) are highly lipophilic substances, which determines the extent of their distribution, including deposition in body fat, while the formulation of parenteral dosage forms (for subcutaneous injection to cattle) influences the plasma concentration profile following the administration of a single dose (200 μg/kg). The commercially available preparations differ in formulation: ivermectin is a non-aqueous (60% propylene glycol/40% glycerol formal) preparation; doramectin is an oil-based preparation containing sesame oil/ethyl oleate (90:10), and moxidectin is an aqueous-based solution. The pharmacokinetic parameters describing the rates of absorption and elimination of these endectocides are compared in Table 2.3 (Lanusse *et al.*, 1997). As the systemic availability (*F*) of the drugs was not determined, the term clearance/systemic availability (Cl_B/F) is used.

Table 2.3 Pharmacokinetic parameters describing the rate of absorption and elimination of ivermectin, doramectin and moxidectin following subcutaneous injection (shoulder region) of single doses (200 μg/kg) of the commercially available preparations to 10-month-old Hereford calves (180–210 kg body weight). Results are expressed as mean ± SEM (*n* = **4**).

Kinetic parameter	Ivermectin	Doramectin	Moxidectin
C_{max} (ng/mL)	42.8 ± 3.8	37.5 ± 3.9	39.4 ± 3.4
t_{max} (days)	4.00 ± 3.94[a]	6.00 ± 1.35	0.32 ± 0.0[c]
$t_{1/2}$ (days)	17.2 ± 4.26[b]	6.25 ± 0.16	14.5 ± 1.20[c]
Cl_B /F (mL/day·kg)	457 ± 52.5[a]	322 ± 164	938 ± 62.5[c]

[a] Mean kinetic parameters for ivermectin are significantly different from those obtained for
[a] moxidectin and [b] doramectin at *P* < 0.05. Mean kinetic parameters for moxidectin are significantly different from those obtained for [c] doramectin at *P* < 0.05.

The intramuscular bioavailability of amoxicillin in pigs is 83%, based on intravenous injection of amoxicillin sodium and intramuscular injection of amoxicillin trihydrate 15% in oil (described as the conventional formulation) in the neck, 10 cm behind the ear, of pigs. The conventional formulation provides slow absorption of amoxicillin (MAT, 7.3 h), C_{max} of 5.1 μg/mL and delays elimination of the drug ($MRT_{i.m.}$ is 8.8 h compared with $MRT_{i.v.}$ of 1.5 h). Administration of the long-acting formulation of amoxicillin trihydrate 15% in mixed oil base at the same intramuscular site provides two peaks, 1.7 µg/mL and 0.8 µg/mL at 1.3 h and 6.6 h, respectively, and considerably prolongs the elimination of the antibiotic ($MRT_{i.m.}$, 66.8 h) (Agerso & Friis, 1998). The two peaks in the plasma concentration–time curve may be ascribed to the mixture of different oil vehicles from which amoxycillin is released at different rates.

The shape of the plasma concentration–time curve and the features describing the curve (C_{max}, t_{max}, AUC and MRT) often vary between different parenteral formulations of the same drug administered by intramuscular injection, even at the same site. Five different parenteral formulations of ampicillin, administered by intramuscular injection in the lateral neck of ruminant calves at a similar dose level (7.7 $\pm$ 1.0 mg/kg), yielded plasma concentration–time curves which varied widely in shape and in the values of C_{max} (0.46–4.8 µg/mL) while bioavailability also differed between the for-mulations (Nouws *et al.*, 1982). Comparison of three parenteral formulations (one conventional and two long-acting) of oxytetracycline (20 mg/kg) administered intramuscularly in the lateral neck of pigs showed statistically significant differences between the formulations in C_{max}, t_{max} and MRT, while AUCs did not differ significantly between the formulations. The use of a 24-h dosage interval would be appropriate for the conventional formulation and a 48-h interval for either of the long-acting formulations (Table 2.4) (Banting & Baggot, 1996).

Table 2.4 Pharmacokinetic parameters describing the absorption and disposition of three oxytetracycline formulations administered intramuscularly (lateral neck) to pigs ($n = 8$) at a dose of 20 mg/kg body weight. Results are expressed as mean $\pm$ SD.

Pharmacokinetic term	Product A[a]	Product B[b]	Product C[c]
C_{max} (µg/mL)	6.27 $\pm$ 1.47	5.77 $\pm$ 1.0	4.68 $\pm$ 0.61
t_{max} (h)	3.0 (2.0–4.0)	0.5 (0.083–2.0)	0.5 (0.083–2.0)
AUC (µg·h/mL)	79.22 $\pm$ 25.02	91.53 $\pm$ 20.84	86.64 $\pm$ 14.21
MRT (h)	11.48 $\pm$ 2.01	25.27 $\pm$ 9.22	37.66 $\pm$ 15.62
$C_{p\ (24h)}$ (µg/mL)	0.81 $\pm$ 0.34	1.01 $\pm$ 0.26	0.97 $\pm$ 0.29
$C_{p\ (48h)}$ (µg/mL)	<LOQ[d]	0.40 $\pm$ 0.17	0.50 $\pm$ 0.09

[a] Engemycine 10% in polyvinylpyrrolidone.
[b] Oxyter LA 20% in dimethylacetamide.
[c] Terramycin LA 20% in pyrrolidone-2 and polyvinylpyrrolidone.
[d] LOQ, limit of quantification (0.1 µg/mL).

Long-acting preparations are designed, by prolonging absorption, to provide an extended dosage interval. A single intramuscular dose (20 mg/kg) of a long-acting preparation of oxytetracycline provides plasma concentrations above 0.5 µg/mL for 48 h in pigs, ruminant calves, cattle, goats, red deer (*Cervus ela-phus*), fallow deer (*Dama dama*) and dromedaries (*Camelus dromedarius*). When considering the clinical efficacy of parenteral preparations (conventional and long-acting) of an antimicrobial agent, it is often useful to compare the areas under the inhibitory plasma concentration–time curves (AUIC = AUC/MIC) for the duration of the recommended dosage interval, because this term indicates the degree of exposure of a microorganism to the drug.

Location of the intramuscular injection site can affect the plasma concentration profile and bioavailability of a drug administered as an aqueous suspension or long-acting (prolonged-release) parenteral dosage form. This is because of differences in blood flow to various muscles and in absorptive surface area. Based on the plasma concentration profile and the systemic availability of amoxycillin (20% aqueous suspension of amoxycillin trihydrate) and of oxytetracycline (10% conventional formulation of oxytetracycline hydrochloride) in cattle, intramuscular injection in the shoulder region (*m. triceps brachii*) or the lateral neck is superior to intramuscular injection in the buttock (*m. semitendineus*) or subcutaneous injection in the lateral neck or the dewlap (Rutgers *et al.*, 1980; Nouws & Vree, 1983). Better antimicrobial absorption from the former sites could be attributed to greater access of drug to a larger absorptive surface area with perhaps greater blood flow. It appears that tissue irritation caused by some parenteral preparations is more severe after subcutaneous than intramuscular injection (Nouws & Vree, 1983; Korsrud *et al.*, 1993). The lateral neck should always be used as the site for intramuscular injection of parenteral preparations in pigs. Age or body weight of calves influences the relative bioavailability, based on comparison of AUCs from time zero to 8 h, of amoxycillin (7 mg/kg) injected intramuscularly as amoxycillin trihydrate 10% aqueous suspension (Marshall & Palmer, 1980). The lower the body weight of calves, the larger the area under the plasma amoxycillin concentration–time curve (i.e. the higher the bioavailability of the antibiotic). When the same parenteral preparation of amoxycillin was administered intramuscularly to different animal species, the trend was for smaller sized animals (cats, dogs, piglets) to show an early high peak plasma concentration followed by a rapid decline, while larger animals (calves, horses) show a lower and relatively constant plasma concentration of amoxycillin over at least an 8-h period after administration of the drug preparation (Fig. 2.8) (Marshall & Palmer, 1980).

Following the injection of procaine penicillin G (20 000 IU/kg) at various intramuscular sites and subcutaneously in the cranial part of the pectoral area in horses, C_{max} and systemic availability of penicillin G were highest when the long-acting preparation was injected intramuscularly in the neck region (*m. serratus ventralis cervicis*). This was followed, in descending order of injection site, by *m. biceps* > *m. pectoralis* > *m. gluteus* or subcutaneously (Fig. 2.9) (Firth *et al.*, 1986). A single dose (25 000 IU/kg) of procaine penicillin G, injected intramuscularly in the lateral neck, will provide effective penicillin concentration in plasma for at least 12 h, and generally for 24 h. Procaine penicillin G (an aqueous suspension containing 300 000 IU/mL) was, until the recent development of oxytetracycline formulated in polyethylene glycol

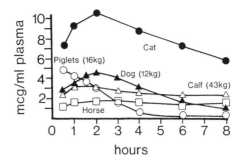

Fig. 2.8 Effect of species and weight on the bioavailability of amoxycillin after intramuscular injection of amoxycillin trihydrate aqueous suspension (100 mg/mL) at the same dose (7 mg/kg) in the various species except cats (10–12 mg/kg).

(indicated for the treatment of equine monocytic ehrlichiosis), the only long-acting parenteral dosage form of an antimicrobial agent suitable for intramuscular administration to horses. The best site for intramuscular injection in the neck of the horse appears to be at the level of the fifth cervical vertebra, ventral to the funicular part of the ligamentum nuchae but dorsal to the brachiocephalic muscle (Boyd, 1987).

Intramuscular injection of ampicillin trihydrate (15% aqueous suspension) in the lateral neck of healthy dwarf goats produces significantly higher plasma ampicillin concentrations than injection of the preparation in the thigh muscle (*m. quadriceps femoris*). Fever, induced with *Escherichia coli* endotoxin, increases the rate of absorption of ampicillin from the thigh (shivering muscles) but decreases ampicillin absorption from the lateral neck (non-shivering muscles) (Groothuis *et al.*, 1980). The effect of fever on the rate of ampicillin absorption

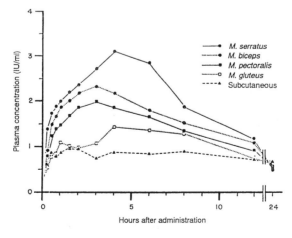

Fig. 2.9 Mean plasma penicillin concentration–time curves after 20 000 IU of procaine penicillin G per kilogram was administered to five animals (four horses and one pony) at five different sites. (Reproduced with permission from Firth *et al.* (1986).)

from the thigh muscle could be attributed to a relative increase in blood flow or more widespread local distribution of the drug preparation in the shivering muscles.

Two potential disadvantages of intramuscular administration are deposition of the drug preparation within intermuscular fascial planes and the production of tissue damage at the site of injection. The latter is more likely to be caused by constituents (such as the vehicle) of the formulation than the drug substance *per se*. While tissue irritation causes discomfort and pain (droperidol–fentanyl combination, ketamine), tissue damage causes persistence of drug residues at the injection site (Rasmussen & Hogh, 1971; Rasmussen & Svendson, 1976; Rasmussen, 1980; Xia *et al.*, 1983; Nouws, 1984, 1990). Useful ante-mortem methods of evaluating the extent of tissue irritation and the rate of resolution at an intramuscular injection site include the echographical examination of muscle tissue in the immediate vicinity of the injection site (Banting & Tranquart, 1991) and the monitoring of plasma creatine kinase (CK) activity (Aktas *et al.*, 1995; Toutain *et al.*, 1995). These methods have the distinct advantage of being applicable to the live animal, and should moderate-to-severe tissue damage be detected the extent of the damage caused and precise nature of the lesion can be described on post-mortem examination. The use of a tissue-damaging parenteral preparation in food-producing animals requires that an appropriate withdrawal period be applied. The withdrawal period for a drug varies with formulation of the dosage form, which should be administered only by the recommended route, and may differ between animal species. While prolonged-release preparations are convenient to use, they have the short-coming of a loss of flexibility in dosage and some, depending on the formulation, cause pain and tissue damage at the intramuscular injection site.

In cats, puppies and piglets, particular attention should be given to the drug concentration in a parenteral preparation and, when giving an intramuscular injection in the thigh (particularly of cats), to avoid causing damage to the sciatic nerve. Because avian and reptilian species appear to have a well developed renal portal system, first-pass renal excretion may decrease the systemic availability of drugs that are mainly eliminated by the kidneys (e.g., β-lactam and aminoglycoside antibiotics) when injected intramuscularly in the thigh of birds or the caudal half of the body of reptiles.

(Note: Parenteral drug administration (by s.c. injection) was introduced by Alexander Wood, a Scottish physician, in 1853).

Bioequivalence

Bioequivalence refers to the comparison made between a generic formulation of a drug, or a product in which a change has been made in one or more of the ingredients or in the manufacturing process, and a reference dosage form of the drug. This comparison is based on the estimation of relative bioavailability together with a measure of the uncertainty (variance) of the estimate.

Relative bioavailability based on comparison of plasma concentration profiles and features describing the curves (C_{max}, C_{max}/AUC, AUC_{0-LOQ}, MRT) involves the assumption that essentially equivalent plasma concentration profiles will yield comparable clinical responses. This assumption is valid only when the following criteria are met:

(1) the active moiety (usually parent drug) goes through the systemic circulation to reach its site of action,
(2) blood is the body compartment that provides the most sensitive discriminator of product inequivalence, and
(3) the study design accurately reflects product relative bioavailability under the conditions of clinical use.

The third criterion is critical in determining the appropriateness of the design of a bioequivalence study.

The fundamental assumption in bioequivalence assessment is that systemic clearance of the drug remains constant across phases of the study (crossover design) or between the animals used in the study (parallel-groups design). This follows from the equation

$$AUC = \frac{F \cdot D}{Cl}$$

where F is the fraction of the administered dose (D) which reaches the systemic circulation unchanged, and Cl is the systemic clearance of the drug. By substituting FD/Cl for AUC, the comparison of systemic clearance becomes

$$\frac{\left[\frac{F \cdot D}{Cl}\right]_{test}}{\left[\frac{F \cdot D}{Cl}\right]_{reference}}$$

To provide an unbiased assessment of the relative systemic availability (F) of a product, both clearance and dose must be constant.

The proposed method of data analysis dictates the design of a bioequivalence study, because design constrains the analysis that can be performed (Metzler, 1989). Bioequivalence studies must satisfy certain criteria which should be taken into account in the study design. The reference product selected should bear the labelling desired (indications, route of administration, animal species) for the generic formulation. The animals used in a bioequivalence study should be healthy and reasonably homogeneous with respect to age and body weight and, whenever practicable, both genders should be equally represented or dairy cows be at the same stage of lactation. Animal management conditions and the time of feeding relative to oral dosing should be standardized and, in ruminant species, both the plane of nutrition and nature (quality and quantity) of the feed should be controlled and feature in the design of bioequivalence studies. The analytical method must be sufficiently sensitive to accurately quantify the drug to a low plasma concentration. Blood samples should be collected at the designated times and be stored under conditions such that loss of the drug (e.g. by degradation or adsorption to storage vials) does not occur. A pilot study, in which a large number of samples are collected and the plasma concentration–time curve tentatively defined, provides useful information on which to base the selection of sampling times for inclusion in the design (sampling protocol) of the definitive study. Blood sampling times should be selected that will characterize the C_{max} and t_{max}, and sample collection should extend for a period corresponding to at least four apparent half-lives of the drug beyond the expected time of the peak plasma concentration. The duration of sampling is important because extrapolation of the measured (observed) plasma concentrations to infinite time is not involved in the analysis of the data; the area under what would otherwise be the extrapolated (terminal) portion of the plasma concentration–time curve should be less than 10% of the total area under the curve. To prevent the occurrence of interaction (carry-over) bias, an appropriate washout period should be allowed to elapse between the phases of a crossover study. It is recommended that 99.9% of the assayed moiety be eliminated from the body before administering any subsequent treatments in a single-dose bioequivalence study. This translates into a washout period equal to ten times the apparent terminal elimination half-life of the drug. Inspection of the data relating to the phases of a crossover study is a simple method of detecting carry-over (interaction) bias (Cleophas, 1990). When carry-over effects are anticipated (e.g. induction or inhibition of drug-metabolizing enzyme activity) or if the duration of the washout period risks changes in drug clearance, the use of a parallel-groups study design should be considered. Under certain justifiable circumstances, such as the use of young rapidly developing animals or the genuine risk of carry-over bias, a parallel-groups design may be preferable to a crossover design.

The principal parameter used to indicate the rate of drug absorption is C_{max}, even though it is also influenced by the extent of absorption; the observed t_{max} is less reliable. Because of the uncertainty associated with C_{max}, it has been suggested (Endrenyi & Yan, 1993; Tozer, 1994) that C_{max}/AUC_{0-LOQ}, where AUC_{0-LOQ} is the area under the curve from time zero to the LOQ of the acceptable analytical method, may more reliably measure the rate of drug absorption, except when multiexponential decline is extensive. Estimation of the terms should be based on the observed (measured) plasma concentration–time data and the use of non-compartmental methods rather than compartmental pharmacokinetic models. MRTs, from time zero to the LOQ of the analytical method, for the test and reference products can be compared, assuming that first-order absorption and disposition of the drug apply (Jackson & Chen, 1987).

In bioequivalence studies, the relative extent of absorption (systemic availability) of the drug is based on the comparison of AUCs from time zero to the LOQ of the acceptable analytical method:

$$F_{relative} = \frac{AUC_{0-LOQ \,(test\,product)}}{AUC_{0-LOQ \,(reference\,product)}}$$

The AUC should generally be estimated by applying the linear trapezoidal rule, but in cases where sampling times are separated by long intervals, logarithmic transformation of the data and application of the log-linear method may be more accurate (Chiou, 1978; Purves, 1992).

The statistical evaluation of bioequivalence studies should be based on confidence interval estimation rather than hypothesis testing (Metzler, 1988, 1989; Westlake, 1988). The 90% confidence interval approach, using $1-2\alpha$ (where $\alpha = 0.05$), should be applied to the individual parameters of interest (i.e. the pharmacokinetic terms that estimate the rate and extent of drug absorption) (Martinez & Berson, 1998). Graphical presentation of the plasma concentration–time curves for averaged data (test vs. reference product) can be misleading, as the curves may appear to be similar even for drug products that are not bioequivalent.

While single-dose studies are generally adequate for assessing product bioequivalence of most immediate-release (conventional) dosage forms, the assessment of some drug products may require multiple dosing. This circumstance applies to drugs that show non-linear (dose-dependent) pharmacokinetic behaviour. Multiple-dose studies are generally required to confirm the bioequivalence of sustained-release preparations labelled for repeated administration (Martinez & Berson, 1998). Dosing should be carried out to beyond the maintenance of steady-state plasma concentrations for two dosage intervals (generally 24 h for sustained-release oral dosage forms used in dogs), which would require the administration, at the recommended dosage interval (usually 12 h in dogs), of 6–8 doses. In order to confirm that steady-state concentrations have been achieved, at least three trough plasma concentrations (C_{min}) should be measured; the first sample of the series for measurement of C_{min} should be collected immediately preceding administration of the fifth dose. The plasma concentration profiles should be compared during the first (provides an estimation of the rate of drug absorption) and the final (estimates the extent of absorption) dosage intervals, as well as over the two dosage intervals at steady-state. The latter provides an accurate assessment of the peak-to-trough (C_{max}/C_{min}) ratio, i.e. the degree of fluctuation in plasma drug concentrations at steady-state. Compared with a conventional dosage form, a sustained-release preparation of the drug should extend the dosage interval and decrease the fluctuation in steady-state plasma concentrations. When linear kinetics apply, the AUC during a dosage interval at steady-state is equal to the *total* AUC (from zero time to infinity) following the administration of a single dose. Comparison of the AUCs at steady-state would provide a more accurate assessment of the relative extent of absorption.

For further discussion of bioequivalence the reader should refer to review of the 1993 Veterinary Drug Bioequivalence Workshop (Martinez & Riviere, 1994), the review paper 'Veterinary drug bioequivalence determination' (Toutain & Koritz, 1997) and the chapter entitled 'Bioavailability bioequivalence assessments' (Martinez & Berson, 1998) in *Development and Formulation of Veterinary Dosage Forms*, 2nd edn.

References

Agerso, H. & Friis, C. (1998) Bioavailability of amoxycillin in pigs. *Journal of Veterinary Pharmacology and Therapeutics*, **21**, 41–46.

Aktas, M., Lefebvre, H.P., Toutain, P.-L. & Braun, J.P. (1995) Disposition of creatine kinase activity in dog plasma following intravenous and intramuscular injection of skeletal muscle homogenates. *Journal of Veterinary Pharmacology and Therapeutics*, **18**, 1–6.

Ali, D.N. & Hennessy, D.R. (1995) The effect of temporarily reduced feed intake on the efficacy of oxfendazole in sheep. *International Journal for Parasitology*, **25**, 71–74.

Ali, D.N. & Hennessy, D.R. (1996) The effect of level of feed intake on the pharmacokinetic disposition and efficacy of ivermectin in sheep. *Journal of Veterinary Pharmacology and Therapeutics*, **19**, 89–94.

Baggot, J.D. (1977) *Principles of Drug Disposition in Domestic Animals: The Basis of Veterinary Clinical Pharmacology*. W.B. Saunders, Philadelphia.

Baggot, J.D., Love, D.N., Stewart, J. & Raus, J. (1988a) Bioavailability and disposition kinetics of amoxicillin in neonatal foals. *Equine Veterinary Journal*, **20**, 125–127.

Baggot, J.D., Wilson, W.D. & Hietala, S. (1988b) Clinical pharmacokinetics of metronidazole in horses. *Journal of Veterinary Pharmacology and Therapeutics*, **11**, 417–420.

Baggot, J.D., Love, D.N., Love, R.J., Raus, J. & Rose, R.J. (1990) Oral dosage of penicillin V in adult horses and foals. *Equine Veterinary Journal*, **22**, 290–291.

Banting, A. de L. & Baggot, J.D. (1996) Comparison of the pharmacokinetics and local tolerance of three injectable oxytetracycline formulations in pigs. *Journal of Veterinary Pharmacology and Therapeutics*, **19**, 50–55.

Banting, A. de L. & Tranquart, F. (1991) Echography as a tool in clinical pharmacology. *Acta Veterinaria Scandinavica*, Suppl. **87**, 215–216.

Baverud, V., Gustafsson, A., Franklin, A., Lindholm, A. & Gunnarsson, A. (1997) *Clostridium difficile* associated with acute colitis in mature horses treated with antibiotics. *Equine Veterinary Journal*, **29**, 279–284.

Baverud, V., Franklin, A., Gunnarsson, A., Gustafsson, A. & Hellander-Edman, A. (1998) *Clostridium difficile* associated with acute colitis in mares when their foals are treated with erythromycin and rifampicin for *Rhodococcus equi* pneumonia. *Equine Veterinary Journal*, **30**, 482–488.

Bevill, R.F., Dittert, L.W. & Bourne, D.W.A. (1977) Disposition of sulfonamides in food-producing animals. IV: Pharmacokinetics of sulfamethazine in cattle following administration of an intravenous dose and three oral dosage forms. *Journal of Pharmaceutical Sciences*, **66**, 619–623.

Boyd, J.S. (1987) Selection of sites for intramuscular injections in the neck of the horse. *Veterinary Record*, **121**, 197–200.

Brown, S.A., Jaglan, P.S. & Banting, A. (1991) Ceftiofur sodium: disposition, protein-binding, metabolism, and residue depletion profile in various species. *Acta Veterinaria Scandinavica*, Suppl. **87**, 97–99.

Chiou, W.L. (1978) Evaluation of the potential error in pharmacokinetic studies of using the linear trapezoidal rule method for the calculation of the area under the plasma level–time curve. *Journal of Pharmacokinetics and Biopharmaceutics*, **6**, 539–546.

Clark, R. & Wessels, J.J. (1952) The influences of the nature of the diet and of starvation on the concentration curve of sulphanilamide in the blood of sheep after oral dosing. *Onderstepoort Journal of Veterinary Research*, **25**, 75–83.

Clarke, C.E., Burrows, G.E., Mac Allister, C.G., Spillers, D.K., Ewing, P. & Lauer, A.K. (1992) Pharmacokinetics of intravenously and orally administered pyrimethamine in horses. *American Journal of Veterinary Research*, **53**, 2292–2295.

Cleophas, T.J.M. (1990) A simple method for the estimation of interaction bias in crossover studies. *Journal of Clinical Pharmacology*, **30**, 1036–1040.

Cook, G., Papich, M.G., Roberts, M.C. & Bowman, K.F. (1997) Pharmacokinetics of cisapride in horses after intravenous and rectal administration. *American Journal of Veterinary Research*, **58**, 1427–1430.

Corveleyn, S., Deprez, P. van der Weken, G., Baeyens, W. & Remon, J.P. (1996) Bioavailability of ketoprofen in horses after rectal administration. *Journal of Veterinary Pharmacology and Therapeutics*, **19**, 359–363.

Courtin, F., Craigmill, A.L., Wetzlich, S.E., Gustafson, C.R. & Arndt, T.S. (1997) Pharmacokinetics of cefiofur and metabolites after single intravenous and intramuscular administration and multiple intramuscular administrations of ceftiofur sodium to dairy goats. *Journal of Veterinary Pharmacology and Therapeutics*, **20**, 368–373.

Craigmill, A.L., Brown, S.A., Wetzlich, S.E., Gustafson, C.R. & Arndt, T.S. (1997) Pharmacokinetics of ceftiofur and metabolites after single intravenous and intramuscular administration and multiple intramuscular administration of ceftiofur sodium to sheep. *Journal of Veterinary Pharmacology and Therapeutics*, **20**, 139–144.

Delbeke, F.T., Debackere, M., Desmet, N. & Stevens, M. (1986) Pharmacokinetics and diuretic effect of bumetanide following intravenous and intramuscular administration to horses. *Journal of Veterinary Pharmacology and Therapeutics*, **9**, 310–317.

Delbeke, F.T., Vynckier, L. & Debackere, M. (1993) The disposition of suxibuzone in the horse. *Journal of Veterinary Pharmacology and Therapeutics*, **16**, 283–290.

De Rick, A., Chakrabarti, S., Belpaire, F. & Bogaert, M. (1979) Bioavailability of three brands of digoxin tablets in dogs. *Journal of Veterinary Pharmacology and Therapeutics*, **2**, 27–29.

Dohoo, S. (1997) Steady-state pharmacokinetics of oral sustained-release morphine sulphate in dogs. *Journal of Veterinary Pharmacology and Therapeutics*, **20**, 129–133.

Duffee, N.E., Stang, B.E. & Schaeffer, D.J. (1997) The pharmacokinetics of cefadroxil over a range of oral doses and animal ages in the foal. *Journal of Veterinary Pharmacology and Therapeutics*, **20**, 427–433.

van Duijkeren, E., Vulto, A.G., Sloet van Oldruitenborgh-Oosterbann, M.M., Mevius, D.J., Kessels, B.G.F., Breukink, H.J. & van Miert, A.S.J.P.A.M. (1994) A comparative study of the pharmacokinetics of intravenous and oral trimethoprim/sulfadiazine formulations in the horse. *Journal of Veterinary Pharmacology and Therapeutics*, **17**, 440–446.

van Duijkeren, E., Vulto, A.G., Sloet van Oldruitenborgh-Oosterbann, M.M., Kessels, B.G.F., van Miert, A.S.J.P.A.M. & Breukink, H.J. (1995) Pharmacokinetics of trimethoprim–sulphachlorpyridazine in horses after oral, nasogastric and intravenous administration. *Journal of Veterinary Pharmacology and Therapeutics*, **18**, 47–53.

Dyke, T.M., Sams, R.A. & Cosgrove, S.B. (1997) Disposition of flunixin after intramuscular administration of flunixin meglumine to horses. *Journal of Veterinary Pharmacology and Therapeutics*, **20**, 330–332.

Endrenyi, L. & Yan, W. (1993) Variation of C_{max} and C_{max}/AUC in investigations of bioequivalence. *International Journal of Clinical Pharmacology, Therapy and Toxicology*, **31**, 184–189.

Ensink, J.M., Barneveld, A., Klein, W.R., van Miert, A.S.J.P.A.M. & Vulto, A.G. (1994) Oral bioavailability of pivampicillin in foals at different ages. *Veterinary Quarterly*, **16**, S113–S116.

Firth, E.C., Nouws, J.F.M., Driessens, F., Schmaetz, P., Peperkamp, K. & Klein, W.R. (1986) Effect of the injection site on the pharmacokinetics of procaine penicillin G in horses. *American Journal of Veterinary Research*, **47**, 2380–2384.

Garg, R.C., Keefe, T.J. & Vig., M.M. (1987) Serum levels and pharmacokinetics of ticarcillin and clavulanic acid in dog following parenteral administration of Timentin®. *Journal of Veterinary Pharmacology and Therapeutics*, **10**, 324–330.

Gibaldi, M. & Perrier, D. (1982) *Pharmacokinetics*, 2nd edn. pp. 433–444. Marcel Dekker, New York.

Gilman, J.M., Davis, L.E., Neff-Davis, C.A., Koritz, G.D. & Baker, G.J. (1987) Plasma concentration of gentamicin after intramuscular or subcutaneous administration to horses. *Journal of Veterinary Pharmacology and Therapeutics*, **10**, 101–103.

Gingerich, D.A., Baggot, J.D. & Yeary, R.A. (1975) Pharmacokinetics and dosage of aspirin in cattle. *Journal of the American Veterinary Medical Association*, **167**, 945–948.

Groothuis, D.G., Werdler, M.E.B., van Miert, A.S.J.P.A.M. & van Duin, C.Th.M. (1980) Factors affecting the absorption of ampicillin administered intramuscularly in dwarf goats. *Research in Veterinary Science*, **29**, 116–117.

Hennessy, D.R., Ali, D.N. & Tremain, S.A. (1995) The partition and fate of soluble and digesta particulate associated oxfendazole and its metabolites in the gastrointestinal tract of sheep. *International Journal for Parasitology*, **24**, 327–333.

Hogben, C.A.M., Tocco, D.J., Brodie, B.B. & Schanker, L.S. (1959) On the mechanism of intestinal absorption of drugs. *Journal of Pharmacology and Experimental Therapeutics*, **125**, 275–282.

Hungate, R.E. (1966) *The Rumen and its Microbes*, p. 218. Academic Press, New York.

Jackson, A.J. & Chen, M.L. (1987) Application of moment analysis in assessing rates of absorption for bioequivalency studies. *Journal of Pharmaceutical Sciences*, **76**, 6–9.

Jacobs, D.E., Fox, M.T., Gowling, G., Foster, J., Pitt, S.R. & Gerrelli, D. (1987) Field evaluation of the oxfendazole pulse release bolus for the chemoprophylaxis of bovine parasitic gastroenteritis: a comparison with three other control strategies. *Journal of Veterinary Pharmacology and Therapeutics*, **10**, 30–36.

Jaglan, P.S., Roof, R.D., Yein, F.S., Arnold, T.S., Brown, S.A. & Gilbertson, T.J. (1994) Concentration of ceftiofur metabolites in the plasma and lungs of horses following intramuscular treatment. *Journal of Veterinary Pharmacology and Therapeutics*, **17**, 24–30.

Klink, P.R., Ferguson, T.H. & Magruder, J.A. (1998) Formulation of veterinary dosage forms. In: *Development and Formulation of Veterinary Dosage Forms*, (eds G.E. Hardee & J.D. Baggot), 2nd edn. pp. 145–229. Marcel Dekker, New York.

Koritz, G.D., McKiernan, B.C., Neff-Davis, C.A. & Munsiff, I.J. (1986) Bioavailability of four slow-release theophylline formulations in the Beagle dog. *Journal of Veterinary Pharmacology and Therapeutics*, **9**, 293–302.

Korsrud, G.O., Boison, J.O., Papich, M.G. *et al.* (1993) Depletion of intramuscularly and subcutaneously injected procaine penicillin G from tissues and plasma of yearling beef steers. *Canadian Journal of Veterinary Research*, **57**, 223–230.

Laby, R.H. (1974) U.S. patent 3 844 284.

Landoni, M.F. & Lees, P. (1995) Influence of formulation on the pharmacokinetics and bioavailability of racemic ketoprofen in horses. *Journal of Veterinary Pharmacology and Therapeutics*, **18**, 446–450.

Lanusse, C. Lifschitz, A., Virkel, G. *et al.*, (1997) Comparative plasma disposition kinetics of ivermectin, moxidectin and doramectin in cattle. *Journal of Veterinary Pharmacology and Therapeutics*, **20**, 91–99.

Loscher, W. & Frey, H.-H. (1981) Pharmacokinetics of diazepam in the dog. *Archives Internationales de Pharmacodynamie et de Therapie*, **254**, 180–195.

Maitho, T.E., Lees, P. & Taylor, J.B. (1986) Absorption and pharmacokinetics of phenylbutazone in Welsh Mountain ponies. *Journal of Veterinary Pharmacology and Therapeutics*, **9**, 26–39.

Marshall, A.B. & Palmer, G.H. (1980) Injection sites and drug bioavailability. In: *Trends in Veterinary Pharmacology and Toxicology*, (eds A.S.J.P.A.M. van Miert, J. Frens and F.W. van der Kreek). pp. 54–60. Elsevier, Amsterdam.

Martinez, M.N. & Berson, M.R. (1998) Bioavailability/bioequivalence assessments. In: *Development and Formulation of Veterinary Dosage Forms*, (eds G.E. Hardee and J.D. Baggot), 2nd edn. pp. 429–467. Marcel Dekker, New York.

Martinez, M.N. & Riviere, J.E. (1994) Review of the 1993 Veterinary Drug Bioequivalence Workshop. *Journal of Veterinary Pharmacology and Therapeutics*, **17**, 85–119.

Masson, M.J. & Phillipson, A.T. (1951) The absorption of acetate, propionate and butyrate from the rumen of sheep. *Journal of Physiology* (London), **113**, 189–206.

Masson, M.J. & Phillipson, A.T. (1952) The composition of the digesta leaving the abomasum of sheep. *Journal of Physiology* (London), **116**, 98–111.

Metzler, C.M. (1988) Statistical methods for deciding bioequivalence of formulations. In: *Oral Sustained-Release Formulations: Design and Evaluation*, (eds A. Yacobi and E. Halperin-Walega), pp. 217–238. Pergamon Press, New York.

Metzler, C.M. (1989) Bioavailability/bioequivalence: study design and statistical issues. *Journal of Clinical Pharmacology*, **29**, 289–292.

Nielsen, P. (1997) The influence of feed on the oral bioavailability of antibiotics/chemotherapeutics in pigs. *Journal of Veterinary Pharmacology and Therapeutics*, **20** (Suppl. 1), 30–31.

Nielsen, P. & Gyrd-Hansen, N. (1998) Bioavailability of spiramycin and lincomycin after oral administration to fed and fasted pigs. *Journal of Veterinary Pharmacology and Therapeutics*, **21**, 251–256.

Nouws, J.F.M. (1984) Irritation, bioavailability and residue aspects of ten oxytetracycline formulations administered intramuscularly to pigs. *Veterinary Quarterly*, **6**, 80–84.

Nouws, J.F.M. (1990) Injection sites and withdrawal times. *Annales de Recherches Vétérinaires*, **21**(Suppl. 1), 145S–150S.

Nouws, J.F.M. & Vree, T.B. (1983) Effect of injection site on the bioavailability of an oxytetracycline formulation in ruminant calves. *Veterinary Quarterly*, **5**, 165–170.

Nouws, J.F.M. van Ginneken, C.A.M., Hekman, P. & Ziv, G. (1982) Comparative plasma ampicillin levels and bioavailability of five parenteral ampicillin formulations in ruminant calves. *Veterinary Quarterly*, **4**, 62–71.

Papich, M.G. & Alcorn, J. (1995) Absorption of diazepam after its rectal administration in dogs. *American Journal of Veterinary Research*, **56**, 1629–1636.

Petersen, M.B. & Friis, C. (2000) Pharmacokinetics of fenbendazole following intravenous and oral administration to pigs. *American Journal of Veterinary Research*, **61**, 573–576.

Phillipson, A.T. & McAnally, R.A. (1942) Studies on the fate of carbohydrates in the rumen of the sheep. *Journal of Experimental Biology*, **19**, 199–214.

Purves, R.D. (1992) Optimum numerical integration methods for estimation of area-under-the-curve (AUC) and area-under-the-moment curve (AUMC). *Journal of Pharmacokinetics and Biopharmaceutics*, **20**, 211–226.

Rasmussen, F. (1980) Tissue damage at the injection site after intramuscular injection of drugs in food-producing animals. In: *Trends in Veterinary Pharmacology and Toxicology*, (eds, A.S.J.P.A.M. van Miert, J. Frens and F.W. van der Kreek), pp. 27–33. Elsevier, Amsterdam.

Rasmussen, F. & Hogh, P. (1971) Irritating effect and concentration at the injection site after intramuscular injection of antibiotic preparations in cows and pigs. *Nordisk Veterinaer-Medicin*, **23**, 593–605.

Rasmussen, F. & Svendsen, O. (1976) Tissue damage and concentration at the injection site after intramuscular injection of chemotherapeutics and vehicles. *Research in Veterinary Science*, **20**, 55–60.

Rowlands, D. ap T., Shepherd, M.T. and Collins, K.R. (1988) The oxfendazole pulse release bolus. *Journal of Veterinary Pharmacology and Therapeutics*, **11**, 405–408.

Rutgers, L.J.E., van Miert, A.S.J.P.A.M., Nouws, J.F.M. & van Ginneken, C.A.M. (1980) Effect of the injection site on the bioavailability of amoxycillin trihydrate in dairy cows. *Journal of Veterinary Pharmacology and Therapeutics*, **3**, 125–132.

Sams, R.A. & Ruoff, Jr., W.W. (1985) Pharmacokinetics and bioavailability of cefazolin in horses. *American Journal of Veterinary Research*, **46**, 348–352.

Sangiah, S., McAllister, C.C. & Amouzadeh, H.R. (1988) Effects of cimetidine and ranitidine on basal gastric pH, free and total acid contents in horses. *Research in Veterinary Science*, **45**, 291–295.

Schwarz, C., Steinmetzer, K. & Caithaml, K. (1926) *Arch. Ges. Physiol.*, **213**, 595. (Cited by Dukes, H.H. (1955) In: *The Physiology of Domestic Animals*, 7th edn., p. 330. Comstock/Cornell University Press, Ithaca, NY.

Snow, D.H., Baxter, P. & Whiting, B. (1981) The pharmacokinetics of meclofenamic acid in the horse. *Journal of Veterinary Pharmacology and Therapeutics*, **4**, 147–156.

Taylor, S.M., Malton, T.R., Blanchflower, J., Kennedy, D.G. & Hewitt, S.A. (1993) Effects of dietary variations on plasma concentrations of oral flukicides in sheep. *Journal of Veterinary Pharmacology and Therapeutics*, **16**, 48–54.

Theeuwes, F. & Bayne, W. (1977) Dosage form index: an objective criterion for evaluation of controlled-release drug delivery systems. *Journal of Pharmaceutical Sciences*, **66**, 1388–1392.

Toutain, P.-L. & Koritz, G.D. (1997) Veterinary drug bioequivalence determination. *Journal of Veterinary Pharmacology and Therapeutics*, **20**, 79–90.

Toutain, P.-L., Lassourd, V., Costes, G., Alvinerie, M., Bret, L., Lefebvre, H.P. & Braun, J.P. (1995) A non-invasive and quantitative method for the study of tissue injury caused by intramuscular injection of drugs in horses. *Journal of Veterinary Pharmacology and Therapeutics*, **18**, 226–235.

Tozer, T.N. (1994) Bioequivalence data analysis: Evaluating the metrics of rate and extent of drug absorption. *Journal of Veterinary Pharmacology and Therapeutics*, **17**, 105.

Vinagre, E., Rodrigue, C., San Andres, M.I., Boggio, J.C., San Andres, M.D. & Encinas, T. (1998) Pharmacokinetics of indomethacin in sheep after intravenous and intramuscular administration. *Journal of Veterinary Pharmacology and Therapeutics*, **21**, 309–314.

Wagner, S.O., Sams, R.A. & Podell, M. (1998) Chronic phenobarbital therapy reduces plasma benzodiazepine concentrations after intravenous and rectal administration of diazepam in the dog. *Journal of Veterinary Pharmacology and Therapeutics*, **21**, 335–341.

Westlake, W.J. (1988) Bioavailability and bioequivalence of pharmaceutical formulations. In: *Biopharmaceutical Statistics for Drug Development*, (ed. K.E. Peace), pp. 329–352. Marcel Dekker, New York.

Wilson, R.C., Duran, S.H., Horton, Jr., C.R. & Wright, L.C. (1989) Bioavailability of gentamicin in dogs after intramuscular or subcutaneous injections. *American Journal of Veterinary Research*, **50**, 1748–1750.

Wilson, W.D., Spensley, M.S., Baggot, J.D., Hietala, S.K. & Pryor, P. (1991) Pharmacokinetics and bioavailability of ticarcillin and clavulanate in foals after intravenous and intramuscular administration. *Journal of Veterinary Pharmacology and Therapeutics*, **14**, 78–89.

Xia, W., Gyrd-Hansen, N. & Nielsen, P. (1983) Comparison of pharmacokinetic parameters for two oxytetracycline preparations in pigs. *Journal of Veterinary Pharmacology and Therapeutics*, **6**, 113–120.

Chapter 3
Interpretation of Changes in Drug Disposition and Interspecies Scaling

Introduction

Following the entry of a drug into the systemic circulation, it is rapidly conveyed throughout the body in the circulating blood. The *free* (unbound) fraction is immediately available for extravascular distribution and for elimination (i.e., biotransformation and excretion). Drug distribution depends on binding to plasma proteins (acidic drugs bind to albumin while some basic drugs mainly bind to α_1-acid glycoprotein) and to extravascular macromolecules (tissue constituents), and on the capacity of the drug to penetrate cellular barriers and to accumulate (ion trapping effect) in certain body fluids (such as ruminal fluid). The extent of distribution is determined by the chemical nature and related physicochemical properties (pK_a and lipid solubility) of the drug, and is quantitatively expressed by the pharmacokinetic parameter apparent volume of distribution (V_d). A high degree of lipid solubility and either low binding to plasma proteins or high binding to extravascular macromolecules are associated with extensive tissue distribution ($V_d > 0.7\,\text{L/kg}$). Examples of drugs that extensively distribute in tissues include digoxin, propranolol, xylazine, pethidine (meperidine), diazepam, macrolide antibiotics and ivermectin. Because of their high degree of ionization in plasma and extensive ($>80\%$) binding to plasma albumin, the non-steroidal anti-inflammatory drugs have limited distribution ($V_d < 0.3\,\text{L/kg}$), while relatively low solubility in lipid limits the extravascular distribution of aminoglycoside antibiotics (polar organic bases). Despite their limited distribution, aminoglycosides selectively bind to the basolateal membranes of proximal renal tubular epithelium (renal cortex) and cochlear tissue (inner ear) because of the disproportionately high content of phosphatidylinositol in these tissues (Hauser & Eichberg, 1973). Selective tissue binding of aminoglycosides contributes to their potential nephrotoxicity and ototoxicity and accounts for their prolonged terminal elimination from the body.

Disposition is the term used to describe the simultaneous effects of distribution and elimination, that is, the processes that occur subsequent to the absorption of a drug into the systemic circulation. The disposition of a drug is largely influenced by the chemical nature, molecular structure and physio-chemical properties of the drug. Other factors which affect drug disposition include: the extent of binding to plasma proteins and extravascular macro-molecules (tissue constituents), blood flow to the organs of elimination (usually the liver and kidneys), the activity of drug-metabolizing enzymes (determines the capacity of metabolic pathways), and the efficiency of excretion (mainly renal) mechanisms. The relative influence of these factors will vary with the drug in accordance with the fraction of the amount in the body which is bound and the contribution of biotransformation or excretion to elimination. Parti-cularly for drugs that undergo extensive biotransformation, disposition varies between species. These differences are quantified by comparing the pharma-cokinetic properties of a drug in various species. The volume of distribution measures the *apparent* space in the body available to contain the drug. It affects the half-life of the drug and the fluctuation in steady-state concentrations on multiple dosing, but not the average steady-state plasma concentration. The systemic clearance, which represents the sum of the clearances by the organs of elimination, measures the ability of the body to eliminate the drug. It is influ-enced by the availability of the drug to the eliminating organs and their ability to remove the drug from blood. Systemic clearance determines the average steady-state plasma concentration that is attained on multiple dosing, and is probably the most important pharmacokinetic parameter to consider in the design of a dosage regimen. Half-life measures the overall rate of drug elimination. Because half-life expresses the relationship between volume of distribution (area method) and systemic clearance of the drug, it is a composite (hybrid) pharmacokinetic parameter. The principal application of half-life is in selection of the dosage interval, and it determines the time required to reach steady-state concentrations of the drug.

Changes in drug disposition

Some disease states (e.g. fever, dehydration, impaired renal function, uraemia, chronic liver diseases, hypoalbuminaemia, hyperbilirubinaemia, congestive heart failure, oedema), prolonged (> 48 h) fasting, certain physiological condi-tions (such as the neonatal period), or pharmacokinetic-based drug interactions may affect the disposition of drugs. In order to interpret the changes that occur, comparison should be made of the plasma concentration profile, the volume of distribution at steady-state ($V_{d(ss)}$) (Klotz, 1976), which is more relevant than $V_{d(area)}$, the systemic clearance (Cl_B) and the half-life ($t_{1/2}$) of the drug in healthy and diseased animals. The comparison of pharmacokinetic parameters is most informative when based on studies performed in the same animals under healthy and induced disease conditions. Dosage adjustment, if required, in a diseased animal can be based on the anticipated changes in pharmacokinetic parameters, the monitoring of plasma concentrations of drugs with a narrow margin of safety or wide individual (inter-animal) variation (e.g., digoxin, gentamicin, phenobarbitone), clinical assessment of the health status (liver and kidney function, presence of fever, state of hydration) of the animal and severity of the disease state, and close observation of the effects produced by the drug. It is only after administering at least four doses at a constant dosage interval that maximum effects of a drug are produced.

Febrile state

In the presence of *Escherichia coli* endotoxin-induced fever in dogs and etio-cholanolone-stimulated fever in human beings, the serum concentrations of gentamicin are lower than in the afebrile state (Fig. 3.1) (Pennington *et al.*, 1975). This could be attributed to increased extravascular distribution of gentamicin, although renal clearance and the half-life of the antibiotic were not significantly

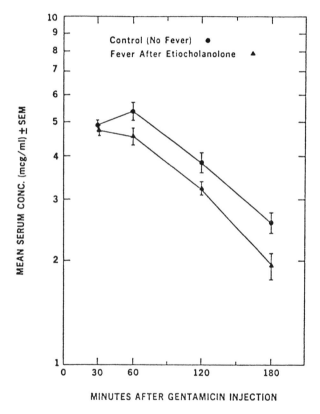

MINUTES AFTER GENTAMICIN INJECTION

Fig. 3.1 Comparison of the mean serum gentamicin concentration–time curves in control (afebrile) and etiocholanolone-induced febrile subjects ($n = 6$) following the intramuscular injection of a single dose of gentamicin sulfate (1.5 mg/kg). Note the lower serum gentamicin concentrations in the presence of fever. Neither the renal clearance nor the half-life of gentamicin were significantly changed (Reproduced with permission from Pennington *et al.* (1975).)

changed. It is known that penicillin G (benzylpenicillin) distributes more widely in tissues during the febrile state. Based on the microconstants associated with the two-compartment pharmacokinetic model describing the disposition of penicillin G in normal (afebrile) and streptococcal-induced febrile dogs, the simulated (analogue computer-generated) curves depicting penicillin levels in the central (serum) and peripheral (tissue) compartments of the model illustrate the effect of fever (Fig. 3.2) (Baggot, 1980). Inspection of the tissue level curves shows that the peak tissue level in the febrile dogs represents 21% of the dose, compared with 7% in normal dogs. This indicates that extra-vascular distribution of penicillin G is increased during the febrile state. Enhanced penetration of the blood–brain barrier during the acute febrile stage of infection may substantially contribute to the clinical effectiveness of penicillin G in the treatment of meningitis caused by penicillin-sensitive bacterial pathogens.

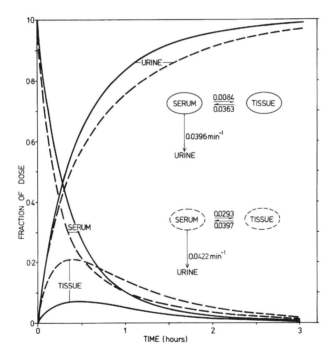

Fig. 3.2 Analogue computer-generated curves showing the levels (as fraction of the intravenous dose) of benzylpenicillin in the central (serum) and peripheral (tissue) compartments of the two-compartment pharmacokinetic model and the cumulative amount excreted unchanged in the urine as a function of time. The curves are based on the first-order rate constants (k_{12}, k_{21}, k_{el}) associated with the compartmental pharmacokinetic model. Note the higher tissue level curve in the febrile (- - - -) compared with the control (———) dogs. The tissue-to-serum level ratios (k_{12}/k_{21}) at the time of attainment of pseudo-distribution equilibrium (peak of tissue level curves) were 0.74 and 0.23 in the febrile and control dogs, respectively. (Reproduced with permission from Baggot (1980).)

During the acute febrile stage of falciparum malaria, the plasma concentrations of quinine (administered orally as quinine sulphate) are significantly higher than in healthy subjects and the logarithmic decline in plasma concentrations is non-linear (Trenholme *et al.*, 1976). The elevated plasma quinine concentrations could be attributed to a relative decrease in tissue distribution of the drug, because it is unlikely that gastrointestinal absorption is increased, while the slower decline in plasma concentrations (associated with the changed elimination kinetics) suggests impaired hepatic metabolism of quinine in the presence of fever.

The effect of experimentally induced bacterial infections, all of which have in common the presence of fever, on the disposition of various antimicrobial agents in pigs is presented in Table 3.1. In the infected pigs, the apparent volume of distribution of penicillin G, ampicillin and, to a lesser extent, trimethoprim is increased, of enrofloxacin and sulphonamides remains unchanged, and of oxytetracycline is decreased. The systemic clearance of penicillin G, ampicillin and trimethoprim is increased, of sulphamethoxazole and sulphadimethoxine remains unchanged, and of sulphadimidine,

Table 3.1 Comparison of the disposition kinetics of some antimicrobial agents in healthy and experimentally infected (febrile) pigs. Results are expressed as mean $\pm$ SD; n = no. of animals in each group.

Antimicrobial agent	Healthy	Infected	Level of significance
Ampicillin (10 mg/kg, i.v.)[a] . *Streptococcus suum*			
n	8	8	
$V_{d\,(ss)}$ (L/kg)	0.51 ± 0.02	0.68 ± 0.06	$P<0.01$
Cl_B (L/h·kg)	0.52 ± 0.07	0.62 ± 0.10	$P<0.05$
$t_{1/2}$ (h)	0.69 ± 0.08	0.72 ± 0.15	NS
Penicillin G (15 000 i.u./kg, i.m.)[b] ; *Streptococcus suis*			
n	8	6	
$V_{d\,(area)}$ (L/kg)	0.67 ± 0.24	1.22 ± 0.34	$P<0.01$
Cl_B (L/h·kg)	0.32 ± 0.06	0.48 ± 0.08	$P<0.01$
$t_{1/2}$ (h)	0.87 ± 0.25	1.08 ± 0.36	NS
Enrofloxacin (2.5 mg/kg, i.v.)[c] . *Escherichia coli*			
n	7	7	
$V_{d\,(area)}$ (L/kg)	3.34 ± 0.69	2.81 ± 1.06	NS
Cl_B (L/h·kg)	0.42 ± 0.04	0.15 ± 0.04	$P<0.05$
$t_{1/2}$ (h)	3.45 ± 0.85	9.13 ± 5.37	$P<0.05$
Trimethoprim (5 mg/kg, i.v.)[d] ; *Actinobacillus pleuropneumoniae* toxins			
n	6	6	
$V_{d\,(area)}$ (L/kg)	1.21 ± 0.13	1.49 ± 0.15	$P<0.05$
Cl_B (L/h·kg)	0.31 ± 0.03	0.39 ± 0.02	$P<0.05$
$t_{1/2}$ (h)	2.7 ± 0.22	2.6 ± 0.21	NS

Contd.

Table 3.1 *Contd.*

Antimicrobial agent	Healthy	Infected	Level of significance
Sulphamethoxazole (25 mg/kg, i.v.)[d] ; *Actinobacillus pleuropneumoniae* toxins			
n	4	4	
$V_{d\ (area\ )}$ (L/kg)	0.35 ± 0.03	0.40 ± 0.02	NS
Cl_B (L/h·kg)	0.10 ± 0.01	0.10 ± 0.01	NS
$t_{1/2}$ (h)	2.5 ± 0.18	2.7 ± 0.11	NS
Sulphadimethoxine (25 mg/kg, i.v.)[d] ; *Actinobacillus pleuropneumoniae* toxins			
n	6	6	
$V_{d\ (area\ )}$ (L/kg)	0.25 ± 0.01	0.24 ± 0.01	NS
Cl_B (L/h·kg)	0.013 ± 0.001	0.013 ± 0.001	NS
$t_{1/2}$ (h)	12.9 ± 0.5	13.4 ± 1.0	NS
Sulphadimidine (50 mg/kg i.v.)[a] ; *Streptococcus suum*			
n	7	7	
$V_{d\ (ss\ )}$ (L/kg)	0.50 ± 0.08	0.52 ± 0.04	NS
Cl_B (L/h·kg)	0.023 ± 0.003	0.017 ± 0.003	$P < 0.05$
$t_{1/2}$ (h)	15 ± 3	20 ± 7	$P < 0.05$
Oxytetracycline (10 mg/kg, i.v.)[e] ; *Actinobacillus pleuropneumoniae* toxins			
n	6	6	
$V_{d\ (ss\ )}$ (L/kg)	1.84 ± 0.18	1.44 ± 0.19	$P < 0.05$
Cl_B (L/h·kg)	0.218 ± 0.020	0.194 ± 0.015	$P < 0.05$
$t_{1/2}$ (h)	5.86 ± 0.21	5.11 ± 0.36	$P < 0.05$

[a] Yuan *et al.* (1997).
[b] Zeng & Fung (1990).
[c] Zeng & Fung (1997).
[d] Mengelers *et al.* (1995).
[e] Pijpers *et al.* (1990).

enrofloxacin and oxytetracycline is decreased. Because of the changes in volume of distribution and systemic clearance, the half-life of sulphadimidine and enrofloxacin is increased, of penicillin G, ampicillin and trimethoprim is not significantly changed, and of oxytetracycline is decreased. Fever had no effect on the disposition of sulphamethoxazole and sulphadimethoxine in pigs.

In dwarf goats infected with *Ehrlichia phagocytophila* (now known as *Cytoecetes phagocytophila*), the systemic clearance of trimethoprim and, though not significantly, of ampicillin is increased, while the clearance of sulphadimidine and oxytetracycline is decreased. The half-life of trimethoprim and ampicillin is not changed, while the half-life of sulphadimidine and oxytetracycline is significantly increased (Anika *et al.*, 1986). Apart from the opposite effect on the half-life of oxytetracycline, the pattern of changes in the disposition of the antimicrobial agents is similar in dwarf goats infected with *C. phagocytophila* and pigs infected with various bacterial pathogens. Fever induced with *E. coli* endotoxin in neonatal calves (24–32h old) did not change any of the pharmacokinetic parameters describing the disposition of phenylbutazone (Semrad *et al.*, 1993). The extent of distribution and rate of elimination of sulphadimidine remain unchanged in *Pasteurella multocida*-infected New Zealand white rabbits (Yuan & Fung, 1990) and in bacterial (*E. coli* and *Staphylococcus aureus*)-induced febrile dogs (Riffat *et al.*, 1982).

Even though infectious diseases have in common the presence of fever, the effect of fever on drug disposition varies with the drug and may be influenced by the pathophysiology of the disease. In a study of the disposition of the antiprotozoal drug imidocarb in healthy and infected goats, it was observed that the various infections caused significant changes in both $V_{d(ss)}$ and Cl_B of imidocarb, while the $t_{1/2}$ of the drug did not significantly change (Abdullah & Baggot, 1986a). Fever induced with *E. coli* endotoxin or infectious bovine rhinotracheitis (IBR) virus caused a similar pattern of changes in the disposition of imidocarb, while the changes caused by *Trypanosoma evansi* infection are distinctly different (Table 3.2). The altered disposition of a drug caused by disease states can be due to changes in either or both of the basic pharmacokinetic parameters, volume of distribution and systemic clearance; half-life, which is a composite derived parameter, will not necessarily reflect an anticipated change in drug elimination and, consequently, cannot be used as the sole indicator of altered disposition.

Table 3.2 The disposition kinetics of imidocarb (4 mg/kg, i.v.) in healthy and experimentally infected (febrile) goats. Results are expressed as mean $\pm$ SD.

Pharmacokinetic parameter	Healthy (*n* = 8)	*E. coli* endotoxin (*n* = 6)	IBR[a] virus (*n* = 6)	*T. evansi* (*n* = 6)	Significance[b]
$V_{d\ (ss)}$ (mL/kg)	492 $\pm$ 82	222 $\pm$ 29	257 $\pm$ 41	1295 $\pm$ 333	$P < 0.01$
$V_{d\ (area)}$ (mL/kg)	544 $\pm$ 88	322 $\pm$ 183	276 $\pm$ 49	1398 $\pm$ 351	$P < 0.01$
Cl_B (mL/min·kg)	1.62 $\pm$ 0.50	0.76 $\pm$ 0.28	0.92 $\pm$ 0.09	4.10 $\pm$ 1.20	$P < 0.01$
$t_{1/2}$ (min)	251 $\pm$ 94	370 $\pm$ 391	208 $\pm$ 31	254 $\pm$ 91	NS

[a] IBR, infectious bovine rhinotracheitis.
[b] Using analysis of variance and *F* test to determine significance.

In monogastric species, fever generally decreases the rate, but not necessarily the extent, of drug absorption from the gastrointestinal tract. This effect is due to delayed gastric emptying. In *E. coli* endotoxin-induced febrile pigs, the rate of absorption of orally administered antipyrine (150 mg/kg) and trimethoprim (20 mg/kg) is decreased twofold (Ladefoged, 1979). Because of the decreased rate of absorption, the larger volume of distribution and unchanged clearance of these drugs in the febrile pigs, the apparent half-life is significantly increased. Orally administered enrofloxacin (2.5 mg/kg) appears to be completely available systemically in healthy and *E. coli*-infected pigs, but the average half-life of the drug is increased from 6.9 h in healthy pigs to 15.8 h in infected pigs (Zeng & Fung, 1997). It has been shown that *E. coli* endotoxin is a strong inhibitor of reticulo-ruminal contractions in sheep, goats and cattle (Leek & van Miert, 1971; van Miert, 1971). Orally administered amoxycillin (as trihydrate) is more slowly absorbed in *E. coli* endotoxin-induced febrile calves (3–4-week old) than in healthy (afebrile) calves (Groothuis *et al.*, 1978). However, the rate of absorption of orally administered sulphonamides is not decreased in febrile goats (van Gogh & van Miert, 1977).

Altered plasma protein binding

In the systemic circulation, drugs are partly bound to plasma proteins. Although the effects produced by a drug that acts reversibly are closely related to the free (unbound) concentration at the site of action, it is the total (free plus bound) drug concentration in plasma that is usually measured and to which the therapeutic concentration range refers. The extent of drug binding to plasma proteins, which is expressed as a percentage of the total drug concentration in the plasma, is determined *in vitro* using either equilibrium dialysis or ultra-filtration; it varies with the concentrations of drug and plasma protein, the affinity between drug-binding protein and drug, and the number of binding sites per molecule. Within the range of therapeutic concentrations, the extent of binding in healthy animals is characteristic of the drug, is independent of the drug concentration for the majority of drugs but concentration-dependent for some (e.g. salicylate, naproxen, valproic acid, disopyramide, ceftriaxone, cefoperazone), and can be broadly classified as extensive (>80%), moderate (50–80%) or low (<50%).

Albumin largely accounts for the binding of acidic drugs (e.g. β-lactam antibiotics, sulphonamides, non-steroidal anti-inflammatory drugs) in plasma. Basic drugs (e.g. macrolides and lincosamides, trimethoprim, propranolol, quinidine, lignocaine, pethidine) often associate more avidly with other proteins, particularly α_1-acid glycoprotein, than with albumin (Piafsky, 1980). The range of total plasma/serum protein concentration is similar (6.0–8.5 g/dL) in domestic animals and humans, but is lower (3.8–5.2 g/dL, due to relatively lower albumin concentration) in Galliformes. Although the extent of plasma protein binding of a drug varies between domestic animal species, the range of binding is reasonably narrow in the collective species (Table 3.3). Protein binding in humans is often at the upper end or somewhat above the range of binding in domestic animals: ketamine and doxycycline are exceptions. Species variation in the binding of acidic drugs might be mainly attributable to differences in the conformation of plasma albumin that would affect the binding capacity of the protein. Plasma protein (albumin) binding of salicylate is unusual in that mammalian species can be separated into two distinct groups. One group, comprising horse, dog, baboon, rat and mouse, shows a low protein-binding capacity for the drug, while the other group (man, Rhesus

Table 3.3 Range of binding of some drugs, at therapeutic concentrations, to plasma proteins in domestic animal species and, for comparison, the average percentage bound in the human.

Drug	Domestic animals range of binding (%)	Human average bound (%)
Nitroxynil[a]	97–98	–
Furosemide	85–95	99
Digitoxin	88–93	97
Quinidine	82–92	87
Sulphadimethoxine	78–88	–
Phenytoin	73–85	89
Ketamine	35–55	12
Amphetamine	20–40	26
Digoxin	18–30	25
Morphine	12–25	34

[a] Cattle, sheep and rabbits.

monkey, rabbit and guinea pig) possesses a high protein-binding affinity for salicylate (Sturman & Smith, 1967; Kucera & Bullock, 1969). Moreover, protein binding of salicylate is concentration-dependent: the percentage bound decreases as the total plasma salicylate concentration increases.

Protein binding of individual drugs within the same chemical class (e.g. penicillins, cephalosporins, sulphonamides, tetracyclines) can differ widely in the same animal species. Even though protein binding is readily reversible, extensive binding decreases the antimicrobial concentration at sites of infection or the concentration of a pharmacological agent at its site of action. The concentration attained in cerebrospinal fluid by a lipid-soluble drug (e.g., thiopental, amphetamine) is approximately equal to the free (unbound) concentration of the drug in plasma. The effect of protein binding on drug elimination depends on the process involved. Extensive binding to plasma proteins invariably decreases renal excretion when glomerular filtration is the sole mechanism of elimination, whereas it may either hinder or facilitate drug elimination when proximal renal tubular secretion or hepatic metabolism is the predominant elimination mechanism. Whether elimination is delayed or enhanced appears to depend on the extraction ratio (blood clearance/organ blood flow) for the drug by the organ of elimination.

In clinical pharmacology the fraction unbound ($f_u = 1 - f_b$) is of greater interest than the fraction bound (f_b) to plasma proteins, because it is the free drug in plasma that distributes extravascularly and interacts (activates or inhibits) with drug receptors at the site(s) of action. An increase in the fraction unbound, which may occur in certain disease states (such as hypoalbuminaemia and uraemia) or be due to competitive displacement from albumin binding sites, can increase the intensity of the effect produced. This is of particular concern for drugs that bind extensively to plasma proteins (Table 3.4) and have a narrow margin of safety or range of therapeutic plasma concentrations.

In chronic liver disease, especially cirrhosis with associated hypoalbumi-naemia, the extent of plasma protein binding of acidic drugs and of only some bases (e.g., diazepam, theophylline, quinidine) is decreased. In chronic heart failure, decreased protein binding of acidic drugs may be mainly attributed to an increased plasma concentration of endogenous binding competitors, such as free fatty acids (palmitate and oleate) that arise from mobilization of adipose tissue. Gram-negative bacterial infections may cause an elevated free fatty acid concentration in plasma that results in decreased albumin binding of acidic drugs (Craig *et al.*, 1976). In chronic renal failure, decreased binding of acidic drugs can be attributed to the combined effect of uraemia which, due to accumulation of endogenous competitor substances, other than free fatty acids, in plasma, decreases the apparent affinity of albumin for binding acidic drugs (Sjoholm *et al.*, 1976) and to the accompanying hypoalbuminaemia. The complementarity of these effects can markedly decrease plasma albumin binding of virtually all acidic drugs. The increased sensitivity (lower dosage requirement) of uraemic dogs to pentobarbital sodium could be at least partly due to decreased protein (albumin) binding of the anaesthetic. Impaired renal

Table 3.4 Drugs that extensively bind to plasma proteins and anticipated effect of hypoalbuminaemia or uraemia on the fraction bound.

Drug	Principal pharmacological effect	Effect of hypoalbuminaemia	Uraemia
Phenylbutazone	Anti-inflammatory	↓	↓
Furosemide	Diuretic	↓	↓
Propranolol	β-Adrenoceptor antagonist; dysrhythmic	↔	↔/↑
Quinidine	Anti-arrythmic; myocardial depressant	↓	↔/↑ [a]
Diazepam	Sedative; anti-convulsant	↓	↓
Phenytoin	Anti-convulsant; anti-arrythmic	↓	↓
Valproic acid	Anti-convulsant	↓	↓
Doxycycline	Antimicrobial	(↓)	↓
Cloxacillin	Antimicrobial		↓
Clindamycin	Antimicrobial	↔	↔
Ceftriaxone	Antimicrobial	↓	
Sulphadimethoxine	Antimicrobial	↓	↓

[a] Percentage bound is increased in the presence of inflammatory diseases.

function does not affect the overall rate of elimination (half-life) of pento-barbital. Apart from a few exceptions, notably diazepam (Kober *et al.*, 1979) and triamterene (Reidenberg & Affrime, 1973), the binding of bases does not appear to be altered in renal disease (Piafsky, 1980). On the contrary, plasma protein binding of basic drugs may be increased (fentanyl, oxazepam, propranolol, quinidine) in chronic renal failure with associated inflammatory disease. The increased binding could be attributed to increased plasma concentrations of α_1-acid glycoprotein and lipoproteins to which basic drugs mainly bind (Pacifici *et al.*, 1986). Drug metabolites are more polar than the parent drugs, hence less widely distributed and, under normal circumstances, are rapidly excreted by the kidneys. In the presence of renal impairment, drug metabolite concentrations in plasma may increase to a level at which competition occurs between a metabolite and the parent drug for albumin binding sites. Oxy-phenbutazone, the primary metabolite of phenylbutazone, is an example. Uraemia not only decreases the binding of acidic drugs to plasma albumin but also reduces the activity of some metabolic pathways, in particular hydrolysis by plasma pseudocholinesterase, non-bacterial reductive reactions and acetylation (Reidenberg, 1971).

Plasma concentrations of α_1-acid glycoprotein and other acute-phase proteins are elevated during the acute phase of various diseases, such as rheumatoid arthritis, ulcerative colitis, neoplasia, and under stress conditions (Piafsky, 1980; van Miert, 1995). The binding of basic drugs that interact with these proteins would be expected to increase in these conditions. Plasma protein binding of quinidine is significantly increased in patients with chronic respiratory failure (Perez-Mateo & Erill, 1977). In dogs showing a four- to fivefold elevation in α_1-acid glycoprotein and concurrent hypoalbuminaemia associated with inflammatory disease, the percentage *free* drug is significantly lower for drugs that bind mainly to α_1-acid glycoprotein (lignocaine, oxpre-nolol, propranolol), whereas for drugs that bind to albumin it is unchanged (phenytoin) or significantly higher (digitoxin, diazepam) than in healthy dogs (Table 3.5) (Belpaire *et al.*, 1987).

Plasma albumin concentration is decreased in the presence of hepatic cir-rhosis, liver abscess, acute pancreatitis, gastrointestinal disease, the nephrotic syndrome and chronic renal failure. Hypoalbuminaemia is a characteristic of neonatal animals, apart from foals, whereas the plasma concentration of α_1-acid glycoprotein is markedly elevated in newborn piglets. Hyperbilirubinaemia could further decrease the albumin binding capacity of acidic drugs and some basic drugs in neonatal animals.

Drug displacement

An unrelated drug or a metabolite formed, or increased plasma concentrations of endogenous substances such as free fatty acids or bilirubin, can compete with the principal drug (particularly organic acids) for binding sites on plasma

Table 3.5 Erythrocyte sedimentation rate (ESR), drug-binding protein concentrations and percentage free drug in serum of 21 healthy dogs and 21 dogs with inflammatory diseases. Results are expressed as mean ± SEM (Data from Belpaire *et al.* (1987).

Substance measured	Healthy dogs	Dogs with inflammation	Level of significance[a]
ESR (mm/h)	0.21 ± 0.09	23.3 ± 4.4	$P<0.001$
Total protein (g/L)	71.6 ± 0.9	72.3 ± 2.4	NS
Albumin (g/L)	31.3 ± 0.5	27.6 ± 1.0	$P<0.001$
α-Acid glycoprotein (mg/L)	374 ± 37	1632 ± 266	$P<0.001$
Percentage free (unbound) drug in serum			
Lidocaine	43.5 ± 2.4	11.7 ± 1.8	$P<0.01$
Oxprenolol	27.8 ± 2.0	9.3 ± 1.4	$P<0.01$
Propranolol	11.0 ± 0.7	4.8 ± 0.6	$P<0.01$
Phenytoin	18.1 ± 0.3	17.6 ± 0.6	NS
Digitoxin	15.5 ± 0.5	18.9 ± 0.6	$P<0.01$
Diazepam	1.57 ± 0.06	2.78 ± 0.34	$P<0.05$

[a] Mann–Whitney *U*-test.

albumin. The competition results in displacement or a decrease in the apparent binding affinity of albumin for the drug. The invariable outcome is an increased concentration of free drug in the plasma which can give rise to an enhanced, even toxic, effect. Decreased binding assumes clinical importance only when the fraction unbound (i.e. the free drug concentration) is significantly increased, which may occur with drugs that very extensively bind ($\geq 92\%$ to plasma albumin. Examples include naproxen (concentration-dependent), ibuprofen, ketoprofen, phenylbutazone, diazepam, desmethyldiazepam, oxazepam, furosemide, digitoxin (but not digoxin), valproate, warfarin, ceftriaxone (concentration-dependent), cloxacillin, dicloxacillin, ketoconazole and itraconazole. The concomitant administration of phenylbutazone and warfarin in dogs causes an increase (due to displacement) in the fraction unbound of warfarin from 2.6 to 8.0%. The increased anticoagulant effect (hypoprothrombinaemia) of warfarin, which has a low extraction ratio and small volume of distribution, is accompanied by a twofold decrease in the half-life (from 18.4 to 9.6 h) of the drug (Bachmann & Burkman, 1975).

Whether decreased protein binding (due to hypoalbuminaemia, uraemia, competition for binding sites or displacement) will affect the half-life of drugs that *extensively* bind to plasma proteins depends on the effect of the decrease in binding on both the volume of distribution and clearance of the drug. For a drug with a low extraction ratio ($E<0.3$) and small volume of distribution ($V_d<0.3$ L/kg), the half-life may be decreased (due to increased clearance), whereas for a drug with a high extraction ratio ($E>0.6$) and large volume of distribution ($V_d>0.7$ L/kg), the half-life may be increased (due to an increased volume of distribution). The half-lives of drugs with either a high extraction ratio and small volume of distribution or a low extraction ratio and large volume of distribution would not be expected to change (Tozer, 1984). Selection of the dosage interval for drugs with decreased protein binding should be based on the anticipated change in the half-life with the objective of minimizing fluctuations in steady-state plasma concentration of the drug while maintaining the therapeutic effect. The situation is more complicated for drugs showing concentration-dependent protein binding, because the values of clearance, volume of distribution and half-life change with concentration of drug in the plasma.

   Although albumin, with its extensive distribution into intenstinal fluids, may quantitatively be the principal drug binding protein, some drugs avidly bind to other tissue constituents. Digoxin, for example, distributes widely in tissues and binds with high affinity to cell membranes, particularly of the myocardium where it inhibits Na^+, K^+-ATPase. The extent of digoxin binding to plasma protein (albumin) in domestic animals is in the range 18–36%. When quinidine is administered to an animal on maintenance therapy with digoxin, displacement of digoxin from tissue binding sites causes a marked decrease in its volume of distribution that could lead to an increase in plasma digoxin concentration with resultant toxity.

Hepatic disease

The liver metabolizes lipid-soluble drugs by various biotransformation reactions, depending on the functional groups in the drug molecule, and quantitative differences in the capacity of the metabolic pathways account for variation between species in the amounts of the metabolities formed. In addition to converting several drugs to polar metabolites (often conjugates) for excretion in urine and/or bile, the liver performs a variety of physiological functions which include the synthesis of amino acids, plasma albumin, fibrinogen, prothrombin and primary bile acids, conversion of glycogen to glucose (glycogenolysis), gluconeogenesis, and metabolism of endogenous substances (bilirubin, insulin, thyroid and steroid hormones) which facilitates their excretion. Hepatic disease comprises an assortment of inflammatory or degenerative lesions that may affect the capacity of synthetic and metabolic functions or the efficiency of biliary excretion. An alteration in the activity of hepatic microsomal drug-metabolizing enzymes, which mediate a variety of oxidative reactions and glucoronide conjugation, will influence the rate of biotransformation of several lipid-soluble drugs, while change in liver blood flow may affect the clearance of drugs that are mainly eliminated by hepatic biotransformation. However, as the liver possesses considerable reserve capacity and regenerative ability, even a moderate degree of cellular damage might not be reflected by measurable changes in its metabolic and synthetic functions. In the presence of hepatic disease, the pharmacological effect produced by a drug, particularly when multiple doses are administered, may be enhanced. This could be attributed to a decreased rate of biotransformation, a higher fraction of free (unbound) drug in the plasma (due to hypoalbuminaemia, with or without hyperbilirubinaemia), or reduced hepatic blood flow.

The hepatic clearance (Cl_H) of a drug, which indicates the volume of blood cleared of the drug per unit time (mL/min·kg), is the product of blood flow to the liver (Q_H) and the hepatic extraction ratio (E_H) of the drug:

$$Cl_H = Q_H \cdot E_H$$

Variables in addition to liver blood flow that may influence the capacity of the liver to extract a drug from the blood for elimination by hepatic processes (biotransformation and/or biliary excretion of unchanged drug) are the unbound fraction in blood and the hepatic intrinsic clearance, which is a measure of the maximal ability of the liver to eliminate the drug. The hepatic clearance (with respect to blood concentrations) is determined by the following relationship between the variables which affect drug elimination by the liver:

$$Cl_H = Q_H \cdot \frac{f_u \cdot Cl_{int}}{Q_H + (f_u \cdot Cl_{int})}$$

where Q_H is liver blood flow, f_u is the unbound fraction of drug in blood and Cl_{int} is the hepatic intrinsic clearance for the drug. These physiological variables differ between species and may be influenced not only by hepatic disease but also by some other disease states (e.g. chronic renal disease, congestive heart failure, fever) and could be affected by the concomitant use of another drug.

In order to predict the likely effect of disease on the hepatic clearance of a drug, it is useful to categorize drugs that are mainly eliminated by the liver according to their hepatic extraction ratio as low ($E_H < 0.3$), intermediate (E_H, 0.3–0.6) or high ($E_H > 0.6$) (Table 3.6), while acknowledging that the category to which a particular drug belongs could differ between species, for example, diazepam (Klotz *et al.*, 1976).

Either acute or chronic liver disease can alter the disposition of drugs that are poorly extracted ($E_H < 0.3$) by the liver. Hepatic clearance of poorly extracted drugs that are mainly eliminated by biotransformation is affected by the unbound fraction in blood and the activity of drug-metabolizing enzymes. Because hypoalbuminaemia is a consistent feature of chronic liver disease, the unbound fraction, at least of acidic drugs and some basic drugs, is increased. In icteric and uraemic animals, endogenous albumin-binding competitor substances such as bilirubin (hepatic disease), free fatty acids and other substances (renal function impairment), accumulate in the blood and generally increase the unbound fraction. For drugs with a low extraction ratio, the effect of an increase in the unbound fraction on half-life depends on the volume of distribution (*vide supra*). The difference in half-life of valproate, which has a low extraction ratio and small volume of distribution, between humans ($t_{1/2} = 14$ h) and dogs $t_{1/2} = 2$ h) is largely due to the variation in clearance and the species difference in the unbound fraction of the drug (Loscher, 1978).

Table 3.6 Categorization of drugs that are mainly eliminated by the liver on the basis of their hepatic extraction ratio (E_H).

Low ($E_H < 0.3$)	Intermediate (E_H 0.3–0.6)	High ($E > 0.6$)
Antipyrine	Codeine	Bromsulphalein
Indocyanine green (dog)	Salicylate	Indocyanine green (human)
Diazepam (human)	Metronidazole	Diazepam (dog)
Phenobarbitone	Trimethoprim	Lignocaine
Phenylbutazone		Morphine
Naproxen		Pentazocine
Quinidine		Pethidine
Rifampin		Propoxyphene
Theophylline		Propranolol
Thiopental		Xylazine
Valproic acid		

The significant decrease in the half-life of warfarin, resulting from albumin-binding displacement of warfarin by phenylbutazone, is associated with increased hepatic clearance of warfarin. In contrast, the rate of elimination of warfarin in uraemic rabbits is significantly decreased (half-life increased) compared with healthy rabbits (Tvedegaard *et al.*, 1981). In the uraemic rabbits there were significant changes in plasma creatinine concentration (increased) and plasma albumin concentration (decreased). Even though the unbound fraction in blood is increased and more free drug is available for extravascular distribution and for elimination (by hepatic biotransformation), the volume of distribution remained unchanged, while the systemic (which reflects hepatic) clearance of warfarin was significantly lower in the uraemic rabbits and decreased further as uraemia progressed. The lower clearance can be attributed to the suppressant effect of uraemia on the activity of the microsomal metabolic pathway(s) for warfarin in the liver of rabbits. The activity of drug-metabolizing enzymes can only be assessed by the use of marker substances (which serve as model substances) for the various metabolic pathways. Drug-metabolizing enzyme activity can either be based on the disposition kinetics of the marker substances or be measured *in vitro* using liver biopsy specimens. There is evidence that when hepatic synthetic functions are impaired, the activity of drug metabolic pathways in the liver is reduced.

The galactose elimination capacity is a useful method of estimating the functioning liver mass (Tygstrup, 1964). A significant correlation was found between the apparent elimination rate constant for phenylbutazone (the plasma half-life) and the galactose elimination capacity ($r = 0.868$, $P < 0.05$) in cirrhotic patients (Hvidberg *et al.*, 1974).

The hepatic clearance of highly extracted drugs ($E_H > 0.6$) is mainly affected by changes in liver blood flow. As the hepatic extraction ratio approaches unity, the blood flow to the liver becomes the limiting factor governing clearance. The difference in systemic clearance, which reflects hepatic clearance, of propranolol between humans (15 mL/min·kg) and dogs (34 mL/min·kg) can be attributed to liver blood flow, which is 24 mL/min·kg and 42 mL/min·kg in humans and dogs, respectively (Evans *et al.*, 1973). Blood flow to the liver may be reduced in chronic liver disease and in congestive heart failure or be a secondary pharmacological effect of some drugs (e.g. racemic propranolol or the $S(-)$ enantiomer). The half-life of lignocaine (lidocaine) is 50% longer in dogs medicated with racemic propranolol than in non-medicated dogs (Branch *et al.*, 1973). The increased half-life is due to the significantly decreased systemic (hepatic) clearance of lignocaine which results from reduced cardiac output and liver blood flow caused by propranolol. When liver blood flow is reduced (as in chronic liver disease), the clearance of highly extracted drugs is decreased and, since volume of distribution generally remains unchanged, the half-life is increased.

The hepatic clearance of drugs with an intermediate extraction ratio (E_H, 0.3–0.6) is affected by all three physiological variables: blood flow to the liver, the unbound fraction in blood and the activity of hepatic drug-metabolizing enzymes. Disease-induced changes in the disposition of these drugs is least predictable.

Measurement of the clearances of antipyrine and indocyanine green (marker substances) can be used to assess different aspects of liver function. Antipyrine (phenazone) has a low extraction ratio ($E_H < 0.3$), binds to plasma proteins to a low extent ($< 20\%$) and is eliminated by hepatic microsomal oxidation. Indocyanine green has a high extraction ratio ($E_H > 0.6$), binds extensively to plasma proteins (mainly liproteins), is eliminated unchanged in the bile and does not undergo enterohepatic circulation. Values of pharmacokinetic parameters describing the disposition of antipyrine and indocyanine green in healthy human subjects and in patients with chronic liver disease (serum albumin concentration < 3 g/dL; normal range, 6.0–8.4 g/dL) are compared in Table 3.7 (Branch *et al.*, 1976). A highly significant decrease in the systemic clearance of both marker substances occurs in the presence of chronic liver disease, while volume of distribution is not significantly changed. Because of the relationship between volume of distribution ($V_{d(area)}$) and systemic clearance (Cl_B), the half-life of both substances is increased. Half-life, rather than clearance, of antipyrine is the parameter generally used to assess hepatic microsomal oxidative activity in the presence of liver disease and to compare the activity in different animal species. As the clearance of antipyrine is independent of changes in liver blood flow and the fraction bound to plasma proteins is very low, the decreased clearance may be attributed to a reduction in the mass of drug-metabolizing enzymes resulting in decreased hepatic microsomal oxidative activity. In addition to determining the clearance and half-life, a useful refinement would be to measure the rate of formation of antipyrine metabolites (4-hydroxyantipyrine, 3-methyhydrox-

Table 3.7 Pharmacokinetic parameters (mean ± SEM) describing the disposition of antipyrine and indocyanine green in healthy human subjects ($n = 6$) and in patients ($n = 9$) with chronic liver disease (serum albumin concentration <3 g/dL).

Kinetic parameter	Healthy	Liver disease	Significance
Antipyrine (E_H <0.3)			
$V_{d\ (area)}$ (L)	33.3 ± 2.8	41.3 ± 3.2	NS
Cl_B (mL/min)	38.4 ± 4.4	10.3 ± 1.6	$P < 0.001$[a]
$t_{1/2}$ (h)	10.3 ± 0.6	53.1 ± 7.5	$P < 0.001$[a]
Indocyanine green (E_H >0.6)			
$V_{d\ (area)}$ (L)	3.5 ± 0.41	5.3 ± 0.67	NS
Cl_B (mL/min)	1215 ± 190	182 ± 55	$P < 0.001$[a]
$t_{1/2}$ (min)	3.5 ± 0.33	44.7 ± 16.3	$P < 0.01$[b]

[a] Student's unpaired *t*-test.
[b] Wilcoxon rank test.

yantipyrine and norantipyrine) since this would indicate the activity of selective cytochrome P-450 isoenzymes (Wensing *et al.*, 1990). The decreased clearance of indocyanine green in human patients with chronic liver disease could indicate reduced liver blood flow and/or reduced hepatobiliary transport of the marker substance.

Unlike in humans, the extraction ratio of indocyanine green (low dose, 0.5 mg/kg i.v.) is low (E_H <0.3) in dogs. This implies that decreased clearance of the marker substance could be due to decreased binding to plasma proteins (mainly lipoproteins) or reduced capacity of the liver to eliminate (biliary secretion) indocyanine green. In dogs with dimethylnitrosamine-induced liver damage, which closely resembles natural chronic hepatic disease, the clearance of indocyanine green is significantly decreased (compared with healthy dogs) in the presence of moderate or severe, but not mild, damage. Neither the extent of plasma protein binding nor the volume of distribution at steady-state is changed (Boothe *et al.*, 1992). Predictably, the mean residence time ($MRT_{i.v.} = V_{d(ss)}/Cl_B$) is significantly increased when the hepatic damage is moderate or severe. The chemically-induced liver damage, regardless of the extent of the damage produced, significantly decreases serum albumin concentration. The clearance of antipyrine (20 mg/kg, i.v.) is significantly decreased in dogs with moderate or severe, but not mild, liver damage induced with dimethylnitrosamine (Boothe *et al.*, 1994). These results indicate that hepatic microsomal oxidative activity is reduced in the presence of moderate or severe liver damage. The extent of the damage, as judged by the character of microscopic lesions (histological grade), is not reflected in the magnitude of the decrease in antipyrine clearance. Moderate or severe liver damage reduces the intrinsic capacity of the liver to eliminate antipyrine (microsomal oxidation) and indocyanine green (biliary secretion).

Effect of fasting on hepatic function

Fasting induces hyperbilirubinaemia (increased plasma unconjugated bilirubin concentration) in healthy individuals and patients with hepatic dysfunction, and in healthy horses (Gronwall & Mia, 1972) and ponies (Gronwall, 1975; Gronwall *et al.*, 1980). The lower clearance of bilirubin appears to be related to decreased biliary secretion, rather than increased production or redistribution from extravascular sites. Biliary secretion of sulphobromophthalein (brom-sulphalein, BSP) and indocyanine green (ICG), like bilirubin, is carrier-mediated. Following the uptake of these organic anions from hepatic sinusoids, bilirubin undergoes conjugation with glucuronic acid and BSP with glutathione, whereas ICG is excreted unchanged. As the clearance of bilirubin, BSP and ICG is decreased in horses fasted for 72 h, with free access to water, it seems likely that both liver blood flow and hepatobiliary transport of the organic anions are affected by fasting (Engelking *et al.*, 1985). The half-life of BSP in healthy horses under normal feeding conditions is in the range 2.1–3.5 min: a half-life exceeding 4.5 min is considered to be highly suggestive of decreased hepatic function. Because bilirubin competes with BSP for hepatobiliary transport, the half-life of BSP is increased in horses with hyperbilirubinaemia: in horses fasted for 72 h with water available *ad libitum*, the average half-life of BSP is 4.8 min (Engelking *et al.*, 1985). The presence of fever, even a slight elevation in body temperature, may increase the half-life of BSP. Consequently, caution must be exercised when half-life is the only parameter of BSP disposition used to indicate a change in hepatic function. The half-life of BSP in healthy koalas is significantly shorter (range 0.8–1.5 min) than in marsupial and eutherian herbivores (Blanshard, 1994). Koalas are strictly folivorous and exist almost exclusively on the leaves of certain *Eucalyptus* spp. which, under natural conditions, adequately meet the water and energy needs of these animals. Antipyrine, acetaminophen (paracetamol) and lidocaine (lignocaine) are eliminated by hepatic biotransformation. In horses fasted for 72 h, with free access to water, the clearance (based on measurement of plasma concentrations) of these three unrelated drugs is decreased, although to a lesser degree than clearance of the organic anions (Table 3.8) (Engelking *et al.*, 1987). Based on the composite results it could be concluded that both reduced liver blood flow and decreased eliminating capacity of the liver (hepatic intrinsic clearance) contribute to the fasting-induced hyperbilirubinaemia and the lower systemic clearance of drugs.

In a study of the disposition of antipyrine (20 mg/kg, i.v.) in eight healthy Standardbred mares aged between six and nine years, the following values (mean $\pm$ SD or median (range)) were obtained for the major pharmacokinetic parameters: $V_{d(ss)}$ (mL/kg) 864 (731–952), Cl_B (mL/min·kg) 6.2 (4.3–8.6), MRT (h) 2.3 (1.7–3.5), and the overall elimination rate constant (per hour) 0.37 $\pm$ 0.09 (Dyke *et al.*, 1998). It was established that renal clearance accounts for <2% of systemic clearance, which implies that hepatic clearance exceeds 98%, and that 4-hydroxyantipyrine (formed by hepatic microsomal oxidation) is the major

Table 3.8 Comparison of the systemic clearance (mL/min·kg) of bilirubin, marker substances and some drugs eliminated by the liver in horses fed and fasted for 72 h. Results are expressed as mean ± SD.

Substance	n	Fed	Fasted	Percentage change[a]
Bilirubin[b]	4	0.54 ± 0.06	0.26 ± 0.06	−52
Indocyanine green[c]	10	3.53 ± 0.67	1.58 ± 0.57	−55
Sulfobromophthalein[c]	10	8.65 ± 1.02	4.51 ± 1.08	−48
Antipyrine[d]	3	5.83 ± 2.21	4.57 ± 1.73	−22
Acetaminophen[d]	3	4.84 ± 0.64	3.93 ± 0.62	−19
Lidocaine[d]	3	52.0 ± 11.7	43.7 ± 8.5	−16

[a] Percentage change = 100 [(mean fasted/mean fed) − 1].
[b] Gronwall & Mia (1972).
[c] Engelking *et al.* (1985).
[d] Engelking *et al.* (1987).

metabolite. Pretreatment of horses with phenobarbitone (induces hepatic microsomal oxidative activity) significantly increases the clearance of antipyrine, whereas pretreatment with carbon disulphide (reduces the mass of hepatic drug-metabolizing enzymes) significantly decreases the clearance of antipyrine. Neither induction nor inhibition changes the steady-state volume of distribution of antipyrine.

In goats fasted for 66 h but with free access to water, the systemic clearance of chloramphenicol was significantly lower than in the same goats fed cut grass (fed, 3.78 ± 2.19 mL/min·kg; fasted, 1.36 ± 0.95 mL/min·kg; $P < 0.05$) (Abdullah & Baggot, 1986b). The volume of distribution was not significantly changed, while the half-life of chloramphenicol increased almost threefold. The fraction of dose excreted unchanged in urine over a 12-h period was similar, but the urine collection period corresponded to eight half-lives in fed goats and three half-lives in fasted goats. As chloramphenicol is a poorly extracted drug, is bound to a low extent to plasma proteins (30% in goats), and a larger fraction of the dose is ultimately excreted unchanged in urine of fasted than of fed goats, it is reasonable to conclude that prolonged fasting decreases the rate of hepatic biotransformation (mainly microsomal-mediated glucuronide conjugation) of chloramphenicol.

Because of its influence on the dissolution of benzimidazole anthelmintics, the rate of passage of digesta along the gastrointestinal tract (particularly from the rumen to the abomasum) of ruminant animals determines the plasma concentration profile of the sulphoxide metabolite formed by first-pass metabolism following oral or intraruminal administration of albendazole or febendazole. A decrease in the gastrointestinal transit rate increases the time available for dissolution of the parent drug, the amount absorbed and the systemic availability (both peak plasma concentration and area under the curve) of the anthelmintically active sulphoxide metabolite. Compared with cattle fed *ad libitum*, a 48-h period of fasting preceding the intraruminal administration of albendazole micronized suspension (100 mg/mL) at a dose of 10 mg/kg to cattle significantly increased the peak plasma concentration and the total area under the curve of albendazole sulphoxide, and prolonged its elimination (Fig. 3.3) (Sanchez *et al.*, 1997). The plasma concentration profile of the sulphone metabolite, formed from the sulphoxide by hepatic microsomal oxidation, follows a generally similar pattern, but the apparent half-life of this

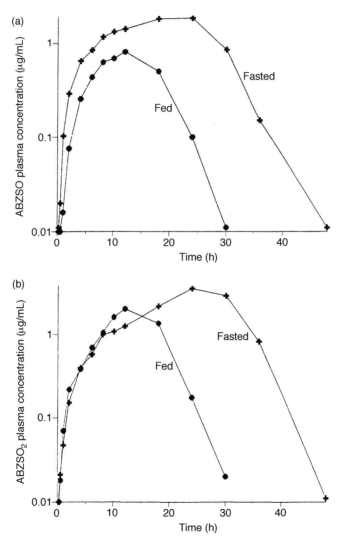

Fig. 3.3 Mean (*n* = 6) plasma concentrations of (A) albendazole sulphoxide (ABZSO) and (B) albendazole sulphone (ABZSO$_2$), obtained after the intraruminal administration of albendazole (10 mg/kg) to fed and fasted calves. (Reproduced with permission from Sanchez *et al.* (1997).)

metabolite is not increased. Because fasting did not change the disposition (volume of distribution and systemic clearance) of albendazole administered intravenously, the fasting-induced change (increase) in the formation of albendazole sulphoxide can be attributed to an increased extent of absorption of the parent drug from the gastrointestinal tract.

Prolonged (>48 h) fasting causes hyperbilirubinaemia, reduces liver blood flow and decreases drug elimination capacity of the liver, in that the hepatic clearance of drugs is lower and their half-life longer. As fasting and fever (Blaschke *et al.*, 1973) independently affect the intrahepatic handling and biliary secretion of sulphobromophthalein, a study of their combined effect on the disposition (including hepatic intrinsic clearance) of antimicrobial agents that are mainly eliminated by the liver (e.g., nafcillin, cefoperazone, clindamycin, trimethoprim, pyrimethamine, rifampin) would be of clinical interest.

Renal disease

Renal disease decreases the rate of elimination of drugs that are removed from the body predominantly by excretion of unchanged drug in the urine (e.g. aminoglycosides, most penicillins, cephalosporins and tetracyclines, most diuretics, digoxin, non-depolarizing neuromuscular blocking agents). The elimination of drugs that undergo hepatic biotransformation and are partly excreted unchanged may also be affected, particularly weak organic acids or bases that may be passively reabsorbed in the distal nephron (e.g. sulphona-mides, trimethoprim, phenobarbitone, amphetamine). Renal disease causes the accumulation in plasma of drug metabolites, some of which are pharmacolo-gically active (e.g. oxyphenbutazone, *N*-acetylprocainamide, alloxanthine, desmethyldiazepam and oxazepam) or toxic (normeperidine may lead to central nervous system excitation, metabolite of nitrofurantoin), and of endo-genous substances (free fatty acids and other substances) that compete for plasma albumin binding sites. In chronic renal disease and the nephrotic syndrome the concentration of plasma albumin is decreased, whereas in inflammatory diseases the plasma concentration of α_1-acid glycoprotein is increased.

Renal blood flow affects all three renal excretion mechanisms: glomerular filtration, carrier-mediated proximal tubular secretion and pH-dependent passive reabsorption from tubular fluid in the distal nephron. Changes in renal blood flow have more pronounced effects on tubular secretion and reabsorp-tion than on glomerular filtration. Drugs and drug metabolites that are excreted by the kidneys and have high renal extraction ratios (e.g. β-lactam antibiotics, glucuronide and sulphate conjugates of several drugs) are more dependent on renal blood flow than drugs with low extraction ratios (e.g. aminoglycosides, tetracyclines, sulphafurazole, digoxin, acetazolamide). The degree to which decreased renal function will affect drug elimination depends on the fraction of the dose that is normally excreted unchanged (as parent drug) in the urine. The systemic clearance of ampicillin considerably decreases in the presence of renal impairment and the half-life of the antibiotic increases, because the volume of distribution remains unchanged. Plasma protein (albumin) binding of ampicillin is low (about 20%) and not affected by uraemia. The half-life of ampicillin is 1.3 h in normal subjects, while in anephric patients ampicillin half-life is 12.7 h (Jusko *et al.*, 1973). The suppressed renal tubular secretion of furosemide in azotaemic dogs may partially account for the reduced therapeutic efficacy of the diuretic in renal disease accompanied by azotaemia (Rose *et al.*, 1976).

Reduced glomerular filtration rate and dehydration cause accumulation of aminoglycosides and thereby enhance their nephro- and ototoxicity. Because tetracyclines (apart from doxycycline) are eliminated by glomerular filtration, although slowly due to enterohepatic circulation, their clearance could be affected by a decrease in renal function. However, the effect of decreased renal function on the clearance of tetracyclines would be influenced by changes in extravascular (tissue) distribution. Digoxin has a very large volume of distribution (due to tissue binding) and, because the drug undergoes enterohepatic circulation, it is slowly excreted by glomerular filtration. In azotaemic dogs, the volume of distribution, the renal and systemic clearances, and the cumulative amount of the drug excreted in urine collected over a six-day period are significantly decreased (Table 3.9) (Gierke *et al.*, 1978). Even though the average half-life of digoxin is not significantly changed, variation between individual dogs is wider during azotaemia, and because of decreased systemic clearance the average steady-state plasma concentration that the usual dosage rate would attain would be increased and toxicity could ensue. The lower volume of distribution of digoxin in azotaemic dogs could be attributed to decreased tissue binding of the drug.

Renal disease (uraemia) may increase the volume of distribution of acidic drugs that extensively bind to plasma albumin (e.g., phenytoin, valproic acid, naproxen, phenylbutazone, furosemide). As decreased protein binding would increase the unbound (free) fraction in the plasma, the therapeutic concentration range (based on total drug concentration) would be lower than the usual

Table 3.9 Pharmacokinetic parameters describing the disposition of digoxin (0.05 mg/kg, i.v.) in dogs before and during azotaemia and the cumulative amount of the drug excreted in urine collected over a 6-day period. Results are expressed as mean $\pm$ SD; $n = 7$.

Kinetic parameter	Normal	Azotaemic	Significance[a]
$V_{d \text{ (area)}}$ (L/kg)	9.46 ± 1.66	7.91 ± 1.06	$P < 0.05$
Cl_B (mL/min·kg)	3.94 ± 0.67	2.69 ± 0.67	$P < 0.001$
Cl_R (mL/min·kg)	1.76 ± 0.57	0.69 ± 0.31	$P < 0.01$
Cl_{Cr} (mL/min·kg)	2.15 ± 0.52	0.78 ± 0.25	$P < 0.001$
$t_{1/2}$ (h)	28.0 ± 4.0	36.2 ± 11.5	NS
Amount excreted (ng)	416 ± 49	223 ± 42	$P < 0.01$

[a] Student's *t*-test for paired data.

range. Whether the dosage rate would require adjustment depends on the systemic clearance of the drug and whether the liver or the kidney is the eliminating organ. Uraemia does not affect the extent of protein binding of basic drugs that mainly bind to α_1-acid glycoprotein (e.g. propranolol, quinidine, trimethoprim). It follows that the effect of renal disease on drug–protein binding depends on the binding protein and the extent of binding to albumin.

In the presence of uraemia the activity of some biotransformation pathways (e.g. reductive and hydrolytic reactions, and acetylation) is decreased, whereas the activity of other pathways (hepatic microsomal oxidative reactions and glucuronide conjugation) appears to be unaffected (Reidenberg & Drayer, 1980). Even though the distribution of morphine is not changed and the drug is mainly eliminated by glucuronide conjugation, respiratory depression associated with higher than expected total plasma concentrations may occur in uraemic patients. This has been attributed to regeneration of the parent drug by hydrolysis of the accumulated glucuronide conjugate (Verbeeck, 1982). The increased sensitivity of uraemic animals to acidic drugs which act on the central nervous system is probably due to decreased binding to plasma albumin, although uraemia could conceivably increase the permeability of the blood–brain barrier.

The systemic availability of some orally administered drugs is increased in the presence of renal disease. The increased systemic availability of propranolol (Bianchetti *et al.*, 1978) and propoxyphene (Gibson *et al.*, 1980) has been attributed to decreased pre-systemic biotransformation (first-pass effect). Although the systemic availability of orally administered digoxin is not affected by renal disease, because the drug is not subject to the first-pass effect, the peak plasma concentration is higher and more slowly reached (Ohnhaus *et al.*, 1979). The higher peak plasma concentration may be due to the combined effect of the smaller volume of distribution (decreased tissue binding) and the lower systemic clearance of digoxin caused by decreased renal function.

Renal clearance

The renal clearance of a drug represents the net effect of glomerular filtration and the renal tubular processes that may be involved in the renal handling of the drug:

$$Cl_R = (Cl_{RF} + Cl_{RS})(1 - f_{RA})$$

where Cl_{RF} is renal filtration clearance, Cl_{RS} is renal secretion clearance and f_{RA} is the fraction of drug that is reabsorbed from the renal tubules (distal nephron). Renal blood flow can influence all of these processes, but changes in renal blood flow are likely to have a more pronounced effect on the tubular processes (secretion and reabsorption) than on glomerular filtration. Factors that influence glomerular filtration are the extent of drug binding to plasma proteins, the integrity of the glomerular membrane (disrupted in the nephrotic syndrome), the number of functioning nephrons and renal blood flow. As only the unbound (free) drug in the systemic circulation can pass through the glomerular capillary pores, extensive binding to plasma proteins limits the availability of a drug for glomerular filtration and thereby influences the renal filtration clearance:

$$Cl_{RF} = f_u \cdot GFR$$

where f_u is the unbound fraction of drug in the plasma and GFR is the glomerular filtration rate. While inulin clearance provides a more accurate measurement of GFR, endogenous creatinine clearance satisfactorily estimates GFR in dogs. The procedure entails the measurement of creatinine concentrations in plasma (P_{Cr}) and in urine (U_{Cr}) collected over a fixed period of time, and measurement of the total volume of urine formed during the collection period (V, mL/min). The values obtained allow calculation of renal clearance (mL/min):

$$Cl_{Cr} = \frac{U_{Cr} \cdot V}{P_{Cr}}$$

For comparative purposes, GFR is expressed on a unit body weight basis (mL/min·kg). In dogs with decreased renal function (GFR < 3 mL/min·kg), the reciprocal of plasma creatinine concentration provides a clinically useful estimation of the glomerular filtration rate that could serve as a guide for dosage interval adjustment for drugs with a narrow margin of safety and are excreted by the kidney (e.g. aminoglycoside antibiotics, digoxin) (Finco *et al.*, 1995).

Halothane anaesthesia changes the disposition of gentamicin (4 mg/kg, i.v.) in horses (Smith *et al.*, 1988). The systemic clearance in particular and the volume of distribution of gentamicin are significantly decreased by halothane (Table 3.10). The longer half-life (4.03 ± 1.69 h in halothane-anaesthetized horses; 2.01 ± 0.35 h in the same six horses not anaesthetized) and higher plasma gentamicin concentrations at 8 h after administration of the drug could

Table 3.10 Pharmacokinetic parameters showing the influence of halothane anaesthesia on the disposition of gentamicin (4 mg/kg, i.v.) in horses. Results are expressed as mean $\pm$ SD; $n = 6$.

Pharmacokinetic parameter	Gentamicin	Gentamicin + halothane	Significance[a]
$V_{d \, (area)}$ (L/kg)	261 ± 24.4	248 ± 29.6	$P < 0.05$
Cl_B (mL/min·kg)	1.54 ± 0.27	0.81 ± 0.32	$P < 0.01$
$t_{1/2}$ (h)	2.01 ± 0.35	4.03 ± 1.69	$P < 0.05$
$C_{p \, (8h)}$ (µg/mL)	1.26 ± 0.84	4.75 ± 2.15	$P < 0.01$

[a] Student's *t*-test for paired data.

be mainly attributed to the decreased clearance of gentamicin caused by the effect of halothane on renal blood flow.

Renal tubular processes are influenced by renal blood flow and by the chemical nature and physicochemical properties (polarity, degree of ionization and lipid solubility) of the drug or drug metabolite. Plasma protein binding does not directly influence tubular secretion, presumably due to rapid dissociation of the drug–protein complex. It follows that tubular secretion is generally a function of *total* plasma drug concentration. Active, carrier-mediated secretion of organic acids and bases into the tubular lumen takes place in the proximal renal tubule. There are separate transport systems for organic acids (anions) and organic bases (cations) (Table 1.9). Drugs of a similar chemical nature (anions or cations) have the potential to compete for the transport carrier that mediates tubular secretion. Probenecid is perhaps the best known substance which competes with organic acids for tubular secretion. The concomitant use of probenecid and penicillin G prolongs the duration of effective plasma concentrations of penicillin by markedly decreasing the rate of penicillin elimination. A similar degree of effect (increased half-life due to lower renal clearance of penicillin) may be produced by phenylbutazone. The concomitant use of organic anions and methotrexate has serious clinical implications (Aherne *et al.*, 1978). Much less is known about the competition between organic cations for renal tubular secretion. The concomitant use of cimetidine and procainamide significantly increases the area under the plasma concentration–time curve for procainamide and the average plasma concentration of N-acetylprocainamide (active metabolite). Both increases are quantitatively consistent with the measured decreases in renal clearance of the parent drug and active metabolite (Somogyi *et al.*, 1983). To avoid adverse effects, it may be necessary to reduce the dose of procainamide when the dysrhythmic drug is used concomitantly with cimetidine.

While a drug may enter tubular fluid both by glomerular filtration and proximal tubular secretion, its renal clearance may also be influenced by reabsorption from the distal nephron (which refers to the distal convoluted tubule and collecting tubule). As tubular reabsorption takes place by passive diffusion, it is influenced by lipid solubility and concentration of the drug in distal tubular fluid, and by the pK_a/pH determined degree of ionization of weak organic acids and bases. The reabsorption of weak organic acids and bases is confined to the non-ionized, lipid-soluble form of these drugs. Because of the highly efficient reabsorption of water from the glomerular filtrate in the proximal tubule, a high concentration gradient generally exists between drug in distal tubular fluid and in plasma water (i.e. unbound in the blood). It is, however, influenced by urine flow rate (i.e. the rate of formation of urine). Urinary pH reflects the pH of distal tubular fluid and is mainly determined by the composition of the diet. It is generally acidic (pH 5.5–7.0) in carnivorous species, alkaline (pH 7.2–8.4) in herbivorous species and varies over a wide range (pH 4.5–8.0) in omnivorous species, including human beings. Neonatal animals of all species excrete acidic urine. In monogastric species and preruminant animals, urinary pH can be intentionally changed by orally administering a urinary acidifying agent (e.g. ammonium chloride, hexamine and sodium acid phosphate, ascorbic acid) or an alkalinizing agent (sodium bicarbonate). Alteration of urinary pH, which can be clinically useful in the management of drug intoxication, may affect the excretion rate of weak organic acids (pK_a 3.5–7.2) and bases (pK_a 7.6–10). The urine pH-excretion rate dependency is considerable only when a significant fraction (> 20%) of the dose is normally excreted unchanged in the urine and the non-ionized moiety in distal tubular fluid is lipid-soluble. Because of their high degree of ionization in distal tubular fluid and low solubility in lipid, changing urinary pH does not affect the rate of elimination of penicillins (Sarasola *et al.*, 1992). For drugs that are eliminated both by hepatic biotransformation and renal excretion, the fraction of dose excreted unchanged in the urine can vary widely between species; it is generally lower in the herbivorous species due to more rapid biotransformation of lipid-soluble drugs in herbivorous than in carnivorous species and human beings. The fraction of trimethoprim (organic base, pK_a 7.3) excreted unchanged in urine is less than 5% in cattle and goats, 10% in horses, 20% in dogs and $69 \pm 17\%$ in human beings. Urinary acidification promotes the reabsorption from distal tubular fluid of weak organic acids and enhances the renal excretion of weak organic bases. The urinary pH affects the contribution of renal clearance to the systemic (body) clearance of amphetamine (organic base, pK_a 9.8) and the half-life of the drug. At a urinary pH of 6.5, approximately 35% of the dose of amphetamine is eliminated by renal excretion in humans, dogs and cats, and the half-life is 15 h in humans, 4.5 h in dogs and 6.5 h in cats. By changing the urinary pH from 6.5 to 5.5 in humans the half-life decreases to 8 h. As less than 5% of the dose is eliminated by renal excretion in horses, changes in urinary pH do not affect the half-life of amphetamine (1.4 h) in horses (Baggot *et al.*, 1972). Alkalinization of the urine, by favouring ionization of organic acids (salicylate, pK_a 3.5; sulphadiazine, pK_a 6.4; phenobarbitone, pK_a 7.2) in distal tubular fluid, may increase their elimination depending on the fraction of dose that is excreted by the kidney. Because tubular reabsorption is also influenced by urine flow, the induction of alkaline diuresis (mannitol in conjunction with an alkalinizing agent) will further increase the rate of excretion of weak organic acids.

A renal clearance value greater than the GFR indicates that the drug is actively secreted, but a value less than the GFR does not preclude active secretion because tubular reabsorption takes place in the distal nephron. Competitive inhibition provides the only conclusive evidence that a transport process is carrier-mediated; for example, probenecid decreases proximal tubular secretion of penicillin G.

Drug interactions

In this section, mention will be made only of pharmacokinetic-based drug interactions arising from the co-administration or concomitant use of two drugs, one of which alters the absorption or changes the disposition of the other. Although the mechanism of the interaction may be known, it is difficult to predict the degree to which the effect produced by the affected drug will be altered, particularly in the presence of a disease state. Whenever a drug interaction is suspected, a pharmacokinetic mechanism must be excluded before speculating that the interaction has a pharmacodynamic basis.

Drug interactions which affect absorption from the gastrointestinal tract may alter either the rate or the extent of absorption and only some are of clinical importance. By promoting gastric emptying, metoclopramide may increase the rate of absorption of orally administered non-steroidal anti-inflammatory drugs in monogastric species. In contrast, opioids and antichlolinergic drugs, by decreasing gastrointestinal motility, can decrease the rate of drug absorption. However, the absorption of poorly water-soluble drugs can be increased by allowing more time for dissolution to occur. Chelation with divalent cations (Ca^{2+}, Mg^{2+}, Fe^{2+}) or with Al^{3+}, especially in milk and antacids, decreases the extent of absorption of tetracyclines. By adsorbing a wide variety of drugs (e.g. paracetamol, aspirin, phenobarbitone, theophylline) and poisonous substances, activated charcoal prevents their absorption from the gastrointestinal tract. Cholestyramine resin, which should be given in the feed or water, interrupts the enterohepatic circulation of drugs (such as digitoxin) by binding (adsorbing) them in the lumen of the intestine; it also binds bile acids and endotoxins. The addition of adrenaline (epinephrine) hydrochloride, to give a concentration of $10\,\mu g/mL$ (1:100 000) in the final solution, to a local anaesthetic (such as lignocaine) prolongs the duration of field (infiltration nerve) block by delaying the absorption (α-adrenoceptor mediated local vasoconstriction) of the local anaesthetic. Procaine penicillin G, which should only be administered by intramuscular injection (preferably in the neck of horses), extends the dosage interval for the penicillin to 12 or 24 h.

Plasma protein (albumin)-binding displacement is the most common type of interaction which mostly affects the disposition of acidic drugs. Displacement causes an increase in the concentration of free drug (unbound fraction) in the plasma, but is clinically significant only for drugs that are very extensively bound (>92%) to plasma albumin and have a small volume of distribution (<0.3 L/kg). Drugs which meet these criteria include naproxen, ketoprofen, phenylbutazone, oxyphenbutazone, furosemide, valproic acid, phenytoin and warfarin. When a drug is displaced from its plasma protein-binding sites by a single dose of the displacer (more avidly bound drug), the increase in the unbound fraction is transient and the enhanced pharmacological effect is short-lived. When, however, the displacer and the displaced drug are given concurrently on a multiple-dose regimen, the influence of displacement on the unbound (free) drug concentration at steady-state will depend on the extraction ratio of the drug. For a drug with a low extraction ratio ($E_H < 0.3$), the systemic clearance is influenced by the unbound fraction. Displacement causes an increase in the unbound fraction which, in turn, increases the rate of elimination (i.e. the half-life decreases) and the total plasma concentration falls.

When a new steady-state is achieved, the concentration of free drug in plasma is at the original value, but the total plasma concentration of the drug is lower. The pharmacological response is unaffected. This scenario applies to the displacement of warfarin by phenylbutazone and of phenytoin by a displacing drug (e.g. valproic acid should these anticonvulsants be administered concurrently). As the therapeutic range relates to total drug concentrations in plasma, it should be noted with regard to phenytoin that the displacement interaction lowers the range of therapeutic plasma concentrations. For a drug with a high extraction ratio, neither the systemic clearance nor the total plasma concentration at steady-state are affected by the increased unbound fraction of the drug. Consequently a greater pharmacological response may be produced by the displaced drug, which may require a reduction in the maintenance dosage.

The displacement of digoxin from tissue binding sites (apart from those of the heart) by quinidine causes a marked decrease in the volume of distribution that could lead to an increase in plasma digoxin concentration. Because, in addition to displacement, the renal clearance of digoxin is decreased in humans (Hager *et al.*, 1979; Doering *et al.*, 1982) and horses but apparently not in dogs (Gibson & Nelson, 1980), plasma digoxin concentrations will probably be increased to a greater degree in humans and horses than in dogs.

Enhancement (induction) or inhibition of drug biotransformation mainly applies to hepatic microsomal oxidative reactions. An enhanced drug-metabolizing capacity is due to an increase in the amount of smooth-surfaced endoplasmic reticulum in hepatocytes and the content of cytochrome P450 and cytochrome *c* reductase, rather than increased microsomal activity *per se* (Conney & Burns, 1972). A wide variety of drugs (e.g. phenobarbitone, phenytoin, phenylbutazone, rifampin, methimazole), the chlorinated hydrocarbon insecticides (such as dichlorodiphenyl-trichloroethane (DDT), dieldrin) and environmental pollutants (notably the polychlorinated biphenyls (PCBs)) are capable of inducing hepatic microsomal enzymes. A high degree of lipid solubility is the only physicochemical property that these structurally unrelated compounds have in common. The effect of enhanced biotransformation on the pharmacokinetic properties of an extensively metabolized drug varies with the hepatic extraction ratio of the drug. For drugs with a low extraction ratio, the clearance increases and half-life decreases, but oral bioavailability generally remains unchanged. Induction with phenobarbitone or phenytoin decreases the half-life of quinidine, while rifampin induction lowers the average steady-state concentration of quinidine in plasma. Induction with phenobarbitone or rifampin decreases the half-life of digitoxin. Phenobarbitone and rifampin increase hepatic microsomal oxidative activity within 48–72 h. Cytochrome P450 isoenzymes show different substrate specificities and may be separately inducible. For example, cytochrome P450 2BI is induced by chronic (1–2 weeks) administration of phenobarbitone (i.e. the administration of multiple doses of phenobarbitone at a constant dosage interval for 1–2 weeks), whereas cytochrome P450 IAI is induced by polycyclic aromatic hydrocarbons.

Induction increases the rate of biotransformation of drugs that have a low extraction ratio and, consequently, decreases their duration of action except when an active metabolite is formed. The clearance and half-life of a drug with a high extraction ratio remain essentially unchanged, while oral bioavailability is reduced.

Inhibition of drug-metabolizing enzymes prolongs the duration of action of drugs that undergo biotransformation by the inhibited metabolic pathways. Clearance of the affected drug is decreased, half-life is increased and oral bioavailability may be increased. Resulting from the changes in pharmacokinetic parameters, the average steady-state plasma concentration may be increased. Various drugs (e.g. chloramphenicol, cimetidine, phenylbutazone) cause a general inhibition of the hepatic microsomal oxidative pathways. Drugs that may be affected by inhibition of microsomal oxidation include phenytoin, carbamazepine, diazepam, lignocaine, propranolol, theophylline and antipyrine, the marker substance for microsomal oxidation. Norfloxacin, enrofloxacin and ciprofloxacin significantly decrease the systemic clearance of theophylline, due to selective inhibition of cytochrome P450 isoenzymes partially responsible for the metabolism of theophylline (Prince *et al.*, 1989; Intorre *et al.*, 1995). The administration of enrofloxacin (5 mg/kg, i.v. once a day) during maintenance dosage with an oral sustained-release theophylline formulation (20 mg/kg at 12-h intervals) progressively and significantly increased the mean trough concentrations of theophylline in plasma of Beagle dogs. The pharmacokinetic-based interaction indicates that plasma theophylline concentrations should be monitored and used as the basis for adjustment of theophylline dosage.

A flavin-containing mono-oxygenase (FMO) could be responsible for the reversible oxidation of albendazole to the anthelmintically active sulphoxide metabolite (Galtier *et al.*, 1986), while the cytochrome P450 mono-oxygenase system is thought to be involved in the slower, irreversible conversion of albendazole sulphoxide to the inactive sulphone (Souhaili El Amri *et al.*, 1988). The co-administration of netobimin (oral zwitterion suspension) and methimazole, either orally or by intramuscular injection, to sheep significantly increased the amount of albendazole sulphoxide formed during first-pass metabolism and decreased the rate of its elimination by delaying microsomal oxidative conversion to albendazole sulphone (Lanusse *et al.*, 1992). The clinical implication of the drug interaction is that the changed plasma concentration profile for albendazole sulphoxide may enhance the efficacy of netobimin.

Certain drugs inhibit non-microsomal metabolic pathways. Metronidazole, like disulfiram, inhibits aldehyde dehydrogenase, the enzyme that normally oxidizes acetaldehyde to acetic acid in the metabolic pathway for ethanol. Allopurinol inhibits xanthine oxidase, the enzyme that catalyses the oxidation of hypoxanthine to xanthine and xanthine to uric acid. Because azathioprine and 6-mercaptopurine are metabolized by xanthine oxidase, the dosage of these drugs (synthetic xanthine analogues), when used concomitantly with allopurinol, should be reduced to avoid toxicity. The use of allopurinol may be indicated in Dalmatian dogs with the objective of reducing the excessive amount of uric acid excreted by the kidney and formation of the sparingly soluble ammonium urate. As organophosphorus compounds 'irreversibly' inhibit plasma pseudocholinesterase, the metabolism of drugs that are hydrolysed by this enzyme (e.g. succinylcholine) would be considerably reduced.

Drugs or disease states that reduce cardiac output decrease liver blood flow and may change the hepatic clearance of drugs with a high extraction ratio ($E_H > 0.6$). Propranolol decreases its own clearance (Nies *et al.*, 1973) as well as the clearance of lignocaine (Ochs *et al.*, 1980). The decreased clearance of propranolol co-administered with cimetidine has a dual basis, in that liver blood flow is reduced by propranolol and hepatic microsomal oxidation of propranolol is inhibited by cimetidine (Feely *et al.*, 1981). Liver blood flow varies between species, but is directly proportional to the weight (mass) of the liver and is approximately equal to 1.5 L/min per kilogram liver weight (Boxenbaum, 1980). The weight of the liver, expressed as a percentage of live body weight, is 1.3 in horses, 2.3 in dogs and 2.6 in humans. Average values generally quoted for liver blood flow (mL/min per kilogram body weight) are 24 in humans, 25 in horses and 42 in dogs.

Because drug combinations are commonly used for pre-anaesthetic medication and general anaesthesia, the potential exists for drug interactions to occur. In xylazine pre-medicated female ruminant calves, the duration of ketamine anaesthesia is significantly prolonged (Table 3.11) (Waterman, 1984). This effect is associated with significant decreases in both the volume of distribution and the systemic clearance of ketamine, while the half-life is not significantly changed but varies more widely between individual calves when the two drugs are used. The lower clearance of ketamine, a highly extracted drug, in the xylazine pre-medicated calves could be due to reduced

Table 3.11 Pharmacokinetic parameters showing the influence of xylazine premedication (0.2 mg/kg, i.m.) on the disposition of ketamine (5 mg/kg, i.v.) and the duration of anaesthesia in female ruminant calves. Results are expressed as mean $\pm$ SEM; $n = 4$.

Pharmacokinetic parameter	Ketamine	Xylazine + ketamine	Significance[a]
$V_{d\ (area)}$ (L/kg)	4.04 $\pm$ 0.66	1.41 $\pm$ 0.32	$P < 0.01$
Cl_B (mL/min·kg)	40.39 $\pm$ 6.6	21.25 $\pm$ 5.4	$P < 0.05$
$t_{1/2}$ (min)	60.5 $\pm$ 5.4	54.2 $\pm$ 11.4	NS
Duration of anaesthesia	9.8 $\pm$ 1.7	22.3 $\pm$ 2.5	$P < 0.01$
range (min)	6–14	17–26	

[a] Student's *t*-test unpaired data.

liver blood flow resulting from the decrease in cardiac output caused by xylazine.

Probenecid competes with organic acids (anions) for carrier-mediated proximal tubular secretion and decreases the elimination rate of acidic drugs that are substantially excreted by this active process (e.g. penicillin, methotrexate). Although phenylbutazone undergoes proximal tubular secretion and delays the elimination of penicillin G, it is mainly eliminated by hepatic biotransformation in horses and dogs. The co-administration of probenecid (50 mg/kg as an aqueous suspension via nasogastric tube at 12-h intervals) and phenylbutazone (4 mg/kg, i.v.) to horses significantly decreased the steady-state volume of distribution of phenylbutazone, and the plasma phenylbutazone concentration at 12 h post-administration was significantly increased (Zertuche *et al.*, 1992). The mean systemic clearance was decreased, although not significantly, and the half-life remained unchanged.

The concurrent use of an organic anion and methotrexate enhances the toxicity of methotrexate. The toxicity of gentamicin (excreted by glomerular filtration) is enhanced by the presence of dehydration or the concurrent use of furosemide.

Interspecies scaling

The drug disposition-related pharmacokinetic parameters (half-life, clearance, volume of distribution) may be used for interspecies scaling, which is based on the mathematical relationship that exists between the selected parameter and the body weight of various animal species. The relationship between a pharmacokinetic parameter, like that between the weight of an organ (e.g. the liver) or a physiological variable (e.g. cardiac output, liver blood flow, glomerular filtration rate), and species body weight is described by the allometric equation (Adolph, 1949):

$$Y = aW^b$$

where Y, the dependent variable, is the pharmacokinetic parameter (organ weight or physiological variable) of interest; W, the independent variable, is the average body weight of the animal species; and a and b are the allometric coefficient and exponent, respectively. The value of the exponent b, which denotes the fractional power to which the independent variable W is raised, has special significance. For most physiological processes and for physiologically-based pharmacokinetic parameters (clearance, volume of distribution), the value of b generally lies between 0.67 and unity. The empirical allometric exponent used for interspecies scaling of body surface area (m^2) in relation to body weight (kg) of eutherian mammalian species is 0.75 (Calder, 1984). For physiological periods (such as cardiac circulation (which refers to mean residence time of blood in the vascular system), heartbeat duration and length of respiratory cycle) and for drug half-lives, the value of b is generally close to

0.25, which represents that for energy expenditure in mammalian species (Kleiber, 1975) and the turnover time of endogenous processes (Boxenbaum, 1982). In theory, mammals have four heartbeats during each respiratory cycle as the value of the exponent *b* is the same, while that of the allometric coefficient *a* differs by a factor of four.

Logarithmic transformation of the heterogonic equation yields:

$$\log Y = \log a + b \log W$$

where *a* is the Y-intercept and *b* is the slope of the straight line on the double logarithmic plot. The values of both *a* and *b* vary with the drug. Interspecies scaling should be performed only on a precisely measured dependent variable determined in at least four animal species representing a wide range of body weight, expressed as log body weight ratio. The procedure entails linear regression analysis of the logarithmically transformed variables, which provides values of the allometric coefficient and exponent, and the construction of a double logarithmic plot to verify the linearity of the relationship and identify any non-conforming (outlying) species for possible subsequent exclusion from the scaling procedure. Whether interspecies scaling can feasibly be applied depends on both the elimination process for the drug and the precision of measurement of the selected pharmacokinetic parameter. Non-conformity by a species may be genuine in that it reflects a peculiar feature of the distribution, or more often biotransformation, of the drug that is unique to the animal species, or be an artifact attributable to imprecise measurement of the parameter under consideration.

Interspecies scaling of drug elimination, using half-life or systemic clearance, would be expected to have greatest application to drugs that are eliminated by a single process, in particular glomerular filtration. Although renal blood flow is 22–24% of cardiac output in mammalian species, the excretion of a drug by glomerular filtration is influenced by extensive binding to plasma proteins. The allometric equations relating GFR (mL/min), based on inulin clearance, and systemic clearance (mL/min) of gentamicin to the body weight (kg) of domestic animal species and human beings are:

$$\text{GFR} = 4.13W^{0.86}$$

$$r = 0.989\,(P < 0.001)$$

$$\text{Gentamicin clearance} = 2.60W^{0.86}$$

$$r = 0.970\,(P < 0.001)$$

The quotient of these allometric equations shows that gentamicin clearance is approximately 63% of GFR. As gentamicin binds to a negligible extent (<10%) to plasma proteins, the relatively lower value of gentamicin clearance is suggestive of renal tubular reabsorption which is independent of urinary pH and could be partly attributed to selective kidney tissue binding. The GFR (mL/min) in avian species is $0.4(\text{body weight})^{0.06}$ times that of mammalian species; the mammal:bird ratio of inulin clearance is $2.5\,(\text{body weight})^{-0.06}$

(Calder, 1981). Average values of GFR (mL/min·kg) in normally hydrated ostriches (0.77), chickens (1.23) and turkeys (1.32) are below the range of values in domestic animal species (horse 1.65–dog 3.96), which could be a reflection of the lower filtration efficiency of the reptilian-type nephrons in birds. The clearance (mL/min·kg) of gentamicin in chickens (0.78) and turkeys (0.83) is below the range of gentamicin clearance in domestic animals (horses 1.20–dogs 3.10). The glomerular filtration rate (estimated from inulin and creatinine clearance values combined) in reptiles is lower than in mammals or birds (Edwards, 1975).

The bispyridinium oxime HI-6, which is a powerful reactivator of 'unaged' organophosphate-inhibited acetylcholinesterase, is eliminated by renal excretion. The allometric equations expressing the relationship between pharmacokinetic parameters describing the elimination of HI-6 and body weight of various mammalian species (mouse, rat, rabbit, Rhesus monkey, Beagle dog, sheep and man) are:

Systemic clearance (mL/min). $= 9.80^{0.76}$

$r = 0.986 \, (P < 0.001)$

Half-life(min) $= 23.3 \, W^{0.25}$

$r = 0.926 \, (P < 0.01)$

The log body weight ratio was 3.4.

Double logarithmic plots of the pharmacokinetic parameters vs. body weight show the linearity of the relationship (Fig. 3.4) (Baggot, 1994). The data indicate that allometric scaling of the species studied is feasible and that the use of systemic clearance is preferable to half-life. Data obtained in the same five species (mouse, rat, monkey, dog and human) on methotrexate (Dedrick *et al.*, 1970) and ceftizoxime (Mordenti, 1985), both of which are eliminated by renal excretion (glomerular filtration and tubular secretion), show a strong allometric correlation between systemic clearance of the drugs and body weight of the five species.

Because of the availability in research papers of half-life values for drugs and the composite (hybrid) nature of half-life, this parameter is generally used for interspecies allometric scaling of drug elimination. In a detailed survey of the feasibility of using half-life for interspecies scaling, Riviere *et al.* (1997) showed that a strong allometric correlation exists between half-life and species body weight for 11 of the 44 drugs analysed. The majority of the 11 drugs (ampicillin, carbenicillin, cephapirin, gentamicin, apramycin, tetracycline, oxytetracycline, chlortetracycline, erythromycin, prednisolone and diazepam) to which interspecies allometric scaling using half-life can satisfactorily be applied are antibiotics that are eliminated by renal excretion, although the tetracyclines included undergo enterohepatic circulation and erythromycin is eliminated by the liver in bile. It is likely that the composite nature of half-life allows diazepam to be included in this list of drugs. The average value ($\pm$ SD) of the allometric exponent (*b*) for these 11 drugs was 0.236 ± 0.09, which is close to

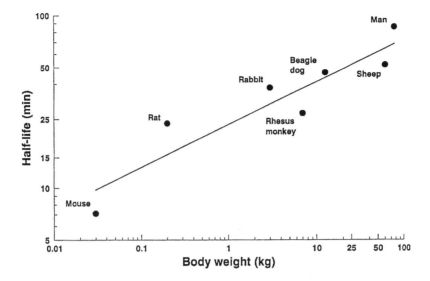

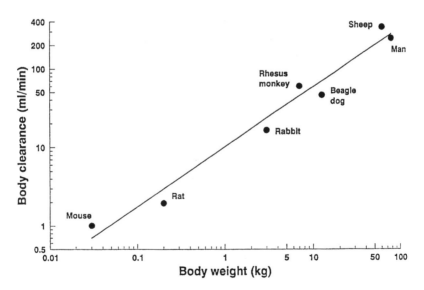

Fig. 3.4 Double logarithmic plots showing the allometric relationship between (a) half-life and (b) body (systemic) clearance of HI-6 and body weight of seven animal species. (Reproduced with permission from Baggot (1994).)

0.25, for the coefficient of determination (r^2) was 0.87 ± 0.09, and for the log body weight ratio was 8.1 ± 2.1. The average number of species, representing a wide range of body weight, per study was 6.2 ± 2.2 (Riviere *et al.*, 1997).

Interspecies scaling of drug elimination based on half-life would be expected to have least application to poorly extracted drugs that are eliminated by a variety of processes which are influenced by plasma protein binding, capacity of metabolic pathways or pK_a/pH-influenced renal tubular reabsorption. The use of systemic clearance or eliminating organ clearance, rather than half-life greatly increases the feasibility of interspecies scaling of some poorly extracted drugs. Cefodizime was studied in five species (mouse, rat, rabbit, monkey and dog) and shows species variation in plasma protein binding and in excretion (renal and biliary). The pharmacokinetic parameter that strongly correlates with body weight is renal clearance of unbound drug (Matsushita *et al.*, 1990). Systemic clearance of antimicrobial agents eliminated by various processes, gentamicin (glomerular filtration), ampicillin (glomerular filtration and tubular secretion), oxytetracycline (glomerular filtration, but undergoes enterohepatic circulation), and enrofloxacin (converted to ciprofloxacin by *N*-deethylation, a microsomal oxidative reaction), shows a high degree of correlation with body weight of several animal species (Table 3.12). Theophylline and antipyrine are poorly extracted drugs that are eliminated by phase I hepatic biotransformation reactions and show weak allometric correlations between half-life and body weight of mammalian species. Based on data obtained in nine species (rat, guinea pig, rabbit, cat, dog, pig, human, cattle and horse), log body weight ratio

Table 3.12 Allometric relationship[a] between clearance (mL/min) of some drugs and body weight (kg) of various mammalian species.

Drug	Elimination process[b]	No. of species	Allometric Coefficient	Allometric Exponent	Correlation coefficient
Gentamicin	E(r)	8[c]	2.60	0.86	0.970
Ampicillin	E(r)	8[d]	5.47	0.94	0.959
Oxytetracycline	E(r)	8[e]	7.96	0.73	0.978
Enrofloxacin	M(h)	8[f]	12.53	0.93	0.984
Theophylline	M(h)	9[g]	1.98	0.83	0.978
Antipyrine	M(h)	10[h]	8.16	0.85	0.989

[a] For each drug the level of significance is $P < 0.001$.
[b] E(r) is excretion (renal); M(h) is metabolism (hepatic).
[c] Cat, dog, goat, sheep, pig, human, cattle, horse
[d] Rabbit, dog, sheep, pig, human, donkey, cattle horse
[e] Rabbit, dog, goat, sheep, pig, donkey, cattle, horse
[f]   Rabbit, cat, dog, sheep, pig, llama, horse, cow
[g] Rat, guinea pig, rabbit, cat, dog, pig, human, cattle, horse
[h] Mouse, rat, guinea pig, rabbit, monkey, dog, goat, sheep, pig, cattle (human is a non-conforming species).

of 3.2, a high degree of correlation was found between systemic clearance of theophylline and body weight of the animal species. Antipyrine binds to a low extent to plasma proteins, distributes in total body water and is eliminated by hepatic microsomal oxidation. Based on data obtained in 11 species (mouse, rat, guinea pig, rabbit, monkey, dog, goat, sheep, pig, human and cattle), log body weight ratio of 5.2, there is a strong allometric correlation between volume of distribution and body weight and, when the human (non-conforming species) is excluded, between hepatic intrinsic clearance (unbound drug) and body weight (Boxenbaum, 1980). The explanation offered by Boxenbaum (1982) for the observation that the hepatic intrinsic clearance of antipyrine in humans is approximately one-seventh of that which would be predicted from the other mammalian species is that oxidative drug-metabolizing capacity is relative to the longevity (maximum life-span potential) of the species. When correction was made for maximum life-span potential, the human could be included with the ten other species in the allometric relationship between unbound antipyrine

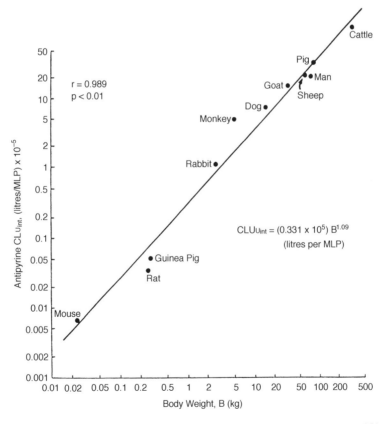

Fig. 3.5 Allometric relationship between unbound antipyrine intrinsic clearance ($Cl_{u(int)}$) per maximum life-span potential (MLP) and body weight. Note that the body weight exponent of the regression equation is close to unity. Units on the ordinate (litres per MLP) are equivalent to $Cl_{u(int)}$ (L/min) $\times$ MLP (min). (Reproduced with permission from Boxenbaum (1982).)

intrinsic clearance per maximum life-span potential and body weight (Fig. 3.5) (Boxenbaum, 1982, 1983). Based on an equation involving brain weight and body weight (Sacher, 1959), maximum life-span potential is much longer in human beings (93 years) than in horses (39 years), dogs (20 years), cats (14 years) and particularly laboratory animal species (Table 3.13). Maximum life-span potential under free-range conditions in red kangaroos, leopards, lions

Table 3.13   Body weight, brain weight and the calculated maximum life-span potential (MLP) for various mammalian species.

Species	Body weight (g)	Brain weight (g)	MLP (years)
Laboratory animals			
Mouse	23	0.33	2.67
Rat	250	1.88	4.68
Guinea pig	1040	5.50	6.73
Rabbit	2550	9.97	8.01
Domestic animals			
Cat	3300	26.0	13.9
Dog	14200	75.4	19.7
Pig	77200	58.2	11.35
Sheep	57000	110	18.3
Goat	39000	113	20.4
Cattle	310000	252	21.2
Donkey	175000	385	31.6
Horse	308000	647	38.7
Primate species			
Rhesus monkey	6710	85	25.2
Baboon	21800	193	32.5
Gorilla	120000	406	35.6
Chimpanzee	45000	360	41.1
Human	70000	1530	93.4
Other species			
Fox	4500	52.0	20.1
Leopard	48000	135	21.7
Lion	150720	241	24.3
Tiger	209000	302	26.0
Llama	70000	215	26.8
Red deer	125530	411	35.5
Eland	560000	480	28.0
Red kangaroo	36000	68	15.0
Giraffe	529000	680	35.4
Camel (Arabian)	400000	760	40.4
Elephant (African)	6 654000	5712	77.4

and African elephants is estimated to be 15 years, 22 years, 24 years and 77 years, respectively.

Because the clearance of highly extracted drugs mainly depends on a single physiological variable (blood flow to the eliminating organ, which is linearly proportional to species body weight to the power of 0.75), the use of clearance as the pharmacokinetic parameter should make interspecies scaling feasible for these drugs. It could be stated that the smaller the number of physiological variables affecting the elimination of a drug, the higher will be the predictive value of interspecies allometric scaling. When hepatic biotransformation is the principal process of elimination, the likelihood of there being a non-conforming species is greatly increased.

The use of half-life incorporates the variables that can influence the rate of drug elimination, those that affect distribution and clearance, whereas the use of systemic clearance focuses on the process of elimination, and corrections can be made for the extent of binding to plasma proteins and for estimated maximum life-span potential. Corrections seem to be justifiable when the human is included in the interspecies scaling technique. The necessity to apply correction factors, however, detracts from the use of allometric scaling for predicting the values of pharmacokinetic parameters.

Interspecies scaling can be applied to the volume of distribution of drugs. The value of the exponent b, like for clearance, is in the range 0.67–1. It would seem preferable to use the volume of distribution at steady-state ($V_{d(ss)}$), which is independent of the rate of drug elimination, rather than $V_{d(area)}$. A large volume of distribution with tissue binding involvement (e.g. digoxin) could interfere with the application of interspecies scaling. In ruminant species, ionic trapping of lipid-soluble organic bases in ruminal fluid (pH 5.5–6.5) could lead to substantially larger volumes of distribution in these animals than in monogastric species. It follows that the elimination process for most drugs and the distribution pattern for some have a significant influence on their suitability for interspecies allometric scaling. The predictive value of allometric scaling is limited by the uncertainty as to which species might be non-conforming. Assuming knowledge of the principal process of elimination of a drug and with the judicious selection of animal species, the allometric technique of interspecies scaling could be most usefully applied during the pre-clinical phase of drug development.

References

Abdullah, A.S. & Baggot, J.D. (1986a) Influence of induced disease states on the disposition kinetics of imidocarb in goats. *Journal of Veterinary Pharmacology and Therapeutics*, **9**, 192–197.

Abdullah, A.S. & Baggot, J.D. (1986b) Effect of short term starvation on disposition kinetics of chloramphenicol in goats. *Research in Veterinary Science*, **40**, 382–385.

Adolph, E.F. (1949) Quantitative relations in the physiological constitutions of mammals. *Science*, **109**, 579–585.

Aherne, G.W., Piall, E., Marks, V. *et al.* (1978) Prolongation and enhancement of serum methotrexate concentrations by probenecid. *British Medical Journal*, **1**, 1097–1099.

Anika, S.M., Nouws, J.F.M., van Gogh, H. *et al.* (1986) Chemotherapy and pharmacokinetics of some antimicrobial agents in healthy dwarf goats and those infected with *Ehrlichia phagocytophila* (tick-borne fever). *Research in Veterinary Science*, **41**, 386–390.

Bachmann, K.A. & Burkman, A.M. (1975) Phenylbutazone–warfarin interaction in the dog. *Journal of Pharmacy and Pharmacology*, **27**, 832–836.

Baggot, J.D. (1980) Distribution of antimicrobial agents in normal and diseased animals. *Journal of the American Veterinary Medical Association*, **176**, 1085–1090.

Baggot, J.D. (1994) Application of interspecies scaling to the bispyridinium oxime HI-6. *American Journal of Veterinary Research*, **55**, 689–691.

Baggot, J.D., Davis, L.E., Murdick, P.W. *et al.* (1972) Certain aspects of amphetamine elimination in the horse. *American Journal of Veterinary Research*, **33**, 1161–1164.

Belpaire, F.M., De Rick, A., Dello, C. *et al.* (1987) Alpha$_1$-acid glycoprotein and serum binding of drugs in healthy and diseased dogs. *Journal of Veterinary Pharmacology and Therapeutics*, **10**, 43–48.

Bianchetti, G., Graziani, G., Brancaccio, D. *et al.* (1978) Pharmacokinetics and effects of propranolol in terminal uraemic patients and in patients undergoing regular dialysis treatment. *Clinical Pharmacokinetics*, **1**, 373–384.

Blanshard, W.H. (1994) Medicine and husbandry of koalas. In: *Wildlife*, Proceedings (No. 233, pp. 547–623) of the Post-graduate Committee in Veterinary Science, University of Sydney.

Blaschke, T.F., Elin, R.J., Berk, P.D. *et al.* (1973) Effect of induced fever on sulfo-bromophthalein kinetics in man. *Annals of Internal Medicine*, **78**, 221–226.

Boothe, D.M., Brown, S.A., Jenkins, W.L. *et al.* (1992) Indocyanine green disposition in healthy dogs and dogs with mild, moderate, or severe dimethylnitrosamine-induced hepatic disease. *American Journal of Veterinary Research*, **53**, 382–388.

Boothe, D.M., Cullen, J.M., Calvin, J.A. *et al.* (1994) Antipyrine and caffeine dispositions in clinically normal dogs and dogs with progressive liver disease. *American Journal of Veterinary Research*, **55**, 254–261.

Boxenbaum, H. (1980) Interspecies variation in liver weight, hepatic blood flow, and antipyrine intrinsic clearance: extrapolation of data to benzodiazepines and phenytoin. *Journal of Pharmacokinetics and Biopharmaceutics*, **8**, 165–176.

Boxenbaum, H. (1982) Interspecies scaling, allometry, physiological time, and the ground plan of pharmacokinetics. *Journal of Pharmacokinetics and Biopharmaceutics*, **10**, 201–227.

Boxenbaum, H. (1983) Evolutionary biology, animal behavior, fourth-dimensional space, and the raison d'être of drug metabolism and pharmacokinetics. *Drug Metabolism Reviews*, **14**, 1057–1097.

Branch, R.A., Shand, D.G., Wilkinson, G.R. & Nies, A.S. (1973) The reduction of lidocaine clearance by *dl*-propranolol: an example of hemodynamic drug interaction. *Journal of Pharmacology and Experimental Therapeutics*, **184**, 515–519.

Branch, R.A., James, J.A. & Read, A.E. (1976) The clearance of antipyrine and indocyanine green in normal subjects and in patients with chronic liver disease. *Clinical Pharmacology and Therapeutics*, **20**, 81–89.

Calder III, W.A. (1981), Scaling of physiological processes in homeothermic animals. *Annual Review of Physiology*, **43**, 301–322.

Calder III, W.A. (1984) *Size, Function and Life History*. Harvard University Press, Cambridge, Mass.

Conney, A.H. & Burns, J.J. (1972) Metabolic interactions among enviromental chemicals and drugs. *Science*, **178**, 576–586.

Craig, W.A., Evenson, M.A. & Ramgopal, V. (1976) The effect of uremia, cardiopulmonary bypass and bacterial infection on serum protein binding. In: *The Effect of Disease States on Drug Pharmacokinetics*, (ed., L.Z. Benet) pp. 125–136. American Pharmaceutical Association, Academy of Pharmaceutical Sciences Washington DC.

Dedrick, R.L., Bischoff, K.B. & Zaharko, D.S. (1970) Interspecies correlation of plasma concentration history of methotrexate (NSC-740). *Cancer Chemotherapy Reports*, (Part 1), **54**, 95–101.

Doering, W., Fichth, B., Hermann, M. & Besenfelder, E. (1982) Quinidine-digoxin interaction: Evidence for involvement of an extrarenal mechanism. *European Journal of Clinical Pharmacology*, **21**, 281–285.

Dyke, T.M., Sams, R.A. & Hinchcliff, K.W. (1998) Antipyrine pharmacokinetics and urinary excretion in female horses. *American Journal of Veterinary Research*, **59**, 280–285.

Edwards, N.A. (1975) Scaling of renal functions in mammals. *Comparative Biochemistry and Physiology*, **52A**, 63–66.

Engelking, L.R., Anwer, M.S. & Lofstedt, J. (1985) Hepatobiliary transport of indocyanine green and sulfobromophthalein in fed and fasted horses. *American Journal of Veterinary Research*, **46**, 2278–2284.

Engelking, L.R., Blyden, G.T., Lofstedt, J. & Greenblatt, D.J. (1987) Pharmacokinetics of antipyrine, acetaminophen and lidocaine in fed and fasted horses. *Journal of Veterinary Pharmacology and Therapeutics*, **10**, 73–82.

Evans, G.H., Nies, A.S. & Shand, D.G. (1973) The disposition of propranolol III. Decreased half-life and volume of distribution as a result of plasma binding in man, monkey, dog and rat. *Journal of Pharmacology and Experimental Therapeutics*, **186**, 114–122.

Feely, J., Wilkinson, G.R. & Wood, A.J.J. (1981) Reduction of liver blood flow and propranolol metabolism by cimetidine. *New England Journal of Medicine*, **304**, 692–695.

Finco, D.R., Brown, S.A., Vaden, S.L. & Ferguson, D.C. (1995) Relationship between plasma creatinine concentration and glomerular filtration rate in dogs. *Journal of Veterinary Pharmacology and Therapeutics*, **18**, 418–421.

Galtier, P., Alviniere, M. & Delatour, P. (1986) *In vitro* sulfoxidation of albendazole by ovine liver microsomes: assay and frequency of various xenobiotics. *American Journal of Veterinary Research*, **47**, 447–450.

Gibson, T.P. & Nelson, H.A. (1980) Digoxin alters quinidine and quinidine alters digoxin pharmacokinetics in dogs. *Journal of Laboratory Clinical Medicine*, **95**, 417–428.

Gibson, T.P., Giacomini, K.M., Briggs, W.A. *et al.* (1980) Propoxyphene and norpropoxyphene plasma concentrations in the anephric patient. *Clinical Pharmacology and Therapeutics*, **27**, 665–670.

Gierke, K.D., Perrier, D., Mayersohn, M. & Marcus, F.I. (1978) Digoxin disposition kinetics in dogs before and during azotemia. *Journal of Pharmacology and Experimental Therapeutics*, **205**, 459–464.

van Gogh, H. & van Miert, A.S.J.P.A.M. (1977) The absorption of sulfonamides from the gastrointestinal tract during pyrogen-induced fever in kids and goats. *Zentrallblatt Veterinar Medizin, Reihe A*, **24**, 503–510.

Gronwall, R. (1975) Effects of fasting on hepatic function in ponies. *American Journal of Veterinary Research*, **36**, 145–148.

Gronwall, R. & Mia, A.S. (1972) Fasting hyperbilirubinemia in horses. *American Journal of Digestive Diseases*, **17**, 473–476.

Gronwall, R., Engelking, L.R. & Noonan, N. (1980) Direct measurement of biliary bilirubin excretion in ponies during fasting. *American Journal of Veterinary Research*, **41**, 125–126.

Groothuis, D.G., van Miert, A.S.J.P.A.M., Ziv, G. & Nouws, J.F.M. (1978) Effects of experimental *Escherichia coli* endotoxaemia on ampicillin: amoxycillin blood levels after oral and parenteral administration in calves. *Journal of Veterinary Pharmacology and Therapeutics*, **1**, 81–84.

Hager, W.D., Fenster, P., Mayersohn, M. *et al.*, (1979) Digoxin–quinidine interaction: pharmacokinetic evaluation. *New England Journal of Medicine*, **300**, 1238–1241.

Hauser, G. & Eichberg, J. (1973) Improved conditions for the preservation and extraction of polyphosphoinositides. *Biochimica et Biophysica Acta*, **326**, 201–209.

Hvidberg, E.F., Andreasen, P.B. & Ranek, L. (1974) Plasma half-life of phenylbutazone in patients with impaired liver function. *Clinical Pharmacology and Therapeutics*, **15**, 171–177.

Intorre, L., Mengozzi, G., Maccheroni, M. *et al.* (1995) Enrofloxacin–theophylline interaction: influence of enrofloxacin on theophylline steady-state pharmacokinetics in the Beagle dog. *Journal of Veterinary Pharmacology and Therapeutics*, **18**, 352–356.

Jusko, W.J., Lewis, G.P. & Schmitt, G.W. (1973) Ampicillin and hetacillin pharmacokinetics in normal and anephric subjects. *Clinical Pharmacology and Therapeutics*, **14**, 90–99.

Kleiber, M. (1975) Metabolic turnover rate: a physiological meaning of the metabolic rate per unit body weight. *Journal of Theoretical Biology*, **53**, 199–204.

Klotz, U. (1976) Pathophysiological and disease-induced changes in drug distribution volume: pharmacokinetic implications. *Clinical Pharmacokinetics*, **1**, 204–218.

Klotz, U., Antonin, K.-H. & Bieck, P.R. (1976) Pharmacokinetics and plasma binding of diazepam in man, dog, rabbit, guinea pig and rat. *Journal of Pharmacology and Experimental Therapeutics*, **199**, 67–73.

Kober, A., Sjoholm, I., Borga, O. & Odar-Cederlof, I. (1979) Protein binding of diazepam and digitoxin in uremic and normal sera. *Biochemical Pharmacology*, **28**, 1037–1042.

Kucera, J.L. & Bullock, F.J. (1969) The binding of salicylate to plasma protein from several animal species. *Journal of Pharmacy and Pharmacology*, **21**, 293–296.

Ladefoged, O. (1979) Pharmacokinetics of antipyrine and trimethoprim in pigs with endotoxin-induced fever. *Journal of Veterinary Pharmacology and Therapeutics*, **2**, 209–214.

Lanusse, C.E., Gascon, L. & Prichard, R.K. (1992) Methimazole-mediated modulation of netobimin biotransformation in sheep: a pharmacokinetic assessment. *Journal of Veterinary Pharmacology and Therapeutics*, **15**, 267–274.

Leek, B.F. & van Miert, A.S.J.P.A.M. (1971) An analysis of the pyrogen-induced inhibition of gastric motility in sheep. *Journal of Physiology*, **215**, 28–29P.

Loscher, W. (1978) Serum protein binding and pharmacokinetics of valproate in man, dog, rat and mouse. *Journal of Pharmacology and Experimental Therapeutics*, **204**, 255–261.

Matsushita, H., Suzuki, H., Sugiyama, Y. *et al.* (1990) Prediction of the pharmacokinetics of cefodizime and cefotetan in humans from pharmacokinetic parameters in animals. *Journal of Pharmacobio-Dynamics*, **13**, 602–611.

Mengelers, M.J.B., van Gogh, E.R., Kuiper, H.A. *et al.* (1995) Pharmacokinetics of sulfadimethoxine and sulfamethoxazole in combination with trimethoprim after intravenous administration to healthy and pneumonic pigs. *Journal of Veterinary Pharmacology and Therapeutics*, **18**, 243–253.

van Miert, A.S.J.P.A.M. (1971) Inhibition of gastric motility by endotoxin (bacterial lipopolysaccharide) in conscious goats and modification of this response by splanchnectomy, adrenalectomy or adrenergic blocking agents. *Archives Internationales de Pharmacodynamie et de Thérapie*, **193**, 405–414.

van Miert, A.S.J.P.A.M. (1995) Pro-inflammatory cytokines in a ruminant model: pathophysiological, pharmacological and therapeutic aspects. *Veterinary Quarterly*, **17**, 41–50.

Mordenti, J. (1985) Pharmacokinetic scale-up: accurate prediction of human pharmacokinetic profiles from animal data. *Journal of Pharmaceutical Sciences*, **74**, 1097–1099.

Nies, A.S., Evans, G.H. & Shand, D.G. (1973) Regional hemodynamic effects of beta-adrenergic blockade with propranolol in the unanesthetized primate. *American Heart Journal*, **85**, 97–102.

Ochs, H.R., Carstens, G. & Greenblatt, D.J. (1980) Reduction in lidocaine clearance during continuous infusion and by coadministration of propranolol. *New England Journal of Medicine*, **303**, 1101–1107.

Ohnhaus, E.E., Vozeh, S. & Nuesch, E. (1979) Absolute bioavailability of digoxin in chronic renal failure. *Clinical Nephrology*, **11**, 302–306.

Pacifici, G.M., Viani, A., Taddeuci-Brunelli, G. *et al.* (1986) Effects of development, ageing, and renal and hepatic insufficiency as well as hemodialysis on the plasma concentrations of albumin and α_1-acid glycoprotein: implication for binding of drugs. *Therapeutic Drug Monitoring*, **8**, 259–263.

Pennington, J.E., Dale, D.C., Reynolds, H.Y. & MacLowry, J.D. (1975) Gentamicin sulfate pharmacokinetics: lower levels of gentamicin in blood during fever. *Journal of Infectious Diseases*, **132**, 270–275.

Perez-Mateo, M. & Erill, S. (1977) Protein binding of salicylate and quinidine in plasma from patients with renal failure, chronic liver disease and chronic respiratory insufficiency. *European Journal of Clinical Pharmacology*, **11**, 225–231.

Piafsky, K.M. (1980) Disease-induced changes in the plasma binding of basic drugs. *Clinical Pharmacokinetics*, **5**, 246–262.

Pijpers, A., Schoevers, E.J., van Gogh, H. *et al.* (1990) The pharmacokinetics of oxytetracycline following intravenous administration in healthy and diseased pigs. *Journal of Veterinary Pharmacology and Therapeutics*, **13**, 320–326.

Prince, R.A., Casabar, E., Adair, C.G. *et al.* (1989) Effect of quinolone antimicrobials on theophylline pharmacokinetics. *Journal of Clinical Pharmacology*, **29**, 650–654.

Reidenberg, M.M. (1971) *Renal Function and Drug Action*, pp. 19–31. W.B. Saunders, Philadelphia.

Reidenberg, M.M. & Affrime, M. (1973) Influence of disease on binding of drugs to plasma proteins. *Annals of the New York Academy of Sciences*, **226**, 115–126.

Reidenberg, M.M. & Drayer, D.E. (1980) Drug therapy in renal failure. *Annual Review of Pharmacology and Toxicology*, **20**, 45–54.

Riffat, S., Nawaz, M. & Rehman, Z. (1982) Pharmacokinetics of sulphadimidine in normal and febrile dogs. *Journal of Veterinary Pharmacology and Therapeutics*, **5**, 131–135.

Riviere, J.E., Martin-Jimenez, T., Sundlof, S.F. & Craigmill, A.L. (1997) Interspecies allometric analysis of the comparative pharmacokinetics of 44 drugs across veterinary and laboratory animal species. *Journal of Veterinary Pharmacology and Therapeutics*, **20**, 453–463.

Rose, H.J., Pruitt, A.W. & McNay, J.H. (1976) Effect of experimental azotemia on renal clearance of furosemide in the dog. *Journal of Pharmacology and Experimental Therapeutics*, **196**, 238–247.

Sacher, G.A. (1959) Relationship of lifespan to brain weight and body weight in mammals. *Ciba Foundation Colloquium on Ageing*, **5**, 115–133.

Sanchez, S.F., Alvarez, L.I. & Lanusse, C.E. (1997) Fasting-induced changes to the pharmacokinetic behaviour of albendazole and its metabolites in calves. *Journal of Veterinary Pharmacology and Therapeutics*, **20**, 38–47.

Sarasola, P., Horspool, L.J.I. & McKellar, Q.A. (1992) Effect of changes in urine pH on plasma pharmacokinetic variables of ampicillin sodium in horses. *American Journal of Veterinary Research*, **53**, 711–715.

Semrad, S.D., McClure, J.T., Sams, R.A. & Kaminski, L.M. (1993) Pharmacokinetics and effects of repeated administration of phenylbutazone in neonatal calves. *American Journal of Veterinary Research*, **54**, 1906–1912.

Sjoholm, I., Kober, A., Odar-Cederlof, I. & Borga, O. (1976) Protein binding of drugs in uremic and normal serum: the role of endogenous inhibitors. *Biochemical Pharmacology*, **25**, 1205–1213.

Smith, C.M., Steffey, E.P., Baggot, J.D. *et al.* (1988) Effects of halothane anaesthesia on the clearance of gentamicin sulfate in horses. *American Journal of Veterinary Research*, **49**, 19–22.

Somogyi, A., McLean, A. & Heinzow, B. (1983) Cimetidine–procainamide pharmacokinetic interaction in man: evidence of competition for tubular secretion of basic drugs. *European Journal of Clinical Pharmacology*, **25**, 339–345.

Souhaili El Amri, H., Mothe, O., Totis, M. *et al.* (1988) Albendazole sulfonation by rat liver cytochrome P-450c. *Journal of Pharmacology and Experimental Therapeutics*, **246**, 758–764.

Sturman, J.A. & Smith, M.J.H. (1967) The binding of salicylate to plasma proteins in different species. *Journal of Pharmacy and Pharmacology*, **19**, 621–623.

Tozer, T.N. (1984) Implications of altered plasma protein binding in disease states. In: *Pharmacokinetic Basis for Drug Treatment*, (eds., L.Z. Benet, N. Massoud & J.G. Gambertoglio), pp. 173–193. Raven Press, New York.

Trenholme, G.M., Williams, R.L., Rieckmann, K.V. *et al.* (1976) Quinine disposition during malaria and during induced fever. *Clinical Pharmacology and Therapeutics*, **19**, 459–467.

Tvedegaard, E., Ladefoged, J. & Ladefoged, O. (1981) Pharmacokinetics of warfarin in rabbits during short-term and long-term uraemia. *Journal of Veterinary Pharmacology and Therapeutics*, **4**, 141–146.

Tygstrup, N. (1964) The galactose elimination capacity in control subjects and in patients with cirrhosis of the liver. *Acta Medica Scandinavica*, **175**, 281–289.

Verbeeck, R.K. (1982) Glucuronidation and disposition of drug glucuronides in patients with renal failure. A review. *Drug Metabolism and Disposition*, **10**, 87–89.

Waterman, A.E. (1984) The pharmacokinetics of ketamine administered intravenously in calves and the modifying effect of premedication with xylazine hydrochloride. *Journal of Veterinary Pharmacology and Therapeutics*, **7**, 125–130.

Wensing, G., Ohnhaus, E.E. & Hoensch, H.P. (1990) Antipyrine elimination and hepatic microsomal enzyme activity in patients with liver disease. *Clinical Pharmacology and Therapeutics*, **47**, 698–705.

Yuan, Z-H. & Fung, K-F. (1990) Pharmacokinetics of sulfadimidine and its N_4-acetyl metabolite in healthy and diseased rabbits infected with *Pasterurella multocida*. *Journal of Veterinary Pharmacology and Therapeutics*, **13**, 192–197.

Yuan, Z.-H., Miao, X.-Q & Yin, Y.-H. (1997) Pharmacokinetics of ampicillin and sulfadimidine in pigs infected experimentally with *Streptococcus suum*. *Journal of Veterinary Pharmacology and Therapeutics*, **20**, 318–322.

Zeng, Z.-L. & Fung K.-F. (1990) Effects of experimentally induced *Streptococcus suis* infection on the pharmacokinetics of penicillin G in pigs. *Journal of Veterinary Pharmacology and Therapeutics*, **13**, 43–48.

Zeng, Z.-L. & Fung, K. (1997) Effects of experimentally induced *Escherichia coli* infection on the pharmacokinetics of enrofloxacin in pigs. *Journal of Veterinary Pharmacology and Therapeutics*, **20** (Suppl. 1), 39–40.

Zertuche, J.M.L., Brown, M.P., Gronwall, R. & Merritt, K. (1992) Effect of probenecid on the pharmacokinetics of flunixin meglumine and phenylbutazone in healthy mares. *American Journal of Veterinary Research*, **53**, 372–374.

Chapter 4
Some Aspects of Dosage, Clinical Selectivity and Stereoisomerism

Introduction

While the clinical use of some drugs (e.g. pre-anaesthetic drugs, intravenous anaesthetic inducing agents) is confined to a single dose, the treatment of disease states requires the administration of multiple doses at intervals appropriate for the drug and the animal species. The formulation of the commercially available dosage form(s) largely determines the route and mode (manner) of administration, as well as the suitability of a drug preparation for use in various animal species. The wide range of body weight of domestic animal species makes solid oral dosage forms (i.e. tablets, capsules) intended for use in dogs and cats cumbersome to administer to horses, while parenteral, particularly prolonged-release, preparations designed for intramuscular administration to ruminant species and pigs are generally unsuitable for use in dogs, and cats and horses. Species (or group of species)-specific dosage forms apply to most, but not all drugs. The clinical efficacy of a drug in a particular species may be influenced by the appropriateness of the dosage form for use in that species.

Dosage regimen

A dosage regimen entails the administration of a series of maintenance (fixed) doses at a constant dosage interval. The design of dosage regimens, particularly for drugs that produce pharmacological effects (therapeutic drugs), represents an important application of pharmacokinetics and requires a knowledge of the therapeutic range of plasma concentrations (see Chapter 1, Table 1.1). The therapeutic range is based on the relationship between plasma drug concentrations (generally total rather than free drug concentration) and the principal pharmacological effect produced by the drug, while due consideration is given to other effects produced. It is generally assumed that the therapeutic concentration range defined for human beings can be applied to domestic animal species. The validity of this assumption largely depends on whether pharmacological activity is entirely associated with the parent drug, as the rate and extent of formation of an active metabolite would probably vary between species. Drugs that are at least partly converted to pharmacologically active metabolites include diazepam, phenylbutazone, primidone, procainamide and lignocaine (lidocaine), while chlorazepate and prazepam (both of which are converted to desmethyldiazepam), enalapril and benazepril (which are converted to enalaprilat and benazeprilat, respectively) are prodrugs.

Pharmacokinetic parameters used in designing a dosage regimen are the volume of distribution, determined by the area method (size of dose), the systemic clearance (dosage rate) and the half-life of the drug (dosage interval). When the drug is administered by an extravascular route (e.g. *per os* or by intramuscular injection), a knowledge of the systemic availability (i.e. the fraction of the administered dose that reaches the systemic circulation unchanged) is required. Values of these pharmacokinetic parameters are obtained, at least initially, in healthy adult animals of the target species. Because disease or physiological states or drug interactions may alter the bioavailability (i.e. the rate and extent of absorption) and the disposition (i.e. the distribution and elimination) of a drug, values of some of the pharmacokinetic parameters could be changed. The margin of safety or therapeutic ratio (i.e. the ratio of the toxic-to-effective plasma concentrations) and the overall rate of elimination (half-life) of a drug are the factors that limit the size of the dose and the duration of action, respectively. The response to treatment is the principal criterion which determines the therapeutic effectiveness (clinical efficacy) of the dosage regimen and the duration of therapy. When the therapeutic effect is a quantifiable physiological variable, such as heart rate or cardiac rhythm, the objective of therapy should be pre-defined and the response monitored to determine whether the objective has been achieved.

Steady-state plasma concentration

The administration of multiple doses of a drug at a constant dosage interval, or drug administration by continuous infusion, causes accumulation of the drug and the attainment of a steady-state plasma concentration. The objective in the design of a dosage regimen may be to maintain either an average steady-state plasma concentration ($C_{p(avg)}$) or plasma concentrations within the limits of the therapeutic range ($C_{p,ss(min)}$)–($C_{p,ss(max)}$) (Fig. 4.1). The therapeutic range defines the minimum effective ($C_{p,ss(min)}$) and the maximum desirable ($C_{p,ss(max)}$) plasma concentrations of a drug at steady-state, i.e. the range of plasma concentrations (relates to measurement of *total* drug) that is safe and therapeutically effective. The width of the range indicates the acceptable degree of fluctuation in steady-state concentrations during a dosage interval, while the units of plasma drug concentration (*e.g.* μg/mL for most drugs or ng/mL for some drugs) reflect the pharmacological activity of the drug.

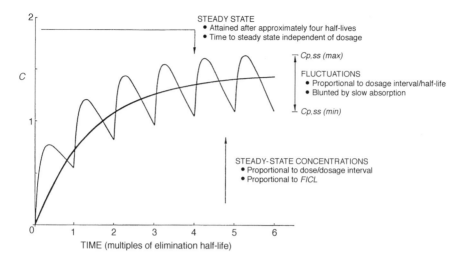

Fig. 4.1 Fundamental pharmacokinetic relationships for repeated administration of drugs. This figure depicts the plasma drug concentrations produced by administering maintenance doses at a constant dosage interval (equal to the half-life of the drug). A plasma concentration within 90% of the eventual steady-state concentration is attained after approximately four half-lives of the drug.

Dosage rate is defined as the systemically available dose divided by the dosage interval

$$\text{Dosage rate} = \frac{F \cdot \text{Dose}}{\text{Dosage interval}}$$

Assuming knowledge of the systemic clearance and the desired average steady-state plasma concentration of a drug, the dosage rate can be calculated from

$$\text{Dosage rate} = Cl_B \cdot C_{P(avg)}$$

Systemic clearance, which measures the ability of the body to eliminate a drug, determines the relationship between the dosage rate and the average steady-state plasma concentration. When multiple (fixed) doses of a drug are administered at a constant dosage interval (τ) the average plasma concentration that will be attained at steady-state can be predicted:

$$C_{P(avg)} = \frac{F \cdot \text{Dose}}{Cl_B \cdot \tau}$$

Because the area under the plasma drug concentration–time curve during a dosage interval at steady-state is equal to the total area under the curve after administering a single intravenous dose, the average plasma concentration at steady-state can be estimated from

$$C_{P(avg)} = \frac{AUC}{\tau}$$

where AUC is the *total* area under the curve after administering a single intravenous dose and τ is the dosage interval associated with a dosage regimen.

The average plasma concentration of a drug at steady-state ($C_{p(avg)}$) is neither the arithmetic nor the geometric mean of the maximum desirable ($C_{p,ss(max)}$) and minimum effective ($C_{p,ss(min)}$) concentrations. Rather, it is a plasma concentration within the therapeutic range which, when multiplied by the dosage interval, corresponds to the total AUC following the administration of a single intravenous dose, or the AUC during a dosage interval at steady-state.

When the usual dose of a conventional dosage form of a drug is known for a species X, the dose that would provide the same average steady-state concentration in another animal species Y can be calculated

$$\text{Dose}_Y = \text{Dose}_X \cdot \frac{F_X}{F_Y} \cdot \frac{Cl_Y}{Cl_X} \cdot \frac{\tau_Y}{\tau_X}$$

where F, Cl and τ are the systemic availability, the clearance and the dosage interval, respectively, in the species of interest.

A disadvantage of basing the design of a dosage regimen on the average plasma concentration at steady-state is that it provides no information regarding the degree of fluctuation in the steady-state concentrations during the dosage interval. This limits the application to drugs that have a relatively wide margin of safety and the selection of a dosage interval approximately equal to the half-life.

When a drug is administered by continuous intravenous infusion, the infusion rate (R_0) required to provide a desired steady-state plasma concentration ($C_{p(ss)}$) is

$$R_0 = C_{P(ss)} \cdot Cl_B$$

Based on this equation, it follows that the concentration at steady-state is directly proportional to the rate of infusion and inversely proportional to the systemic clearance of the drug. While the rate of infusion determines the steady-state concentration that will be attained, the time required to reach steady-state is determined *solely* by the rate of elimination (half-life) of the drug. For practical purposes it can be assumed that a plasma concentration within 90% of the desired steady-state (plateau) concentration will be achieved after continuously infusing the drug solution at a constant rate for a period corresponding to four times the half-life of the drug. An analogous situation, due to drug accumulation, applies to the attainment of steady-state concentrations when multiple doses are administered at a constant dosage interval.

For drugs that have long half-lives, the time to reach steady-state is appreciable. The delay in attaining the desired steady-state concentration can be overcome by administering a loading (or priming) dose. Calculation of the size of the loading dose requires a knowledge of the volume of distribution, which is the proportionality factor that relates the plasma concentration to the total amount of drug in the body:

$$\text{Loading dose} = C_{P(avg)} \cdot V_{d(area)}$$

Depending on the margin of safety, the available dosage forms and oral bioavailability of the drug, the loading dose can either be administered orally as a single entity or increments of the loading dose can be administered at relatively short intervals by *slow* intravenous injection or intravenous infusion.

Application to cardiac drugs

Quinidine is the drug most frequently used to treat supraventricular arrhythmias, especially atrial fibrillation, in horses. The therapeutic range of plasma concentrations. is 2–6 µg/mL and the average half-life (i.v. dose) is 6.5 h, but the half-life of quinidine varies widely between individual horses (McGuirk *et al.*, 1981). The oral bioavailability of quinidine, administered via nasogastric tube as an aqueous suspension of quinidine sulphate, is approximately 50% and the peak plasma concentration is generally reached at 2–2.5 h. In the treatment of supraventricular arrhythmias, a dose (20 mg/kg) of quinidine sulphate is administered via nasogastric tube every 2 h until cardioversion occurs or a total (maximum) of six doses have been given.

Lignocaine (lidocaine) is indicated for the emergency treatment of severe acute ventricular arrhythmias. A parenteral preparation of lignocaine hydrochloride (*without* adrenaline (epinephrine)) must be used. The therapeutic range of plasma concentrations is 1.5–5 µg/mL; an active metabolite, monoethylglycylxylidide, is formed in the liver. In horses, up to four doses (0.5–1 mg/kg) of the drug are administered by slow intravenous injection at 5-min intervals. In dogs, an initial dose (2–4 mg/kg) of lignocaine hydrochloride is administered by slow intravenous injection, followed by intravenous infusion at a rate of 25–75 µg/kg·min.

Oral therapy with procainamide may be used to control ventricular arrhythmias in dogs. Procainamide hydrochloride tablets (conventional dosage form) are administered at a dose of approximately 10 mg/kg at 8-h dosage intervals. Although an oral sustained-release dosage form is available, a dosage regimen for dogs has not been established. The therapeutic range of plasma concentrations is 6–14 µg/mL; an active metabolite, N-acetylprocainamide, is formed in the liver of horses and human beings but not in dogs. In horses, the active metabolite is eliminated (by renal excretion) more slowly than the parent drug (hepatic biotransformation). It is probably because of the inability of dogs to form N-acetylprocainamide that a higher range of plasma concentrations with an average steady-state concentration of 34 µg/mL may be required to control some cardiac arrhythmias (ventricular tachycardia) in dogs (Papich *et al.*, 1986).

Propranolol and sotalol are non-selective β-adrenoceptor antagonists that differ in the relative contributions of their β_1-blocking (decreased atrioventricular nodal conduction, propranolol) and direct membrane (prolonged effective refractory period, sotalol) actions to their anti-arrythmic effect. At therapeutic plasma concentrations (20–80 ng/mL), propranolol slows the heart rate and decreases cardiac contractility. The drug is indicated in dogs for the control of catecholamine-induced suspraventricular arrhythmias and in hyperthyroid cats to prevent tachycardia and cardiac rhythm disturbances. Because propranolol is rapidly metabolized by the liver (half-life in dogs is 1.5 h), the oral bioavailability is low (2–17%) due to the first-pass effect; however, as it has a high extraction ratio ($E_H > 0.6$), its systemic clearance is mainly influenced by liver blood flow. Oral dosage regimens, using conventional tablets or an oral solution, for dogs and cats commence with a low dose (0.25 mg/kg) administered at 8-h intervals, and dosage is increased over 3–5 days to 1 mg/kg for dogs and 0.5 mg/kg for cats, administered at 8-h dosage intervals. Although propranolol is seldom used in horses, the drug (parenteral solution) may be effective in controlling supraventricular arrhythmias; the dose (0.05–0.15 mg/kg) is administered by slow intravenous injection. As non-selective β-adrenoceptor antagonists (propranolol, sotalol) cause blockade of β_2-adrenoceptor in bronchial smooth muscle, an increase in airway resistance (bronchoconstriction) is an important side-effect. The production of this adverse effect may be largely avoided by using a relatively selective β_1-adrenoceptor antagonist, such as atenolol. The oral dosage regimen for the dog is 0.1–0.5 mg/kg administered at 12- or 24-h dosage intervals, depending on the response obtained.

In the treatment of congestive heart failure, the objectives are to adjust cardiac output to meet the needs of the body and to promote the renal excretion of excess fluid. Treatment with digoxin can often meet these objectives, but the therapeutic dosage regimen must be related to the severity of the disease and the response of the animal when steady-state concentrations of the drug have been achieved. The actions of digoxin on the failing heart include: a slowing of the heart rate (due to an increase in the effective vagal tone), a decrease in atrioventricular conduction (antiadrenergic action) and, most importantly, an increased strength of ventricular contraction (positive inotropic effect on myocardial cells). At the molecular level, all therapeutically useful cardiac glycosides inhibit Na^+, K^+-ATPase, the myocardial cell membrane-bound enzyme associated with the sodium pump. The diuretic effect results from the improvement in renal blood flow and the associated decrease in aldosterone secretion by the *zona glomerulosa* cells of the adrenal cortex.

In dogs, digoxin is the drug of choice in the management of congestive heart failure where it is associated with primary or secondary myocardial failure, notably in dilated cardiomyopathy. As digoxin has a narrow margin of safety with a therapeutic plasma concentration range of 0.6–2.4 ng/mL, particular attention must be given both to dosage and the clinical effect produced by the drug. Because of the toxic potential of digoxin and the variation in response between individual animals, dose titration with monitoring of serum digoxin concentrations should be applied. The digitalization state can be achieved either by the rapid method, in which the estimated digitalizing (loading) dose is administered in increments (22 µg/kg at 6-h intervals on the first day of treatment (three doses), or 22 µg/kg at 12-h intervals for 36 h (four doses)) or the slow method, in which the estimated maintenance dose (11 µg/kg at 12-h intervals or 22 µg/kg at 24-h intervals) is administered from the commencement of treatment. The slow method of achieving the digitalization state is based on the principle of accumulation, is slower in onset but more safe, and should generally be used. Because the average half-life of digoxin in dogs is 28 h, a steady-state concentration will be attained on the sixth to eighth day of maintenance dosage. The animal should be carefully examined at this time, the response to therapy assessed and the serum digoxin concentration measured. The earliest evidence of digitalization may be relief from coughing, less laboured breathing and the absence of fatigue upon mild exercise. Other clinical observations include the development of diuresis and the loss of oedema fluid. In dogs with atrial fibrillation, the ventricular rate is a reliable guide to the satisfactoriness of therapy. Because of wide variation in the oral bioavailability of digoxin between different brands of tablet, probably due to dissolution differences, the same brand and strength of tablet should continue to be used in an individual dog. Any change in the maintenance dosage rate would require a further 6–8 days for the response to be fully evident when the new steady-state concentration will be achieved.

In horses, therapy with digoxin may be initiated by administering two doses (20 µg/kg *p.o.* or 5 µg/kg i.v.) 12 h apart and continued with oral maintenance doses (20 µg/kg) administered at 24-h intervals, or attainment of the digitalization state may totally rely on maintenance dosage (10 µg/kg *p.o.* at 12-h dosage intervals). A lesser degree of fluctuation in the steady-state plasma concentrations, which would be attained on the sixth to eighth day of therapy, is associated with the latter dosage regimen and is safer to apply. The oral bioavailability of digoxin in the horse is assumed to be 25%. The administration of quinidine, for the treatment of atrial fibrillation, to horses on maintenance therapy with digoxin increases the average steady-state plasma digoxin concentrations approximately twofold (Fig. 4.2) (Parraga *et al.*, 1995). The basis of the interaction is a decreased volume of distribution of digoxin due to displacement by quinidine from tissue binding sites and, in horses, decreased renal clearance (the principal elimination process) of digoxin. Whenever concomitant use of these drugs is anticipated, maintenance dosage with digoxin should be reduced to one-half for 6–8 days before quinidine therapy.

Captopril, an angiotensin-converting enzyme (ACE) inhibitor, lowers blood pressure principally by decreasing peripheral vascular resistance. This drug acts by inhibiting the enzyme peptidyl dipeptidase that hydrolyses angiotensin I to angiotensin II, a conversion that takes place primarily in the lungs, and inactivates bradykinin (Benowitz, 1992). There is evidence which suggests that ACE inhibitors improve the quality of life in dogs with a moderate degree of congestive heart failure and may improve ventricular diastolic function in cardiomyopathies, especially in cats. As ACE inhibitors are primarily eliminated by renal excretion, renal function should be monitored before and during treatment. Non-steroidal anti-inflammatory drugs may impair the

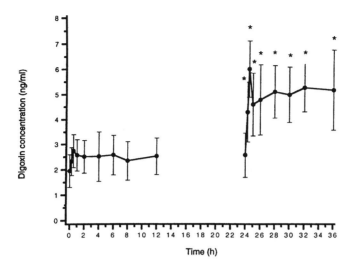

Fig. 4.2 Comparison of mean serum digoxin concentrations pre- and post quinidine administration. Mean ± 1 SD * = *P* < 0.05 vs. baseline. Hours 0–12 are day 6 and hours 24–36 are day 7. (Reproduced with permission from Parraga *et al.* (1995).)

hypotensive effect of captopril (and other ACE inhibitors) by blocking brady-kinin-mediated vasodilation. Enalapril is a prodrug that is converted by de-esterification to an ACE inhibitor enalaprilat (enalaprilic acid), which produces similar effects to captopril. It may be used as an alternative to digoxin for the treatment of mild congestive heart failure in dogs and cats. On the day preceding the commencement of treatment with enalapril, administer two doses (2 mg/kg), 12 h apart, of hydrochlorothiazine, or a single oral dose of furosemide (2 mg/kg). The usual dosage regimen for enalapril maleate (conventional tablet) is 0.5 mg/kg administered at 24-h intervals. Based on the clinical response produced after one week of therapy, the dosage interval may be decreased to 12 h. Since a therapeutic range of plasma concentrations has not been defined for enalaprilat, dosage is empirical and reliant on the clinical response to therapy. It should be borne in mind that once maximal inhibition of the enzyme (ACE) has been achieved, increasing the size of the dose will not increase the therapeutic effect.

   In the treatment of acute myocardial failure with associated pulmonary oedema, the objectives are to improve gas exchange, increase myocardial contractility and reduce the workload of the left ventricle. Dobutamine, a somewhat selective β_1-adrenoceptor agonist, produces a pronounced inotropic effect that results in an increased cardiac output (where contractility is the limiting factor) and an elevation of arterial blood pressure. The drug pre-paration, following appropriate dilution, is administered by continuous intravenous infusion at a rate of 1–5 µg/kg·min. An intravenous dose (0.5 mg/kg) of furosemide (loop diuretic) increases venous capacitance by redistributing venous blood from the lungs to the peripheral circulation, which would contribute towards the relief of pulmonary congestion. This extra-renal effect of furosemide precedes the diuretic effect.

Dobutamine is indicated in dogs for the treatment of dilated cardiomyopathy associated with congestive heart failure (infusion rate 2.5–7.5 μg/kg·min) and in horses for the management of hypotension during anaesthesia (infusion rate of 1 μg/kg·min) with the objective of maintaining mean arterial blood pressure above 70 mmHg (normal is 115 mgHg). Because the drug has a very short half-life (due to rapid biotransformation), a steady-state concentration is achieved within 10 min and can be readily adjusted (by changing the rate of infusion) according to the clinical and haemodynamic responses of the animal. The commercial preparation of dobutamine is a racemic mixture in which the (+)-enantiomer is about ten times more potent as a β-adrenoceptor agonist than the (−)-enantiomer.

Fluctuation in steady-state plasma concentrations

A dosage regimen designed to produce an average steady-state plasma concentration could show wide variation in the steady-state peak ($C_{p,ss(max)}$) and trough ($C_{p,ss(min)}$) concentrations, depending on the dosage interval. A high degree of fluctuation in steady-state concentrations during the dosage interval is unacceptable for drugs that have a narrow range of therapeutic plasma concentrations. At least for these drugs, the maintenance dose should be precisely calculated and a dosage interval be selected with the objective of limiting the degree of fluctuation to a level consistent with maintaining steady-state concentrations within the therapeutic range.

The steady-state trough (minimum effective) plasma concentration obtained after the administration of a maintenance dose is based on the volume of distribution, the fraction of dose remaining ($f_r = e^{-\beta\tau}$), and the fraction of dose eliminated ($f_{el} = 1 - e^{-\beta\tau}$) during the dosage interval. Based on a desired trough plasma concentration ($C_{p,ss(min)}$) at the end of the dosage interval, the maintenance dose that would be required may be calculated as follows:

$$\text{Dose} = C_{P,ss(min)} \cdot V_d \left(e^{+\beta\tau} - 1\right)$$

Selection of the dosage interval (τ) is based on the half-life ($t_{1/2(\beta)}$) and the acceptable degree of fluctuation in the plasma drug concentration at steady-state. The longer the dosage interval relative to the half-life, which is called the relative dosage interval (ε), the greater will be the degree of fluctuation. As the relative dosage interval increases, the extent of drug accumulation on multiple dosing decreases (Table 4.1). The extent of accumulation (R_A), which is reflected by the plasma concentrations at steady-state relative to those occurring after the first dose, is dependent on the fraction of the dose eliminated during the dosage interval (f_{el}):

$$R_A = \frac{1}{f_{el}} = \frac{1}{(1 - e^{-\beta\tau})}$$

Table 4.1 Relationship between the relative dosage interval ($\varepsilon = \tau/t_{1/2}$) and the extent of drug accumulation (R_A) on multiple-dosing.

Relative dosage interval (ε)	Extent of accumulation (R_A)
0.1	14.9
0.5	3.41
1.0	2.00
2.0	1.33
3.0	1.14
4.0	1.07
5.0	1.03

where R_A is the accumulation factor (extent of accumulation), β is the overal elimination rate constant of the drug and τ is the dosage interval (Baggot, 1977). When the dosage interval is equal to the half-life of the drug (i.e. $\varepsilon = 1$), the accumulation factor is 2.00. The administration of maintenance doses at intervals longer than the half-life ($\varepsilon > 1$) gives lower values of the accumulation factor. For example, when the dosage interval is twice the half-life ($\varepsilon = 2$), the accumulation factor is 1.33. The extent of accumulation is a feature of the relative dosage interval rather than a property of the drug.

When designing a dosage regimen to maintain steady-state plasma concentrations within a specified range, the dosage interval corresponding to the length of time for plasma drug concentration to decline from the maximum desirable ($C_{p,ss(max)}$) to the minimum effective ($C_{p,ss(min)}$) concentrations can be calculated:

$$\text{Dosage interval} = \frac{\ln\left(\frac{C_{p,ss(max)}}{C_{p,ss(min)}}\right)}{\beta}$$

where β is the overall elimination rate constant of the drug. A dosage interval close to the calculated value should be selected. The wider the range of therapeutic plasma concentrations the higher the acceptable degree of fluctuation in steady-state plasma concentrations and the longer the dosage interval relative to the rate of elimination (half-life) of the drug. The relationship between the length of the dosage interval and the acceptable degree of fluctuation in steady-state plasma concentrations may be stated in the following way. If the ratio of $C_{p,ss(max)}$ to $C_{p,ss(min)}$ (upper and lower limits of the therapeutic range) for a drug is 2^ε (where ε is the relative dosage interval), then the dosage interval should be ε multiplied by the half-life of the drug. For most drugs, the ratio of the maximum desirable to minimum effective plasma concentrations is less than 8:1. This means that dosage intervals less than three times the half-life have to be used to maintain steady-state plasma concentrations within the therapeutic range. Sustained-release dosage forms will, in many cases, allow less frequent dosing and yield a lower degree of fluctuation in steady-state plasma concentrations.

When the time to approach steady-state by administering maintenance doses is long (approximately four times the half-life of the drug), it may be desirable to initiate therapy with a loading dose. For this type of design, calculation of the loading dose is based on achieving steady-state trough concentrations at the end of the first dosage interval:

$$\text{Loading dose} = C_{P,ss(min)} \cdot V_d \left(e^{+\beta\tau}\right)$$

that is,

$$\text{Loading dose} = \frac{\text{Maintenance dose}}{(1 - e^{-\beta\tau})}$$

A designed dosage regimen allows prediction to be made of the maximum desirable and minimum effective steady-state plasma drug concentrations:

$$C_{P,ss(max)} = \frac{F \cdot \text{Dose}}{V_d \cdot f_{el}}$$

where dose refers to the maintenance dose and f_{el}, the fraction of dose eliminated during a dosage interval, is $(1 - e^{-\beta\tau})$.

$$C_{P,ss(min)} = \frac{F \cdot \text{Dose} \cdot e^{-\beta\tau}}{V_d \left(1 - e^{-\beta\tau}\right)}$$

that is,

$$C_{P,ss(min)} = C_{P,ss(max)} \cdot f_r$$

where f_r, the fraction of dose remaining at the end of the dosage interval, is $e^{-\beta\tau}$.

A dosage regimen consisting of a loading (or priming) dose equal to twice the maintenance dose and a dosage interval of one half-life is satisfactory for drugs with half-lives between 8 and 24 h. Far fewer drugs have half-lives in this range in domestic animals, particularly ruminant species, compared with human beings. A small number of drugs have half-lives longer than 24 h in dogs; examples include digoxin (28 h), phenobarbitone (64 h in mongrel dogs, 32 h in Beagles), and naproxen (74 h in mongrel dogs, 35 h in Beagles). A dosage interval of 12 or 24 h may be used for maintenance therapy with digoxin or phenobarbitone. A lower degree of fluctuation in steady-state plasma concentrations would be associated with the 12-h dosage interval. Nonetheless, plasma concentrations should be monitored and related to the clinical response. Maintenance dosage, without the use of a loading dose, would gradually (about six days for digoxin) achieve a steady-state concentration. Naproxen, if used in dogs, could be administered once daily.

For drugs with half-lives between 3 and 8 h (Table 4.2), selection of the dosage interval must take into account the margin of safety of the drug, the range of therapeutic plasma concentrations, which indicates the degree of fluctuation in steady-state concentrations that would be acceptable, and the

Table 4.2 Drugs that have half-lives between 3 and 8 h in dogs and horses.

Drug	Half-life (h)	
	Dog	Horse
Phenylbutazone	2.5–6.0[a]	4.1–4.7[a]
Flunixin	3.7	1.9
Salicylate	8.6	1.0
Phenytoin	3.5–4.5[a]	8.2
Diazepam	7.6[b]	9.7[b]
Quinidine	5.6	6.5
Procainamide[c]	2.6	3.5
Theophylline	5.7	14.8
Norfloxacin	3.6	6.4
Enrofloxacin[d]	3.4	5.0
Metronidazole	4.5	3.9
Trimethoprim	4.6[e]	3.2
Sulphadiazine	5.6[e]	3.6[e]
Oxytetracycline	6.0	9.6
Doxycycline	7.0	–

[a] Half-life is dose-dependent.
[b] Total benzodiazepine (parent drug and active metabolites).
[c] Procainamide is converted to *N*-acetylprocainamide (active metabolite) in the horse ($t_{1/2} = 6.3$ h), but this metabolite is not formed in the dog.
[d] Enrofloxacin is converted to ciprofloxacin, both of which have antimicrobial activity.
[e] Half-life may be influenced by urinary pH reaction.

convenience or otherwise of repeated dosing. When the margin of safety is narrow or the ratio of the maximum desirable-to-minimum effective plasma concentrations is 4:1, the dosage interval should not exceed twice the half-life (i.e. $\varepsilon = 2$). Drugs that have reasoably high oral bioavailability and half-lives in the range 4–6 h could be suitable for use in dogs as sustained-release oral dosage forms. The dosage regimen for sustained-release anhydrous theophylline tablets (Theo-Dur®) in (Beagle) dogs is 20 mg/kg administered at 12-h dosage intervals, while that for conventional aminophylline tablets is 10 mg/kg administered at 8-h dosage intervals (Koritz *et al.*, 1986). While both dosage regimens will maintain plasma concentrations within the therapeutic range for theophylline (6–16 µg/mL), that for the sustained-release oral dosage form is the more convenient to apply.

For drugs with short half-lives (30 min to 3 h) and a relatively narrow margin of safety, the use of an inconveniently short dosage interval (≤ 6 h) would be required to maintain plasma concentrations within the therapeutic range. This situation applies to carbamazepine and valproic acid (anticonvulsants), which are commercially available as conventional oral dosage forms. For drugs with a wide margin of safety, a longer dosage interval may be selected, but a high degree of fluctuation in steady-state concentrations is an unavoidable consequence. The use of furosemide, administered once or twice daily, provides intermittent rather than continuous therapy and clinical efficacy (as a diuretic) is more closely related to urinary rather than plasma concentration. For drugs with very short half-lives (<30 min), e.g., dobutamine, continuous intravenous infusion is the only satisfactory mode of administration. A steady-state plasma concentration will be achieved within a relatively short period of time (four half-lives of the drug) and fluctuation in steady-state plasma concentrations will be avoided. Based on the clinical response when a steady-state (plateau) concentration has been achieved, either a greater or lesser effect can be produced by adjusting the rate of infusion upward or downward, respectively.

Unlike the estimates of dosage rates and average steady-state plasma concentrations, which may be determined independently of any pharmacokinetic model in that systemic clearance is the only pharmacokinetic parameter used, the prediction of peak and trough steady-state concentrations requires pharmacokinetic compartmental model assumptions. It is assumed that, (i) drug disposition can be adequately described by a one-compartment pharmacokinetic model, (ii) disposition is independent of dose (i.e. linear pharmacokinetics apply), and (iii) the absorption rate is much faster than the rate of elimination of the drug, which is always valid when the drug is administered intravenously. For clinical applications, these assumptions are reasonable.

The administration of a rapidly absorbed drug at intervals exceeding five times the half-life practically constitutes single dosing, because a relative dosage interval (ε) above 5.0 has an accumulation factor (R_A) of less than 1.03. Assuming first-order elimination, the duration of therapeutic plasma concentrations ($t_{Cp(ther)}$) produced by a single dose depends on the size of the administered dose (D_0) relative to the minimum effective dose (D_{min}) and the half-life of the drug:

$$t_{Cp(ther)} = \frac{\ln\left(\frac{D_0}{D_{min}}\right)}{\beta} = \ln\left(\frac{D_0}{D_{min}}\right) \cdot 1.44 \cdot t_{1/2}$$

The relationship between these variables is such that geometric increases in the dose produce linear increases in the duration of therapeutic plasma concentrations. This implies that if twice the minimum effective dose produces therapeutic plasma concentrations for a length of time equal to one half-life of the drug, eight times the minimum effective dose would have to be administered to extend the duration of therapeutic plasma concentrations to three half-lives. The margin of safety of a drug primarily limits the size of dose that can be administered without producing toxic effects. For most pharmacological agents and antimicrobial agents (with the notable exception of penicillins), a dose exceeding five times the minimum effective dose would be likely to produce toxic effects. Moreover, the bulk or volume of prepared dosage forms may make the administration of high doses cumbersome, particularly in large animals. However, the concentration of drug in parenteral dosage forms must be given special attention when estimating the total volume for administration to small animals, particularly cats and toy breeds of dog, or neonatal animals (such as piglets).

Clinical selectivity

Clinical selectivity refers to the clinical use of a drug preparation in a manner such that a desired therapeutic effect is preferentially produced. It is influenced by the action of the drug, the chemical entity (drug *per se* or a derivative) formulated in the dosage form, the route of administration and the dose administered. For therapeutic purposes it is generally desirable to use a drug that interacts with only one type of receptor or, more selectively, a receptor subtype (Table 4.3). Even when such a drug is chosen, a wide range of effects may be produced depending on the tissue distribution of the receptor. By preferential production of a desired effect is meant that the effect is produced either at a lower dose (higher receptor binding affinity) or following administration of the

Table 4.3 Agonists, receptors activated and principal effects produced.

Drug	Receptor(s)	Principal clinical effects
Xylaxine	α_2, (α_1)-Adrenoceptors	Sedation + analgesia
Detomidine	α_2-Adrenoceptor	Sedation + analgesia
Dobutamine	β_1-Adrenoceptor	Increased cardiac output; + inotropic and + chronotropic
Clenbuterol	β_2-Adrenoceptor	Bronchodilation; myometrial relaxation (cows)
Morphine[a]	μ (mainly), δ and κ-Opioid	Profound analgesia; decreased intestinal motility; respiratory depression; sedation (dogs)
Butorphanol	κ-Opioid; inhibits μ-opioid	Analgesia; antitussive
Metoclopramide	Activates muscarinic receptors; inhibits dopamine (DA_e and D_2) receptors	Promotes gastric emptying / Antiemetic
Pilocarpine (ophthalmic)	Muscarinic receptors	Pupillary constriction and spasm of accommodation
Phenylephrine (ophthalmic)	α_1-Adrenoceptor	Pupillary dilation (dogs)

[a] Fentanyl has same action as morphine but is more potent.

dosage form by a particular route (largely limits access of the drug to its receptors in certain tissues).

Dobutamine, a selective β_1-adrenoceptor agonist, is administered by intravenous infusion primarily because of its very short half-life, but this mode of administration has the additional advantage of continuously delivering the drug to its site of action (the heart). Even though the oral bioavailability of atenolol and particularly propranolol is low (due to the first-pass effect) and variable, both drugs are formulated as oral dosage forms for convenience of administration during chronic therapy. They differ in that atenolol (a relatively selective β_1-adrenoceptor antagonist) is cardio-selective in action, whereas propranolol, (a non-selective β-adrenoceptor antagonist) may cause broncho-constriction (β_2 blocking effect) in addition to decreasing cardiac output (β_1 blocking effect) and indirectly increase peripheral vascular resistance (compensatory sympathetic reflex). Use of the ophthalmic preparation (eye drops) confers clinical selectivity on timolol, a non-selective β-adrenoceptor antagonist, for the management of ocular hypertension. However, because some of the drug is absorbed into the systemic circulation, the use of timolol is contra-indicated in patients with congestive heart failure or prone to asthma.

The administration by inhalation of ipratropium (muscarinic receptor antagonist) or clenbuterol (β_2-adrenoceptor agonist) increases the clinical selectivity of these drugs by largely limiting the effect produced, by different mechanisms, to bronchodilation. Propantheline (muscarinic receptor antagonist), administered orally, has a relatively selective action (antispasmodic effect) on smooth muscle of the gastrointestinal tract. It is because ipratropium and propantheline are quarternary ammonium drugs their membrane penetrative capacity, which affects absorption and distribution, is limited relative to atropine, a tertiary ammonium alkaloid. The chemical nature together with the route of administration account for the clinical selectivity of ipratropium and propantheline.

The size of the dose influences the clinical use of atropine (competitive muscarinic receptor antagonist) because the muscarinic receptors at different locations in the body differ in their sensitivity to blockade. When used for pre-anaesthetic medication of dogs, clinical selectivity is more or less achieved by administering a low dose ($44\,\mu g/kg$) of atropine sulphate by subcutaneous injection. Reduced salivation, decreased bronchial secretions and increased luminal diameter of bronchioles collectively comprise the desired effect. Because atropine can markedly decrease intestinal motility in horses, glycopyrronium (glycopyrrolate) ($5\,\mu g/kg$ injected intravenously) is often preferred for pre-anaesthetic medication and prevention of the short-lived second-degree atrioventricular block induced by xylazine. The repeated administration (as required) of high doses of atropine is essential for the management of intoxication with cholinesterase inhibitors, particularly those that have an 'irreversible' action (e.g. organophosphorus compounds). This application avails of the ability of atropine to distribute widely in tissues, including penetration of the blood–brain barrier. It is interesting to relate that

75 years after the observation by Schroff (1852) that some rabbits and their offspring could thrive on a constant diet of atropine-containing plants whereas others fed a similar diet died, it was discovered that the 'resistant' rabbits have a genetically-determined plasma enzyme, atropinase, which hydrolyses atropine into pharmacologically inactive metabolites (Bernheim & Bernheim, 1938).

Xylazine and detomidine readily penetrate the blood–brain barrier (an essential prerequisite for centrally acting drugs) and activate α_2-adrenoceptors in the *locus ceruleus*, which is located in the floor of the fourth ventricle of the brain, to produce sedation and a high degree of analgesia. Detomidine is more potent than xylazine, which means that a lower dose administered by the same route will produce principal effects of similar intensity, and at therapeutic dosage is somewhat more selective in action in that peripheral α_1-adrenoceptors do not appear to be activated by detomidine. The higher potency of detomidine is of less clinical significance than the greater selectivity of action. The clinical indications for use of a drug are often based on its selectivity of action, pharmacokinetic properties that determine access of the drug to its site of action and its rate of elimination, and on the commercially available dosage forms. In some respects, the use of adrenaline (epinephrine) hydrochloride ($20\,\mu g/kg$, injected i.m. or s.c.) for the initial management of acute anaphylactic reactions is an exception, in that advantage is taken of the non-selective action of adrenaline, a mixed (α, β_1 and β_2) adrenoceptor agonist. Furosemide and its analogue bumetanide have the same mechanism of diuretic action, which is inhibition of the $Na^+ - K^+ - 2Cl^-$ cotransport mechanism in the thick ascending limb of the loop of Henle, but differ in potency (relative dose) and in rate of elimination. Both drugs are selective in action and are used clinically in a similar manner (intermittent dosing).

Significance of antagonism

A wide variety of therapeutic agents and antidotal substances owe their action to some form of antagonism, of which there are four types: pharmacological, biochemical, chemical and physiological.

Drugs that act by pharmacological antagonism generally have high affinity for the receptors to which they bind, are *per se* devoid of efficacy (intrinsic activity) and while most act competitively, some are non-competitive in action. The effects resulting from drug receptor blockade may be due to the inability of an endogenous agonist to activate the occupied receptor or to the unopposed (not physiologically counterbalanced) activation of another type (or subtype) of receptor. The former situation is the more usual. If receptor blockade can be overcome by increasing the concentration of the agonist, ultimately achieving the same maximal effect as when unopposed, the antagonism is said to be competitive. This generally applies to antagonists that reversibly bind to the receptor. In competitive antagonism, the antagonistic effect is seen as a reduction in the apparent affinity of the agonist for its receptor site of action; the efficacy of the agonist is unaltered. Spironolactone produces a potassium-sparing diuretic effect by competitively antagonizing the action of aldosterone at mineralocorticoid receptors located in the cortical collecting renal tubule cells. Other drugs that act by competitive antagonism, the receptors to which they reversibly bind and the clinical indications for their use are presented in Table 4.4. While some competitive antagonists are selective in action in that they block a single subtype of receptor, others are non-selective (e.g. propranolol, diphenhydramine).

A non-competitive antagonist prevents the agonist from producing any effect at its receptor site of action. The antagonistic effect may be conceptualized as the removal of receptor or a decreased capacity of the effector system to respond.

Table 4.4 Competitive antagonists, receptors inhibited and principal clinical indications for their use.

Drug	Receptor(s)	Clinical indication(s)
Yohimbine	α_2, (α_1)-Adrenoceptors	Xylazine reversal
Atipamezole	α_2-Adrenoceptor	Detomidine reversal
Tolazoline	α_2-Adrenoceptor	Amitraz toxicity (dogs)
Atenolol	β_1-Adrenoceptor	Supraventricular arrhythmias (dogs and cats)
Propranolol	β_1 and β_2-Adrenoceptors	Supraventricular tachycardia; hypertrophic cardiomyopathy (dogs)
Prazosin[b]	α_1-Adrenoceptor	Congestive heart failure (dogs)
Naloxone	μ, δ and κ-Opioid	Opioid reversal
Diprenorphine	μ, δ and κ-Opioid	Etorphine reversal
Atropine	Muscarinic (M_1, M_2 and M_3) receptors	Pre-anaesthetic medication (dogs); management of organophosphate toxicity
Glycopyrollate	Muscarinic receptors	Pre-anaesthetic medication (horses)
Diphenhydramine	H_1-receptor and muscarinic receptors	Allergic respiratory conditions; relief of pruritis in allergic skin disorders; prevention of motion sickness (dogs)
Cimetidine[a]	H_2-receptor	To reduce gastric secretion of HCl and pepsin

[a] Ranitidine has same action as cimetidine but is more potent.
[b] Use concurrently with digoxin (at reduced maintenance dosage).

The efficacy (i.e. maximal possible effect) of the agonist is reduced, but its affinity for the receptor is not changed. The essential feature of non-competitive antagonism is that the agonist has no influence upon the degree of antagonism or its reversibility. Phenoxybenzamine binds covalently to α-adrenoceptors (somewhat selectively to α_1-adrenoceptors), causing irreversible blockade of long duration. The principal pharmacological effect results from blockade of catecholamine-induced peripheral vasaconstriction. Either log dose-response (LDR) curves or a double reciprocal (the equivalent of the Lineweaver–Burk) plot for an agonist, alone and in the presence of an antagonist, may be used to distinguish between the character of antagonism (Taylor & Insel, 1990).

Selective inhibition of enzymes

Various therapeutic agents act by selective inhibition of certain enzymes (Table 4.5). The inhibition produced by the majority of these drugs is reversible and the duration of action, in common with drugs that reversibly interact with receptors (macromolecular components of tissue), is determined by the rate of drug elimination (half-life) when a single dose is administered or the period of time that plasma drug concentrations are maintained within the therapeutic range, which is a function of the dosage rate, when multiple doses are administered. Drugs with the same mechanism of action (e.g. non-steroidal anti-inflammatory drugs or angiotensin-converting enzyme inhibitors) differ in potency and rate of elimination.

   Inhibition of cyclo-oxygenase (prostaglandin synthase), the enzyme that catalyses the conversion of free arachidonic acid to endoperoxide compounds (initially PGG_2 and PGH_2), is the primary mode of action of non-steroidal anti-inflammatory drugs (NSAIDs). As a result, the biosynthesis of prostaglandins that mediate the inflammatory response (PGE_2 and PGI_2) and fever as well as the formation of thromboxane A_2 are decreased (Vane, 1971). Fever associated with infection is thought to result from the effect on the hypothalamus of bacterial lipopolysaccharide and interleukin-1 stimulated synthesis and release of PGE_2 from migratory cells, such as macrophages. The lipoxygenase pathway that leads to the biosynthesis of leukotrienes is not inhibited by NSAIDs, with the possible exceptions of indomethacin and diclofenac. There is increasing evidence that an action independent of cyclo-oxygenase inhibition may contribute to the range of therapeutic effects produced by NSAIDs (McCormack & Brune, 1991; Twomey & Dale, 1992). It has been established that cyclo-oxygenase exists as two isoforms, COX-1 and COX-2 (Vane & Botting, 1995). COX-1 is a constitutive isoform found in blood vessels (endothelium and platelets), the stomach and the kidneys; it catalyses the synthesis of eicosanoids that perform physiological functions which include cytoprotection, especially of the gastric mucosa, 'fine-tuning' of renal perfusion and control of platelet aggregation. The toxic side-effects produced by NSAIDs are attributable to COX-1 inhibition. COX-2 is induced by cytokines, such as interleukin-1, at sites

Table 4.5 Antagonists that owe that action to inhibition of enzymes.

Drug	Enzyme inhibited	Clinical indication(s)
Aspirin[a]	Cyclo-oxygenases (COX-1 and COX-2)	Anti-inflammatory; analgesic, antipyretic
Theophylline	Cyclic nucleotide phosphodiesterases	Bronchodilation Vasodilation in the presence of
Captopril	Angiotensin-converting enzyme (ACE)	congestive heart failure
Digoxin	Na^+,K^+-ATPase in myocardial cell membrane	Congestive heart failure: slowing of heart rate, decrease in AV condition, positive inotropic effect
Neostigmine	Cholinesterase (reversible)	Reversal of non-deplarizing neuromuscular blockade
Organophosphorus compounds	Cholinesterase (irreversible)	Insecticide; anthelmintic
Acetazolamide	Carbonic anhydrase	Glaucoma (reduces intraocular pressure)
Allopurinol	Xanthine oxidase	Urate calculi (Dalmatian dog)
Tranylcypromine	Monoamine oxidase (MAO)	Antidepressant
Dorzolamide (ophthalmic)	Carbonic anhydrase	Glaucoma
Physostigmine (ophthalmic)	Cholinesterase (reversible)	Glaucoma
Demecarium (ophthalmic)	Cholinesterase (irreversible)	Glaucoma
Diclofenac (ophthalmic)	Cyclo-oxygenase	Pre-operative treatment for cataract extraction
Substances of toxicological significance: Monofluoro-acetate (*Dichapetalum cymosum*)	Aconitase (tricarboxylic acid, Krebs cycle)	No clinical uses Becomes incorporated into fluoroacetyl coenzyme A, which condenses with oxaloacetate to form fluorocitrate ('lethal synthesis')
Pteridium aquilinum	Thiaminase I	–
Dimethyl disulphide; *n*-Propyl disulphide (*Allium cepa*)	Glucose-6-phosphate dehydrogenase (G-6-PD)	–

[a] Phenylbutazone, flunixin, ketroprofen, naproxen have similar action to aspirin but individual NSAID differ in potency and degree of inhibition of cyclo-oxygenase isoforms.

of tissue damage; it catalyses the synthesis of eicosanoids (principally PGE_2) associated with the inflammatory response and fever. Release of the eicosanoids formed by COX-2 together with proteases and other inflammatory mediators (e.g. reactive oxygen radicals) results in inflammation. Reduction in serum thromboxane B_2, which is rapidly formed from thromboxane A_2, is a measure of inhibition of the COX-1 isoform, while decreased inflammatory exudate PGE_2 synthesis indicates inhibition of COX-2. Under experimental conditions, the concentrations of thromboxane B_2 and PGE_2 in serum and inflammatory exudate, respectively, can be measured by radio-immunoassay methods (Sedgwick & Lees, 1986).

Tissue damage stimulates the release of arachidonic acid which serves as substrate for the biosynthesis, catalysed by COX-2 and lipoygenase enzymes, of prostaglandins and leukotrienes. The anti-inflammatory action of glucocorticoids is non-selective in that they inhibit the activity of phospholipase A_2; as a consequence the release of arachidonic acid, which is normally bound in esterified form to cell membrane phospholipids (especially of phagocytes), is greatly reduced. Most currently used NSAIDs either non-selectively inhibit both the COX-1 and COX-2 isoforms of cyclo-oxygenase (naproxen, meloxicam, carprofen) or have modest selectivity for inhibition of the COX-1 isoform (aspirin, phenylbutazone, indomethacin, piroxicam, sulindac sulphide). Carprofen is a weak inhibitor of both isoforms of cyclo-oxygenase. Sulindac, a sulphoxide, is inactive *per se* (prodrug) and undergoes interconversion by hepatic metabolism with the sulphide metabolite, which is active. In contrast to aspirin which, through covalent modification, irreversibly inhibits cyclo-oxygenase, the majority of NSAIDs cause reversible inhibition of the enzyme. Platelets are especially susceptible to cyclo-oxygenase inhibition by aspirin as they have little or no capacity to regenerate the enzyme and consequently remain deprived of cyclo-oxygenase activity for the remainder of their lifespan, which is 8–10 days in humans. Nabumetone, a naphthylacetic acid prodrug, is converted to an active metabolite that is somewhat selective for COX-2 (Meade *et al.*, 1993). The introduction of relatively selective COX-2 inhibitors (nimesulide, rofecoxib) represents an advancement towards producing anti-inflammatory effects with reduced potential to cause gastric and renal side-effects. Wide inter- and intraspecies variations in the overall rate of elimination are a distinctive feature of NSAIDs. The half-lives of individual NSAIDs in horses are: salicylate (1 h), ketoprofen (1.25 h), meclofenamate (1.4 h), flunixin (1.9 h), phenylbutazone (4.1–4.7 h), tolfenamic acid (7.3 h), naproxen (8.3 h) and carprofen (18 h). The range of half-lives is even wider in cattle, from 0.8 h for salicylate to 55 h for phenylbutazone.

The 2-arylpropionic acid NSAIDs (the 'profens') possess a chiral centre at the carbon atom α to the carboxyl function, and it is known that the activity of these drugs resides in the $S(+)$ [*sinister*]-enantiomers while the $R(-)$ [*rectus*]-enantiomers either have low activity or are inactive (Shen, 1981). The NSAIDs of this subclass are formulated as racemic mixtures containing equal quantities of the two enantiomers, with the exception of naproxen which is commercially available as the S(+)-enantiomer. The S(+):R(-) eudismic (or potency) ratio for *in vitro* inhibition of prostaglandin or thromboxane synthesis varies with the drug and is more than 16 for carprofen, 133 for naproxen and 165 for ibuprofen (Evans, 1992). For most of these drugs metabolic inversion of the chiral centre of the R(-)-enantiomers to their S(+) antipodes occurs, but the extent of chiral inversion depends on the individual drug and varies among animal species. The S(+)-enantiomer (eutomer) of the 2-arylpropionic acid NSAIDs generally predominates in the plasma of human beings, while the enantiomer that predominates in plasma of other animal species varies with the drug. After separate intravenous administration of the individual enantiomers of a racemic drug with a single chiral centre, the enantiomeric ratio of the total areas under the plasma concentration–time curves and determination of the extent of chiral inversion are most useful for comparing disposition of the drug in different species. Areas under the curves are used for calculating systemic clearance of the individual enantiomers. A sensitive stereospecific analytical method is required for quantification of the enantiomers in plasma.

Because the organophosphorus compounds irreversibly inhibit acetylcholinesterase (AChE), the duration of their action is dependent upon the rate of biosynthesis of new (replacement) enzyme (AChE). The management of organophosphate toxicity requires the repeated administration of high doses of atropine. Following recent exposure and during the early stage of toxicity, repeated doses of pralidoxime or obidoxime, administered by slow intravenous injection, will hasten the otherwise slow recovery. The oxime regenerates cholinesterase (particularly AChE associated with skeletal neuromuscular junctions) by displacing the phosphate group from the esteratic site on the enzyme, provided the phosphorylated cholinesterase has not 'aged'. The repeated administration of pralidoxime (to regenerate cholinesterase) in conjunction with high doses of atropine (to competitively block the excessive effects of accumulated acetylcholine) provides antidotal treatment of organophosphate toxicity, particularly following recent exposure. The bispyridinium oxime H1–6, used in conjunction with atropine, could be effective for the treatment of poisoning caused by the highly toxic 'nerve gases' (soman, sarin and VX). This oxime is a powerful reactivator of 'unaged' phosphorylated cholinesterase.

Some poisonous plants (e.g. *Pteridium aquilinum, Allium cepa, Dichapetalum cymosum*) owe their toxicity to selective inhibition of enzymes. *D. cymosum* contains monofluoroacetate which *per se* is non-toxic, but is metabolically converted in the body to the highly toxic monofluorocitrate; a process called 'lethal synthesis' (Peters *et al.*, 1953). This change, which occurs in the tricarboxylic acid (Krebs) cycle, depends on fluoroacetate being sterically so similar to acetate that it is accepted by a series of enzymes and undergoes similar enzymatic changes until it becomes fluorocitrate. The toxic effect of fluorocitrate is due to irreversible inhibition of the enzyme aconitase which normally dehydrates citric acid to isocitric acid. The general inhibition of tissue oxidative energy metabolism with accumulation of citrate primarily affects the heart (the ruminant species and horses develop ventricular fibrillation) and central nervous system (dogs become convulsive and die of respiratory paralysis). Under certain circumstances therapeutic advantage can be taken of the process of lethal synthesis. Examples include the antineoplastic action of purine (mercaptopurine) and pyrimidine (fluorouracil and cytarabine) antagonists, the antifungal action of flucytosine, and the activity of acyclovir against susceptible herpes viruses.

As the induction of hepatic microsomal oxidative activity by a lipid-soluble drug (e.g. phenobarbitone) or xenobiotic could decrease the duration of action of therapeutic agents that are mainly eliminated by microsomal oxidation, the effect of induction would be considered a form of biochemical antagonism. Drug-induced inhibition of microsomal oxidative activity, without adjustment of dosage of a concomitantly administered therapeutic agent that undergoes extensive hepatic metabolism, could lead to toxicity. Cimetidine, ketoconazole and chloramphenicol inhibit hepatic microsomal enzyme activity.

Chemical antagonism

Chemical antagonism involves the binding of an active substance by an antagonist, thereby rendering the substance inactive. Protamine, a strongly basic low molecular weight protein that is positively charged at physiological pH, is a specific antagonist of heparin. Protamine sulphate, administered by slow intravenous injection to counteract overdosage with heparin, combines with heparin making it unavailable to exert its anticoagulant effect. Because protamine also interacts with platelets, fibrinogen and other plasma proteins, it may itself cause an anticoagulant effect if overdosed. The minimum amount of protamine required to neutralize the heparin present in the plasma should be administered: approximately 1 mg of protamine will neutralize 100 units of heparin, and the dose should be decreased by 50% for every hour that has elapsed since heparin was administered. The neutralization of excess gastric acid by an antacid substance, such as aluminium hydroxide or sodium bicarbonate, is another example of chemical antagonism.

Chelating agents are used in the antidotal treatment of heavy-metal toxicity. Examples include calcium disodium edetate ($CaNa_2EDTA$), which can be used for the treatment of poisoning by metals that have higher affinity for the chelating agent than does Ca^{2+}; D-penicillamine, copper and lead poisoning; deferoxamine, acute ferric iron toxicity; dimercaprol antagonizes the biological actions of metals that form mercaptides with essential cellular sulphydryl groups, and can be used principally for arsenic and mercury toxicity. Chelating agents (heavy-metal antagonists) are most effective when given shortly after exposure to the metal. A chelate is defined as a coordination complex formed between a metallic ion and a compound containing two or more potential ligands (donor of the electrons necessary to form coordinate covalent bonds with metallic ions). The usefulness of $CaNa_2$ EDTA in the treatment of lead poisoning is due, in part, to the capacity of lead (Pb^{2+}) to displace calcium

(Ca^{2+}) from EDTA in accordance with its 10^7-fold greater affinity for the chelate. Free lead ions are removed from the blood and tissues (directly from bone and indirectly from parenchymatous organs) as the soluble lead chelate formed is rapidly excreted by glomerular filtration. Because of its ionic character, it is unlikely that $CaNa_2EDTA$ significantly penetrates cells; the apparent volume of distribution is numerically similar to the extracellular fluid volume.

Physiological antagonism

Physiological antagonism occurs when two agonists, acting on different receptor types, counterbalance each other by producing opposite effects on the same physiological function. In general, the effects produced by a physiological antagonist are less specific and less easy to control than the effects produced by a pharmacological antagonist. The rationale for using adrenaline (epinephrine) injection in the initial management of acute anaphylactic reactions is to counterbalance the blood pressure lowering effect of histamine (caused mainly by activation of histamine H_1 receptors). Adrenaline, a mixed adrenoceptor agonist (activates α, β_1 and β_2 receptors), quickly reverses the precipitous fall in blood pressure by simultaneously producing peripheral vasoconstriction (α_1-mediated effect) and myocardial stimulation (β_1 effect); in addition, it causes relaxation of bronchial smooth muscle (β_2 effect). The essential feature of physiological antagonism is that opposite effects are produced by the substances that cause and reverse the physiological effect. An antihistaminic drug, H_1-receptor antagonist (e.g. diphenhydramine), may be useful for secondary treatment of anaphylaxis. In this case, pharmacological antagonism is the mechanism involved.

Doxapram (respiratory stimulant that activates peripheral aortic and carotid body chemoreceptors) behaves as a physiological antagonist when used to reverse central respiratory depression caused by barbiturates or inhalational anaesthetic agents.

Synergism

The term synergism refers to the situation in which the conjoint effect of two drugs greatly exceeds the algebraic sum of their individual effects. This type of interaction is mainly applied to chemotherapeutic agents. The drugs, administered either as a combination preparation or concomitantly, may act by complementary mechanisms at different sites, or one of the drugs (the synergist) potentiates the clinical efficacy of the other by altering its distribution (e.g. through plasma protein binding displacement), biotransformation or excretion. The synergistic antimicrobial effect produced by trimethoprim–sulphonamide combinations is due to the sequential blockade of successive steps in the bacterial biosynthetic pathway for folic acid. Other examples of drugs that act synergistically include pyrethrin–piperonyl butoxide (potentiated insecticidal efficacy of pyrethrin) and penicillin–probenecid (increased duration of effective penicillin concentrations). The concomitant use of flucytosine, adminis-tered orally, and amphotericin B, injected intravenously, has a dual basis in that amphotericin B potentiates the antifungal activity of flucytosine while flucy-tosine decreases the maintenance dosage and thereby the nephrotoxicity of amphotericin B. Flucytosine and rifampin are drugs that should always be used concurrently with another systemically-acting antifungal or antimicrobial agent, respectively, to prevent the rapid emergence of resistant mutants.

Antimicrobials and anthelmintics: selectivity and toxicity

The action of antimicrobial agents usually depends on the selective inhibition of biochemical events that occur in and are generally essential to microorgan-isms but not the host animal. Because their action is not confined to pathogenic microorganisms, the balance between the commensal flora can be adversely affected. Oral antimicrobial therapy may cause anorexia and mild-to-moderate diarrhoea in monogastric species. High doses of oral penicillins produce severe diarrhoea in horses. However, pivampicillin, which is hydrolysed to ampicillin in the intestinal mucosa during the absorption process, can safely be used in foals. The commensal flora in the colon of horses are particularly susceptible to disruption by antimicrobial agents. The koala, in common with the horse, is a monogastric hindgut fermenter that relies on microbial digestion of fibrous material in the diet. The fermentation process takes place in the expansive caecum of koalas and can be severely disrupted by various anti-microbial agents. The use of some antimicrobials (e.g. macrolides and linco-samides) is contra-indicated in horses, with the notable exception of oral erythromycin dosage forms in foals. The concomitant use of erythromycin and rifampin is indicated for the treatment of *Rhodococcus equi* pneumonia in foals, but coprophagic behaviour of mares housed with erythromycin-treated foals would lead to ingestion of antibiotic-resistant *Clostridium difficile* and ery-thromycin excreted by the foal and could cause acute colitis in the mare (Baverud *et al.*, 1998). Post-operative stress appears to increase the suscept-ibility of colonic flora to tetracyclines, often resulting in acute colitis. Because ionophore antibiotics are especially toxic to horses (the oral LD_{50} of monensin for horses is 2–3 mg/kg compared with LD_{50}s of 12 mg/kg for sheep and 16 mg/kg for pigs), the utmost care must be taken to prevent accidental incorporation of production enhancing substances into feed for horses. The toxicity of monensin and other ionophores is further increased by drugs that inhibit hepatic microsomal metabolic pathways, such as tiamulin and ery-thromycin. The caeca and rectum of the ostrich form large capacity fermenta-tion chambers in which production of short-chain fatty acids takes place (Skadhauge *et al.*, 1984; Swart *et al.*, 1993). Since this hindgut function resem-bles the digestion of fibrous material in the colon of the horse, the balance between the commensal flora would likely be adversely affected by macrolide and lincosamide antibiotics and by furazolidone. Orally administered anti-microbials can cause digestive disturbances, due to disruption of the ruminal microorganisms, in ruminant species. Some antimicrobials (e.g. chlor-amphenicol and its derivatives, and trimethoprim) are at least partly metabo-lized (inactivated) by ruminal microorganisms. Presystemic metabolism by ruminal microorganisms and by hepatic microsomal oxidative reactions may decrease oral bioavailability to an extent such that effective antimicrobial concentrations are not attained at the site of infection. In ruminant animals, intramuscular injection of parenteral (long-acting) preparations is the most common route of antimicrobial administration and has the advantage of avoiding presystemic metabolism.

Compared to other antimicrobials, diaminopyrimidines (e.g. pyr-imethamine, trimethoprim, baquiloprim) are relatively less selective in action against microorganisms because the enzyme (dihydrofolate reductase) inhib-ited is also present in mammalian cells. The safety of diaminopyrimidines is due to the fact that far higher concentrations would be required to inhibit dihydrofolate reductase in mammalian cells than in susceptible microorgan-isms. Diaminopyrimidines are generally used in combination with sulphona-mides (e.g. trimethoprim–sulphadiazine, trimethoprim–sulphamethoxazole, pyrimethamine–sulphadoxine) because, by blocking successive steps in the biosynthetic pathway for folic acid in microorganisms, their combined action is synergistic. Itraconazole is more selective in action than ketoconazole and is preferred for the treatment of fungal infections in cats.

Apart from a very occasional anaphylactic reaction, antimicrobial agents do not produce clinically observable pharmacological effects unless (acute reac-tion) or until toxicity is manifested. The latter is generally associated with multiple dosing that leads to drug accumulation and can be precipitated by the presence of a concurrent disease state, such as renal function impairment or hepatic dysfunction. Inherent dangers associated with the indiscriminate use of antimicrobials are the widespread development of bacterial resistance and the production of toxicity without premonitory signs.

It should always be borne in mind that there is no drug or drug preparation, with its quota of emulsifiers, solubilizers and stabilizers, that is not capable of causing adverse effects in some proportion of animals treated, no matter how small that proportion may be. Particularly when administered parenterally, penicillins and cephalosporins, due to the similarity of their active moieties, can induce acute anaphylaxis in sensitized individual animals. Far more common, particularly in horses, are central nervous system stimulation and cardiac depression, which can be fatal, produced by procaine following the inadvertent intravenous injection of procaine penicillin G. The too rapid intravenous injection of an antimicrobial preparation can produce an adverse reaction within minutes of administering the drug. Examples include potassium penicillin G (cardiac arrest; the sodium salt of penicillin G is far safer), aminoglycosides which, particularly when used in association with anaesthesia, can cause non-depolarizing (competitive) neuromuscular block-ade (acute skeletal muscular paralysis and apnoea), aminoglycosides and lincosamides (reduced cardiac output), tetracyclines (collapse due to cardio-vascular effects), and trimethoprim–sulphonamide combinations (respiratory failure in horses). Fluoroquinolones, administered by any route, can cause degeneration of articular cartilage in weight-bearing joints of rapidly growing large breeds of dog. This adverse effect could occur in foals and young horses, and fluoroquinolones have the potential to seriously disturb the balance between commensal microbial flora in the colon of the horse. While the more common adverse effects produced by sulphonamides in dogs are renal tubular damage and crystalluria associated with multiple dosing, Doberman Pinschers appear to be more susceptible than other breeds to idiosyncratic (could be hypersensitivity) reactions.

The nephrotoxic potential of aminoglycosides (neomycin > gentamicin, tobramycin and amikacin > kanamycin and streptomycin), amphotericin B (systemic antifungal drug), and the polymyxins (polymyxin B and colistimethate) are related to the dosage rate and duration of antimicrobial therapy with the drug as well as to the renal function status of the animal. When therapy with an aminoglycoside exceeds five days, renal function should be monitored and trough serum or plasma concentrations of the antibiotic measured. In the presence of impaired renal function, the dosage regimen should be adjusted (preferably by increasing the dosage interval in accordance with the decrease in glomerular filtration rate) to avoid drug accumulation with attendant toxic effects (acute tubular necrosis and cochlear damage in dogs or vestibular disturbance in cats). In dogs with decreased renal function (GFR < 3 mL/min·kg; in normal dogs, GFR = 4.07 ± 0.52 mL/min·kg), the reciprocal of serum creatinine concentration provides a clinically useful estimation of the glomerular filtration rate (Finco *et al.*, 1995) that could serve as a guide for dosage interval adjustment. The trough serum or plasma concentration of gentamicin should not be allowed to exceed 2 µg/mL. The concomitant use of furosemide and an aminoglycoside potentiates both the nephro- and ototoxicity of the antibiotic.

Even though amphotericin B (an amphoteric polyene antibiotic) has high nephrotoxic potential, the drug is indicated for the treatment of systemic fungal infections (*Blastomyces*, *Coccidioides*, *Histoplasma*) in dogs and cats, particularly immuno-compromised animals. Some degree of nephrotoxicity inevitably accompanies treatment with amphotericin B. To minimize the extent of renal damage, repeated dosing (by slow intravenous injection or preferably intravenous infusion) should be related to renal function of the animal (Prescott & Baggot, 1993), which must be monitored throughout the course of treatment. Should blood urea nitrogen (BUN) concentration exceed 1.5 times the pretreatment value at any time during treatment with amphotericin B, administration of the drug should be discontinued until the BUN concentration has returned to within the normal range for dogs (10–30 mg/dL). The concurrent use of flucytosine (tentatively 100 mg/kg given orally twice daily) and amphotericin B (0.3 mg/kg administered by slow intravenous injection once per day) may increase clinical efficacy and shorten the overall duration of amphotericin treatment.

As clinically effective alternative antimicrobial agents are available for the treatment of systemic infections caused by Gram-negative aerobic bacteria and because of the high nephrotoxicity of polymyxins (renal tubule epithelial cell damage), there remain few indications for their parenteral administration (by i.m. injection). Nephrotoxicity caused by polymyxins (polymyxin B sulphate and colistimethate sodium) may be due to their surfactant action on renal tubular cells, which is similar to their antibacterial action.

The use of parenteral preparations that cause irritation at intramuscular injection sites should be avoided as they are painful to the animal, are erratically absorbed and residual levels may persist at the injection site. The irritant nature of such preparations may be due either to the drug *per se* or other ingredients of the formulation, or to the pH reaction of the preparation. Even though the absolute bioavailability of clindamycin (as the phosphate), injected intramuscularly in the *quadriceps femoris* muscle mass of dogs, is 87 ± 19%, intramuscular administration cannot be recommended because of the apparent pain induced at the injection site (Budsberg *et al.*, 1992). Clindamycin hydrochloride (in capsules) can be given orally to dogs and cats, but never to horses (use metronidazole), for the treatment of staphylococcal and anaerobic infections of skin, soft tissue and bone. Because horses are particularly sensitive to injection site damage, drug preparations that cause tissue irritation, which include drugs in an oil vehicle, should not be administered to horses, ponies or donkeys.

Anthelmintic drugs have a relatively selective action on helminth parasites in the host animal. To produce activity, an anthelmintic must reach and combine with a receptor site in the parasite; the interruption of a life-requiring function in a concentration- and/or time-dependent manner is the outcome of the drug–receptor interaction. Selectivity of action of anthelmintics refers to the production of toxicity (either lethal effect or inability to survive) in the helminth parasite and depends on the drug receptor being either unique to the parasite or considerably more sensitive (i.e. has much higher affinity for the drug) than a similar type of receptor in the host animal. It is broadly reflected in the margin of safety of an anthelmintic when the dosage form is administered by the recommended route. Apart from organophosphorus compounds (irreversible inhibition of cholinesterase enzymes), levamisole (depolarization of nicotinic receptors) and amitraz (seemingly α_2-adrenoceptor stimulation), the commonly used anthelmintics and insecticides do not normally produce pharmacological effects. Animal species differ in sensitivity to the effects produced by organophosphorus compounds and by levamisole (horses, dogs and cats are more sensitive than other species), while the application of amitraz (ectoparasiticide) to horses and cats is contra-indicated. As fish are unable to detoxify thiophosphate insecticides, contamination of water in rivers and lakes can devastate freshwater fish populations.

While broad spectrum anthelmintics (macrolide endectocides, benzimidazole carbamates, tetrahydropyrimidines) largely overlap in the range of endoparasites (mainly nematodes) they affect, the various anthelmintic classes (based on chemical structure) differ in mechanism of action, degree of activity and in pharmacokinetic properties (bioavailability, tissue distribution and process of elimination). The macrolide endectocides (avermectins and milbe-mycins) are unique in that anthelmintic efficacy is produced at very low doses and they are active against both arthropod and nematode parasites. The dosage form of an anthelmintic determines the route of administration, which largely influences the bioavailability of the drug and the duration of anthelmintic activity. A relationship between plasma concentration of the active moiety (parent drug and/or active metabolite) and clinical efficacy has been estab-lished for most anthelmintic classes; ivermectin (avermectin), albendazole and fenbendazole (benzimidazole carbamates), levamisole (imidazothiazole), diethylcarbamazine (piperazine), clorsulon (benzenedisulphonamide) and closantel (salicylanilide). With the notable exception of macrolide endectocides, species variations in pharmacokinetic properties of broad spectrum anthel-mintics may largely contribute to differences between these drugs in dosage requirement and clinical efficacy. As the benzimidazole anthelmintics undergo extensive hepatic biotransformation, the activity of oxidative enzymes influ-ences their oral bioavailability, rate of elimination and, ultimately, their clinical efficacy. Probenzimidazoles (netobimin and febantel) are dependent on oxidation for their activation. Triclabendazole (flukicide) is completely meta-bolized (first-pass effect) to the active sulphoxide metabolite. The low oral bioavailability of tetrahydropyrimidines (pyrantel in horses, dogs and cats; morantel in ruminant species) limits their clinical efficacy to adult and larval nematodes that are within the gastrointestinal tract. Regardless of the route of administration (oral, subcutaneous injection in ruminant species, in the feed or by subcutaneous injection in the lateral neck of pigs, topical application), ivermectin distributes widely in tissues, apart from the central nervous system, and is slowly eliminated (mainly unchanged) in the bile.

Narrow spectrum anthelmintics refers to drugs that have clinical efficacy for a limited range of economically important parasite species. Examples include piperazine salts (active against some gastrointestinal nematodes in monogastric species), praziquantel (cestodes in dogs and cats), salicylanilides, nitroxynil and clorsulon (trematodes in ruminant species), and triclabendazole (immature and adult *Fasciola* in ruminant species and Equidae). Following oral or intra-muscular administration, praziquantel is well absorbed into the systemic cir-culation and distributes widely in tissues of the body. Widespread distribution is an asset in that activity is produced against adult and larval cestodes. Because of rapid metabolism by the liver, praziquantel has a short duration of action. Oral combination preparations containing praziquantel–pyrantel and febantel–praziquantel–pyrantel are available for use in dogs and cats. These combination preparations provide a broad spectrum of anthelmintic activity.

The salicylanilides (closantel, oxyclozanide and rafoxanide), formulated as oral suspensions, are slowly but well absorbed in ruminant species, have limited extravascular distribution (due to extensive binding to plasma proteins) and are slowly eliminated by excretion in the bile. The difference in clinical efficacy between these drugs appears to be related to the rate of elimination in that oxyclozanide, which has the shortest half-life, is active only against adult trematodes (principally *Fasciola hepatica*). The longer half-life of closantel and rafoxanide might account for their greater efficacy. Nitroxynil, administered by subcutaneous injection to ruminant animals, is partly converted by the liver to an active metabolite and, due to extensive binding to plasma proteins, both the parent drug and metabolite formed are slowly excreted in the bile. The clinical efficacy of nitroxynil may be related to the duration of effective plasma concentrations of the active moieties. Because of metabolic inactivation (reduction of the nitro group in the molecule) by ruminal microorganisms, nitroxynil would be ineffective if administered orally.

Clorsulon, administered orally as a drench to ruminant animals, is active against adult liver fluke (*F. hepatica*). The oral bioavailability of the drug is approximately 55% in goats and 60% in sheep. Extensive binding to plasma proteins and avid binding to carbonic anhydrase in erythrocytes retain the drug within the circulating blood and greatly limit extravascular distribution. The ingestion of blood by adult flukes exposes the parasite to high concentrations of clorsulon. In sheep, the apparent half-life of clorsulon (1 day) is much shorter than that of oxyclozanide (6.4 days), closantel (14.5 days) and rafoxanide (16.6 days). It could be the shorter persistence in blood of clorsulon than of salicylanilides (particularly closantel and rafoxanide) that largely limits the activity of clorsulon to adult *F. hepatica*. A parenteral combination preparation containing clorsulon and ivermectin for administration by subcutaneous injection to cattle is available; the withdrawal period is 28 days.

Pyrethrins and synthetic pyrethroids are among the safest of the topically applied ectoparasiticides, because of their selective toxicity for insects (mammalian-to-insect toxic dose ratio is greater than 1000, compared with 33 for organophosphates and 16 for carbamate insecticides). In contrast to the very wide margin of safety for mammalian species, pyrethroids are toxic to fish. The synergistic action of pyrethrins and piperonyl butoxide (in combination preparations) is due to the inhibition by piperonyl butoxide of the microsomal enzyme system of some arthropods. Preparations of synthetic pyrethroids (permethrin, cypermethrin) often contain a mixture of drug isomers in varying proportions.

Implications of stereoisomerism

Stereoisomerism arises from the occurrence within drug molecules of chiral centres. The number of possible stereoisomers is 2^n, where n is the number (usually unity) of chiral centres. A substantial proportion of the commonly used synthetic drugs contain one or more chiral centres and are commercially available as preparations (dosage forms) containing racemates. Drug preparations containing racemic mixtures have been described as combinations of active drug plus isomeric ballast when one enantiomer produces little or no therapeutic effect (Ariens, 1986). The eudismic or potency ratio is defined as the ratio of the doses (*in vivo* studies) or the concentrations (*in vitro* studies) producing effects of the same intensity. Stereoisomerism has implications in the formulating of dosage forms and, as a chiral environment exists within the body, in determining both the degree of activity and the disposition of race-mates. The dissolution rates of individual enantiomers can differ in a formulation containing a racemic drug and a chiral excipient (e.g. cyclodextrins, cellulose derivatives, phospholipids, ascorbic acid, anhydrous dextrose) (Tomaszewski & Rumore, 1994). Following the administration of a racemic drug with a single chiral centre, the initial 50:50 enantiomeric ratio may continually change in one direction to other ratios that can vary among animal species. The changing proportion assumes clinical significance when the individual enantiomers substantially differ in pharmacodynamic activity (maximal effect, plasma enantiomer concentration that produces 50% of maximal effect) and/or pharmacokinetic behaviour (half-life, systemic clearance, volume of distribution, systemic availability). A racemic mixture containing two enantiomers in equal proportion (50:50) is, in essence, a combination of equal amounts of two drugs that generally produce the same range of pharmacological effects but usually differ in potency (expressed as the eudismic ratio). Examples of racemic drugs for which the enantiomers differ in pharmacodynamic activity are presented in Table 4.6. The more potent enantiomer

Table 4.6 Racemic drugs for which enantiomers differ in pharmacodynamic activity.

Drug	More active enantiomer (eutomer)
Pentobarbital	$S(-)$-enantiomer
Ketamine	$S(+)$-enantiomer
Isoflurane	$(+)$-enantiomer
Morphine (opioids)	$(-)$-enantiomer (analgesic)
	$(+)$-enantiomer (antitussive)
Ketoprofen	$S(+)$-enantiomer
Carprofen	$S(+)$-enantiomer
Ibuprofen	$S(+)$-enantiomer
Naproxen	$S(+)$-enantiomer
Propranolol	$S(-)$-enantiomer
Metroprolol	$S(-)$-enantiomer
Atenolol	$S(-)$-enantiomer
Dobutamine	$(+)$-enantiomer
Captopril	$S(-)$-enantiomer
Verapamil	$S(-)$-enantiomer
Warfarin	$S(-)$-enantiomer
Chlorpheniramine	$S(+)$-enantiomer
Disopyramide	$S(+)$-enantiomer
Amphetamine	*d*-isomer (CNS)
	l > *d*-isomer (CV system)
Cloprostenol	*d*-isomer

is referred to as the eutomer and the other enantiomer as the distomer. The S (*sinister*): R (*rectus*) potency ratio for naproxen, for example, is 133 for *in vitro* inhibition of prostaglandin or thromboxane synthesis, and 28 or 15 for *in vivo* activity depending on the test used for measurement of activity (Evans, 1992). The enantioselective behaviour of drugs used in domestic animals was comprehensively reviewed by Landoni *et al.* (1997). This discussion will focus on the pharmacokinetic behaviour of some chiral drugs.

The occurrence of enantioselective discrimination in drug absorption, distribution, biotransformation and excretion depends on the mechanism of the process. Absorption, extravascular distribution *per se*, passage from the systemic circulation into transcellular fluids and milk, glomerular filtration and renal tubular reabsorption are passive (diffusion) processes that generally do not differentiate between enantiomers. Carrier-mediated renal tubular secretion and transport into bile are likely to be stereoselective processes, but this has not yet been established. The elimination of atenolol, which takes place mainly by renal excretion, may be enantioselective, although the plasma concentration profiles for the $S(-)$- and $R(+)$-enantiomers are similar (Mehvar *et al.*, 1990). The extent of binding to plasma and tissue proteins, and particularly biotransformation reactions are generally stereoselective (Caldwell *et al.*, 1988; Tucker & Lennard, 1990). Stereoselective protein binding could lead to differences between enantiomers in volume of distribution and, consequently, half-life. In the assessment of volume of distribution differences, the use of $V_{d(ss)}$ would be preferable to $V_{d(area)}$. Stereoselective biotransformation would cause differences between enantiomers in systemic clearance and, depending on whether protein binding differs, in half-life. Blood and/or plasma concentrations and pharmacokinetic parameters based on measurement of racemate concentrations often do not reflect those of the active enantiomer (eutomer).

The influence of stereoselective hepatic biotransformation, especially microsomal-mediated oxidative reactions and glucuronide conjugation, on the elimination of extensively metabolized chiral drugs can be related to the distinction between drugs with low and those with high hepatic intrinsic clearances (Walle & Walle, 1986). The hepatic intrinsic clearance reflects solely the inherent ability of the liver to remove a drug from the blood (Wilkinson & Shand, 1975). For drugs with low hepatic intrinsic clearance (such as hexobarbital), the intravenous and oral clearances will be affected similarly by stereoselective hepatic metabolism, with a proportional enantiomeric difference in half-lives. For drugs with high hepatic intrinsic clearance (e.g. propranolol, verapamil), the intravenous clearance and the elimination half-life will not express great stereoselectivity, as both of these parameters are only to a small extent dependent on the activity of drug-metabolizing enzymes. The main difference between the enantiomers for this type of drug will be reflected in the oral clearance and bioavailability (Walle & Walle, 1986).

Because stereoselective processes are species-related, the enantiomeric ratios of plasma concentrations at various times and areas under the plasma concentration–time curves may differ between animal species following the administration of a drug racemate. Chiral inversion, which occurs to a variable extent in different species, can be equivocally established only by administering individual enantiomers to the animal species of interest and measuring, using a sensitive stereospecific analytical method, the enantiomer administered and the optical antipode in biological fluids and tissues. The pharmacokinetic parameters based on plasma concentration–time data for each of the enantiomers can be statistically compared.

The 2-arylpropionic acid ('profen') NSAIDs, each of which contains a single chiral centre, are formulated as racemic (50:50) mixtures of the S(+) and R(−)-enantiomers, with the exception of naproxen which is formulated as the S(+) enantiomer. Based on inhibition of cyclo-oxygenase activity, the S(+)-enantiomer is the eutomer. These drugs differ markedly both in pharmacodynamic activity and pharmacokinetic behaviour and, in addition, enantiomer pharmacokinetics of each drug vary among animal species. Following intravenous administration of racemic ketoprofen to horses, sheep and 20-week-old calves and measurement of individual enantiomers in plasma, significant differences between the enantiomers were found in systemic clearance in horses and in both systemic clearance and volume of distribution in sheep (Table 4.7), while values of the pharmacokinetic parameters in calves did not differ between the enantiomers (Landoni & Lees, 1995a; Jaussaud *et al.*, 1993; Landoni *et al.*, 1995, 1999). The predominant enantiomer in plasma was S(+) in horses, R(−) in sheep, and both enantiomers were present in equal concentrations in calves. The S(+)-to-R(−) ratio of area under the curve (AUC) was 1.35:1 in horses, 0.54:1 in sheep, and 1.05:1 in calves. Following the administration of each enantiomer separately to these species, the extent of chiral inversion from the R(−)- to S(+)-enantiomer was estimated to be 31% in calves, 49% in horses and 5.9% in sheep (Landoni & Lees, 1995b, 1996; Landoni *et al.*, 1999). Unidirectional

Table 4.7 Pharmacokinetic parameters describing disposition of S(+)- and R(−)-enantiomers following intravenous administration of racemic ketoprofen (KTP) to horses (n = 6) and sheep (n = 6). Values are expressed as mean ± SEM.

Pharmacokinetic parameter	Horses[a]		Sheep[b]	
	S(+)-KTP	R(−)-KTP	S(+)-KTP	R(−)-KTP
$t_{1/2\,(\alpha)}$ (h)	0.13 ± 0.03	0.10 ± 0.02	0.14 ± 0.01	0.13 ± 0.03
$t_{1/2\,(\beta)}$ (h)	1.51 ± 0.45	1.09 ± 0.19	0.86 ± 0.08	0.87 ± 0.10
V_d (mL/kg)	491 ± 206	472 ± 146	256 ± 21	168 ± 15[c]
Cl_B (mL/h · kg)	202 ± 22	277 ± 35[c]	351 ± 50	196 ± 32[c]
MRT (h)	2.23 ± 0.15	2.63 ± 0.33	0.79 ± 0.11	0.95 ± 0.13
AUC (µg · h/mL)	5.67 ± 0.47	4.19 ± 0.37[c]	4.74 ± 0.71	8.73 ± 1.22[c]

[a] Data from Landoni & Lees (1995a).
[b] Data from Landoni *et al.* (1999).
[c] Level of significance, P < 0.05.

chiral inversion was estimated to be 49% in Cynomolgus monkeys (*Macaca fascicularis*) (Mauleon *et al.*, 1994), 9% in humans (Rudy *et al.*, 1998) and varied from 27% to 66% in laboratory animal species (Aberg *et al.*, 1995). The oral bioavailability of the S(+)-enantiomer of ketoprofen in Beagle dogs is not affected by the proportion of the R(−)-enantiomer in the oral dosage form, even though considerable (73%) metabolic inversion from the R(−) to the S(+)-enantiomer occurs in dogs (Garcia *et al.*, 1998).

It is usual in humans for the S(+)-enantiomer of 2-arylpropionic acids to predominate in plasma and for the S(+)-to-R(−)-enantiomeric ratio of plasma concentrations to increase with time after administration of the racemate, which is often attributed to metabolic inversion of the chiral centre of the R(−)-enantiomers to their S(+) antipodes (Hutt & Caldwell, 1984). In humans the S(+)- enantiomer is generally eliminated more slowly than the R(−)-enantiomer. The extent of chiral inversion of fenoprofen, which has been attributed to the differential rate of the CoA-thioester by hepatic microsomes (Soraci *et al.*, 1995; Soraci & Benoit, 1996), varies widely among species. It has been estimated to be 90% in dogs (Benoit *et al.*, 1994), 80% in sheep (Soraci *et al.*, 1995), 73% in rabbits (Hayball & Meffin, 1987), 60% in man (Rubin *et al.*, 1985), 42% in rats (Berry & Jamali, 1991), and 38% in horses (Benoit *et al.*, 1994).

Carprofen, a weak inhibitor of cyclo-oxygenase but which produces a significant antioedematous effect in dogs (McKellar *et al.*, 1994) and horses (Lees *et al.*, 1994) and, like fenoprofen, has potent antiplatelet aggregating properties (*in vitro S:R* eudismic ratio > 24), does not appear to undergo chiral inversion in either direction in horses, calves, dogs, cats and humans. Following intravenous or oral administration of racemic carprofen, which contains a 50:50 mixture of the enantiomers, to horses (i.v.), 8–10-week-old calves (i.v.), cats (i.v.) and dogs (p.o.), the R(−)-enantiomer predominated in the plasma and the R(−)-to-S(+) enantiomeric ratio of plasma concentrations increased with time after administration of the racemate. The increasing R(−)-to-S(+) enantiomeric ratio of plasma concentrations with time can be attributed to stereoselective hepatic metabolism, although stereoselective binding to plasma albumin could contribute. In calves both the systemic clearance and volume of distribution of the R(−)-enantiomer were significantly lower than for the S(+)-enantiomer (Delatour *et al.*, 1996), while in cats the systemic clearance of the R(−)-enantiomer was significantly lower and the volume of distribution was lower though not significantly (Taylor *et al.*, 1996). The R(−)-to-S(+) ratio of area under the plasma concentration–time curve (AUC) was 4.5:1 in horses (Lees *et al.*, 1991), 2:1 in cats (Taylor *et al.*, 1996); 1.8:1 in dogs (McKellar *et al.*, 1994), and 1.4:1 in calves (Delatour *et al.*, 1996) following administration of racemic carprofen. A contrasting situation to that which occurs in domestic animals was found in rats and humans, in that the S(+)-enantiomer predominated in plasma and the R(−)-to-S(+) enantiomeric ratio of plasma concentrations decreased (although only slightly in humans) with time after administration of the racemate (Kemmerer *et al.*, 1979; Stoltenberg *et al.*, 1981). AUC enantiomeric ratios in rats and humans were not determined. Caution must be exercised when interpreting pharmacokinetic parameters and calculating dosage of chiral drugs based on plasma concentration–time data that relate to measurement of total (racemic) drug. The half-lives of racemic carprofen in domestic animals are longer than those of the $S(+)$-enantiomer, at least when administered as a racemate. Enantioselective disposition influences the plasma concentration profiles and pharmacokinetic parameters of the enantiomers. Evidence for chiral inversion is obtained by administering individual enantiomers separately and measuring, using a stereoselective analytical method, the enantiomer administered and optical antipode in plasma usually.

Ketamine, which is present in the commercially available preparation as a 50:50 mixture of the $S(+)$- and $R(-)$-enantiomers, is metabolized by hepatic microsomal N-demethylation to the corresponding norketamine (metabolite I) enantiomers. Based on the reported eudismic ratio of $S(+)$-to-$R(-)$ ketamine enantiomers of 2.9:1 and the observed duration of unconsciousness in dogs, the equi-anaesthetic activity provided by 10 mg/kg of racemic ketamine and 6.6 mg/kg of the $S(+)$-enantiomer in Beagle dogs, and the plasma enantiomer concentrations in humans at the time of emergence from anaesthesia, which are 0.5 μg/mL ($S(+)$) and 1.7 μg/mL ($R(-)$), it can be concluded that the $S(+)$-enantiomer is three times more active than the $R(-)$-enantiomer (White *et al.*, 1980; Deleforge *et al.*, 1991; Muir & Hubbell, 1988). Following intravenous injection of racemic ketamine, the $S(+)$-enantiomer of norketamine predominated in the plasma of horses (Delatour *et al.*, 1991a) and dogs (Deleforge *et al.*, 1991). This could be attributed to stereoselective N-demethylation. As the disposition of the individual enantiomers administered separately has not been studied, comment cannot be made regarding the extent of chiral inversion. Systemic clearances of racemic ketamine are 15 mL/min·kg, 28 mL/min·kg and 29 mL/min·kg in humans, horses and dogs, respectively.

Verapamil (calcium channel blocking drug) is administered (usually orally) as a racemic mixture containing equal amounts of $S(-)$-enantiomer and $R(+)$-enantiomer. The range of therapeutic plasma concentrations of racemic verapamil is 80–320 ng/mL. The enantiomers differ considerably in pharmacological activity (negative dromotropic effect on atrioventricular conduction), with $S(-)$-verapamil being 10–20 times more potent than $R(+)$-verapamil in humans (Echizen *et al.*, 1988) and dogs (Satoh *et al.*, 1980). When administered orally verapamil undergoes extensive first-pass metabolism; the $S(-)$-enantiomer is preferentially metabolized leading to predominance of the $R(+)$-enantiomer (distomer) in plasma (Echizen *et al.*, 1985). After oral administration of racemic verapamil to mongrel dogs, the oral clearance, which reflects first-pass hepatic elimination, of $S(-)$-verapamil was over 20 times that of the $R(+)$-enantiomer (Bai *et al.*, 1993). This resulted in a 14-fold difference between the enantiomers in oral bioavailability, which was 1.5% for the $S(-)$-enantiomer and 21% for the $R(+)$-enantiomer. In humans, the differences between the enantiomers in oral clearance (4.9-fold) and oral bioavailability (2.4-fold) are qualitatively similar but quantitatively less pronounced than in dogs (Mikus *et al.*, 1990). The apparent half-life of the two enantiomers was similar in dogs

($S(-)$-verapamil, 2 h; $R(+)$-verapamil, 2.2 h) and in humans ($S(-)$-verapamil, 8.2 h; $R(+)$-verapamil, 8.1 h). Following intravenous administration of racemic verapamil to dogs, both the volume of distribution and systemic clearance of the $S(-)$-enantiomer were approximately 1.5 times higher than for the $R(+)$-enantiomer: the differences were statistically significant for both parameters. The half-life (mean $\pm$ SD, $n = 6$) did not differ between the enantiomers ($S(-)$-verapamil, 2.7 $\pm$ 0.73 h; $R(+)$-verapamil, 2.35 $\pm$ 0.55 h). A similar pattern of enantioselective disposition of verapamil applies to humans (Eichelbaum *et al.*, 1984). The difference between the enantiomers in volume of distribution can be attributed to the difference in extent of plasma protein (α_1-acid glycoprotein) binding in humans ($S(-)$-enantiomer, 88%; $R(+)$-enantiomer, 94%), which represents a twofold difference in the free fraction in plasma, whereas it appears to be mainly due to stereoselective tissue binding in dogs, as plasma protein binding was lower in dogs ($S(-)$-enantiomer, 68%; $R(+)$-enantiomer, 72%) and the difference in the free fraction of less consequence. Oral bioavailability of racemic verapamil in dogs is 15% and the apparent half-life of the racemate is 2.5 h (Bai *et al.*, 1993).

The $S(-)$-enantiomer of propranolol is about 100 times more potent as a β-adrenoceptor antagonist than the $R(+)$-enantiomer, and is believed to be largely responsible for the clinical effects produced by the racemic drug. After oral administration of racemic propranolol to humans and dogs, the ratios of area under the plasma concentration–time curves for $S(-)$-to-$R(+)$ propranolol and for $S(-)$-to-$R(+)$ propranolol glucuronide were 1.4 and 3.4, respectively, in humans, and 0.5 and 3.1, respectively, in dogs (Silber & Riegelman, 1980). These results show that oral bioavailability of $S(-)$-propranolol (eutomer) is 1.4 times higher than for its optical antipode in humans, whereas oral bioavailability of the eutomer is 50% of that for $R(+)$-propranolol (distomer) in dogs. It follows that the stereoselectivity of first-pass hepatic microsomal oxidation of propranolol is opposite in humans and dogs. The route-dependent difference in response at equal plasma concentrations of racemic propranolol in humans can be attributed to the higher oral bioavailability and lower oral clearance of the $S(-)$-enantiomer. The range of therapeutic plasma concentrations of racemic propranolol is 20–80 ng/mL. Oral bioavailability of racemic propranolol in dogs is 2–17% and the apparent half-life of the racemate is 1.1 h (Kates *et al.*, 1979). Because of low oral bioavailability and stereoselective first-pass metabolism, the use of an oral dosage form containing $S(-)$-propranolol only is indicated especially for dogs.

Albendazole and fenbendazole, prochiral sulphide benzimidazole anthelmintics, are metabolically converted (sulphoxidation) to the corresponding active sulphoxide metabolites, each of which exists in the plasma as two enantiomers. Sulphoxide benzimidazoles have a chiral centre around the sulphur atom in their molecules. The sulphoxide metabolites (enantiomers) are irreversibly metabolized (sulphonation) to inactive sulphones. This pathway of hepatic biotransformation has been shown to occur both in ruminant (sheep, goats, cattle) and monogastric (man, dogs, rats) species (Delatour *et al.*, 1991b, c). A flavin-containing mono-oxygenase could be responsible for catalysing the initial oxidative reaction (sulphoxidation) (Galtier *et al.*, 1986), whereas cytochrome P450 mono-oxygenase (mixed function oxidase) is responsible for sulphonation (Souhali El Amri *et al.*, 1988). After oral administration of fenbendazole to sheep, the rate of evolution of the enantiomeric ratio was 0.2%/h, while after orally administered albendazole it was 0.6%/h. Consequently, the plasma enantiomeric concentration ratio differs between fenbendazole sulphoxide (oxfendazole) and albendazole sulphoxide, and for both enantiomers changes in the same direction with time. The ratio of fenbendazole sulphoxide (+) to (−) enantiomers changed from 1.8:1 at 3 h to 6.7:1 at 120 h, while for albendazole sulphoxide enantiomers the plasma concentration ratio changed from 3.3:1 at 3 h to 24:1 at 120 h. AUC enantiomeric ratios were 2.85:1 for fenbendazole sulphoxide and 6.1:1 for albendazole sulphoxide (Delatour *et al.*, 1990a, b). The difference between the enantiomeric ratios of fenbendazole sulphoxide and albendazole sulphoxide is probably due to stereoselective cytochrome P450-mediated sulphonation.

   After oral administration of albendazole (parent drug) there are marked species differences in the disposition of albendazole sulphoxide enantiomers. The plasma enantiomeric concentration ratios (+) to (−) increased linearly with time in man and dogs, but decreased in rats. The (+)-enantiomer represented 80%, 70% and 41% of the area under the plasma concentration–time curve for total albendazole sulphoxide in man, dogs and rats, respectively (Delatour *et al.*, 1991c). The (+)-enantiomer predominated in plasma of sheep, goats and cattle, and represented 86%, 80% and 91%, respectively, of the AUC for total albendazole sulphoxide (Delatour *et al.*, 1991b). The relative anthelmintic activity (eudismic ratio) of the sulphoxide enantiomers of albendazole and fenbendazole is not known at the present time; it could influence the anthelmintic efficacy of both the parent drugs and the prodrugs netobimin (which is converted to albendazole) and febantel (which is converted to fenbendazole). Whether chiral inversion occurs and to what extent in various species remain to be determined.

   In another study it was found that the ratios of (+) to (−) enantiomers of albendazole sulphoxide changed in goats after the administration of albendazole on each of three successive occasions at 24-h intervals. The predominant (+)-enantiomer represented 76%, 91% and 92% of the AUC for total albendazole sulphoxide on occasions 1, 2 and 3, respectively (Benoit *et al.*, 1992). The change in enantiomer proportions could be attributable to induction of drug-metabolizing enzymes. The enantioselectivity of the enzymes responsible for sulphoxidation (flavin-containing mono-oxygenase) and for sulphonation (cytochrome P450 mono-oxygenase) are different, in that the flavin mono-oxygenase produces the (+)-sulphoxide enantiomer whereas the cytochrome P450 mono-oxygenase specifically uses the (−)-sulphoxide enantiomer as substrate. The cytochrome system is induced by albendazole whereas the flavin system is not. Consequently, on repeated administration of the parent sulphide, the plasma concentration ratio of (+) to (−) sulphoxide enantiomers at time zero (obtained by back-extrapolation) increased from approximately 1.5:1 on the first occasion to 3.5:1 and 4.9:1 on the second and third occasions, respectively (Benoit *et al.*, 1992).

The *d* (dextro), *l* (laevo) designation applied to isomers relates to rotation of polarized light, which depends on electronic properties around the chiral atom, while the *R*, *S* classification depends on mass assignments around the chiral atom. Levamisole, an anthelmintic and 'immuno-stimulant' drug is the *l*-isomer of the racemate *dl*-tetramisole. Because anthelmintic activity resides almost entirely in the *l*-isomer and the isomers are equally toxic, preparations of levamisole have a relatively wider margin of safety than tetramisole preparations. Levamisole is indicated for use as an anthelmintic (oral solution, parenteral solution for administration by subcutaenous injection, 'pour-on' solution for cattle) in cattle and sheep but not in goats, and, with caution, as an immunostimulant (oral solution) to restore depressed T-cell function in horses and dogs. Dextropropoxyphene is an analgesic drug while its mirror-image isomer, levopropoxyphene, is an antitussive agent devoid of analgesic activity.

Synthetic pyrethroids are geometric isomers with *cis*, *trans* configurations. Commercially available preparations of cypermethrin contain a mixture of *cis* and *trans* isomers in various proportions, for example, 60:40 and 80:20. Cypermethrin (*cis:trans* 60:40) 2.5% solution is equivalent to cypermethrin (*cis:trans* 80:20) 1.25% solution for 'pour-on' application to sheep. Permethrin, which is the active ingredient incorporated in ear tags for cattle and insecticidal collars for dogs and cats, contains a mixture of *cis* and *trans* isomers in the proportion 40:60.

Whether a racemate or an enantiomer of a chiral drug should be used in formulating dosage forms depends on the relative pharmacodynamic activity (eudismic ratio) and the potential toxicity (or side-effects produced) of the individual enantiomers, their pharmacokinetic profiles and, importantly, the proportions formed over time in the target animal species. Binding to plasma and tissue proteins, hepatic microsomal oxidative reactions and probably glucuronide conjugation and carrier-mediated excretion processes are stereoselective and vary among animal species. First-pass metabolism may influence oral bioavailability of the enantiomers of chiral drugs that are highly extracted by the liver and administered as racemic mixtures. When both enantiomers of a drug with a single chiral centre show distinct and desirable effects (e.g. most opioids, dobutamine, bupivacaine), even though they differ in pharmacodynamic activity, or when their action and the effects produced are not stereoselective, the formulating of racemic mixtures may be entirely justifiable (Caldwell, 1992). Nonetheless, because of species variations, pharmacokinetic profiles of the individual enantiomers should be determined using stereospecific analytical methods (Foster & Jamali, 1987; Delatour *et al.*, 1991b; Pasutto, 1992; Carr *et al.*, 1992) to calculate optimum dosage for the various animal species. Use of the more active enantiomer (eutomer) in formulating dosage forms should be considered when the enantiomers differ widely in pharmacodynamic activity (e.g. $S(-)$-propranolol, the $S(+)$-enantiomer of the

2-arylpropionic acid NSAIDs, *d*-propoxyphene) or toxic potential (levamisole rather than tetramisole). To selectively produce a certain effect a distomer (less potent enantiomer) could be formulated as a particular dosage form, e.g. *R*(+)-timolol as eye drops to reduce intraocular pressure (glaucoma), *R*(+)-verapamil as a parenteral or oral dosage form for the treatment of angina (Drayer, 1986). The use of an enantiomer, a single chemical entity, would increase selectivity of action, reduce total exposure to the racemate, and simplify dose–response relationships. Whenever an enantiomer is used in formulating dosage forms, it must be optically pure. Bioequivalence assessment of a generic drug preparation requires that the generic preparation contain the racemic drug or the enantiomer corresponding to whichever is present in the innovator (reference) dosage form.

References

Aberg, G., Ciofalo, V.B., Pendleton, R.G., Ray, G. & Weddle, D. (1995) Inversion of (*R*)- to (*S*)-ketoprofen in eight animal species. *Chirality* **7**, 383–387.

Ariens, E.J. (1986) Chirality in bioactive agents and its pitfalls. *Trends in Pharmacological Sciences*, **7**, 200–205.

Baggot, J.D. (1977) *Principles of Drug Disposition in Domestic Animals: The Basis of Veterinary Clinical Pharmacology*, pp. 190–218. W.B. Saunders, Philadelphia.

Bai, S.A., Lankford, S.M. & Johnson, L.M. (1993) Pharmacokinetics of the enantiomers of verapamil in the dog. *Chirality*, **5**, 436–442.

Baverud, V., Franklin, A., Gunnarsson, A., Gustafsson, A. & Hellander-Edman, A. (1998) *Clostridium difficile* associated with acute colitis in mares when their foals are treated with erythromycin and rifampin for *Rhodococcus equi* pneumonia. *Equine Veterinary Journal*, **30**, 482–488.

Benoit, E., Besse, S. & Delatour, P. (1992) Effect of repeated doses of albendazole on enantiomerism of its sulfoxide metabolite in goats. *American Journal of Veterinary Research*, **53**, 1663–1665.

Benoit, E., Soraci, A. & Delatour, P. (1994) Chiral inversion as a parameter for inter-species and intercompound discrepancies in enantiospecific pharmacokinetics. *6th International Congress of the European Association for Veterinary Pharmacology and Toxicology*, Edinburgh. Blackwell Science, Oxford.

Benowitz, N.L. (1992) Antihypertensive Agents. In: *Basic and Clinical Pharmacology*, (ed. B.G. Katzung), 5th edn. pp. 139–161. Appleton and Lange, Norwalk, Conn.

Bernheim, E. & Bernheim, M.L.C. (1938) The hydrolysis of homatropine and atropine by various tissues. *Journal of Pharmacology and Experimental Therapeutics*, **64**, 209–216.

Berry, B.W. & Jamali, F. (1991) Presystemic and systemic chiral inversion of *R*(−)-fenoprofen in the rat. *Journal of Pharmacology and Experimental Therapeutics*, **258**, 695–701.

Budsberg, S.C., Kemp, D.T. & Wolski, N. (1992) Pharmacokinetics of clindamycin phosphate in dogs after single intravenous and intramuscular administrations. *American Journal of Veterinary Research*, **53**, 2333–2336.

Caldwell, J. (1992) The importance of stereochemistry in drug action and disposition. *Journal of Clinical Pharmacology*, **32**, 925–929.

Caldwell, J., Hutt, A.J. & Fournel-Gigleux, S. (1988) The metabolic chiral inversion and dispositional enantioselectivity of the 2-arylpropionic acids and their biological consequences. *Biochemical Pharmacology*, **37**, 105–114.

Carr, R.A., Foster, R.T., Lewanczuk, R.Z. & Hamilton, P.G. (1992) Pharmacokinetics of sotalol enantiomers in humans. *Journal of Clinical Pharmacology*, **32**, 1105–1109.

Delatour, P., Benoit, E., Caude, M. & Tambute, A. (1990a) Species differences in the generation of the chiral sulphoxide metabolite of albendazole in sheep and rats. *Chirality*, **2**, 156–160.

Delatour, P., Benoit, E., Garnier, F. and Besse, S. (1990b) Chirality of the sulphoxide metabolites of fenbendazole and albendazole in sheep. *Journal of Veterinary Pharmacology and Therapeutics*, **13**, 361–366.

Delatour, P., Jaussaud, P., Courtot, D. & Fau, D. (1991a). Enantioselective N-demethylation of ketamine in the horse. *Journal of Veterinary Pharmacology and Therapeutics*, **14**, 209–212.

Delatour, P., Garnier, F., Benoit, E. & Caude, I. (1991b) Chiral behaviour of the metabolite albendazole sulphoxide in sheep, goats and cattle. *Research in Veterinary Science*, **50**, 134–138.

Delatour, P., Benoit, E., Besse, S. & Boukraa, A. (1991c) Comparative enantioselectivity in the sulphoxidation of albendazole in man, dogs and rats. *Xenobiotica*, **21**, 217–221.

Delatour, P., Foot, R., Foster, A.P., Baggot, D. & Lees, P. (1996) Pharmacodynamics and chiral pharmacokinetics of carprofen in calves. *British Veterinary Journal*, **152**, 183–198.

Deleforge, J., Davot, J.L., Boisrame, B. & Delatour, P. (1991) Enantioselectivity in the anaesthetic effect of ketamine in dogs. *Journal of Veterinary Pharmacology and Therapeutics*, **14**, 418–420.

Drayer, D.E. (1986) Pharmacodynamic and pharmacokinetic differences between drug enantiomers in humans: an overview. *Clinical Pharmacology and Therapeutics*, **40**, 125–133.

Eichelbaum, M., Mikus, G. & Vogelgesang, B. (1984) Pharmacokinetics of (+)-, (−) and (±)-verapamil after intravenous administration. *British Journal of Clinical Pharmacology*, **17**, 453–458.

Eichizen, H., Vogelgesang, B. & Eichelbaum, M. (1985) Effects of *d*, *l*-verapamil on atrioventricular conduction in relation to its stereoselective first-pass metabolism. *Clinical Pharmacology and Therapeutics*, **38**, 71–76.

Echizen, H., Manz, M. & Eichelbaum, M. (1988) Electrophysiologic effects of dextro and levo verapamil on sinus node and AV function in humans. *Journal of Cardiovascular Pharmacology*, **12**, 543–546.

Evans, A.M. (1992) Enantioselective pharmacodynamics and pharmacokinetics of chiral non-steroidal anti-inflammatory drugs. *European Journal of Clinical Pharmacology*, **42**, 237–256.

Finco, D.R., Brown, S.A., Vaden, S.L. & Ferguson, D.C. (1995) Relationship between plasma creatinine concentration and glomerular filtration rate in dogs. *Journal of Veterinary Pharmacology and Therapeutics*, **18**, 418–421.

Foster, R.T. & Jamali, F. (1987) High-performance liquid chromatographic assay of ketoprofen enantiomers in human plasma and urine. *Journal of Chromatography*, **416**, 388–393.

Galtier, P., Alvinerie, M. & Delatour, P. (1986) *In vitro* sulfoxidation of albendazole by ovine liver microsomes: assay and frequency of various xenobiotics. *American Journal of Veterinary Research*, **47**, 447–450.

Garcia, M.L., Tost, D., Vilageliu, J., Lopez, S., Carganico, G. & Mauleon, D. (1998) Bioavailability of S(+)-ketoprofen after oral administration of different mixtures of ketoprofen enantiomers to dogs. *Journal of Clinical Pharmacology*, **38**, 22S–26S.

Hayball, P.J. & Meffin, P.J. (1987) Enantioselective disposition of 2-arylpropionic acid nonsteroidal anti-inflammatory drugs. III. Fenoprofen disposition. *Journal of Pharmacology and Experimental Therapeutics*, **240**, 631–636.

Hutt, A.J. & Caldwell, J. (1984) The importance of stereochemistry in the clinical pharmacokinetics of the 2-arylpropionic acid non-steroidal anti-inflammatory drugs. *Clinical Pharmacokinetics*, **9**, 371–373.

Jaussaud, P., Bellon, C., Besse, S., Courtot, D. & Delatour, P. (1993) Enantioselective pharmacokinetics of ketoprofen in horses. *Journal of Veterinary Pharmacology and Therapeutics*, **16**, 373–376.

Kates, R.E., Keene, B.W. & Hamlin, R.L. (1979) Pharmacokinetics of propranolol in the dog. *Journal of Veterinary Pharmacology and Therapeutics*, **2**, 21–26.

Kemmerer, J.M., Rubio, F.A., McClain, R.M. & Koechlin, B.A. (1979) Stereospecific assay and stereospecific disposition of racemic carprofen in rats. *Journal of Pharmaceutical Sciences*, **68**, 1274–1280.

Koritz, G.D., McKiernan, B.C., Neff-Davis, C.A. & Munsiff, I.J. (1986) Bioavailability of four slow-release theophylline formulations in the Beagle dog. *Journal of Veterinary Pharmacology and Therapeutics*, **9**, 293–302.

Landoni, M.F. & Lees, P. (1995a) Comparison of the anti-inflammatory actions of flunixin and ketoprofen in horses applying PK/PD modelling. *Equine Veterinary Journal*, **27**, 247–256.

Landoni, M.F. & Lees, P. (1995b) Pharmacokinetics and pharmacodynamics of ketoprofen enantiomers in calves. *Chirality*, **7**, 586–597.

Landoni, M.F. & Lees, P. (1996) Pharmacokinetics and pharmacodynamics of ketoprofen enantiomers in the horse. *Journal of Veterinary Pharmacology and Therapeutics*, **19**, 466–474.

Landoni, M.F., Cunningham, F.M. & Lees, P. (1995) Pharmacokinetics and pharmacodynamics of ketoprofen in calves applying PK/PD modelling. *Journal of Veterinary Pharmacology and Therapeutics*, **18**, 315–324.

Landoni, M.F., Soraci, A.L., Delatour, P. & Lees, P. (1997) Enantioselective behaviour of drugs used in domestic animals: a review. *Journal of Veterinary Pharmacology and Therapeutics*, **20**, 1–16.

Landoni, M.F., Comas, W., Mucci, N. *et al.*, (1999) Enantiospecific pharmacokinetics and pharmacodynamics of ketoprofen in sheep. *Journal of Veterinary Pharmacology and Therapeutics*, **22**, 349–359.

Lees, P., Delatour, P., Benoit, E. & Foster, A.P. (1991) Pharmacokinetics of carprofen enantiomers in the horse. *Acta Veterinaria Scandinavica*, Suppl. **87**, 249–251.

Lees, P., McKellar, Q.A., May, S. & Ludwig, B. (1994) Pharmacodynamics and pharmacokinetics of carprofen in the horse. *Equine Veterinary Journal*, **23**, 203–208.

McCormack, K. & Brune, K. (1991) Dissociation between the antinociceptive and anti-inflammatory effects of the nonsteroidal anti-inflammatory drugs: a survey of their analgesic efficacy. *Drugs*, **41**, 533–547.

McGuirk, S.M., Muir, W.M. & Sams, R.A. (1981) Pharmacokinetic analysis of intravenously and orally administered quinidine in horses. *American Journal of Veterinary Research*, **42**, 938–942.

McKellar, Q.A., Delatour, P. & Lees, P. (1994) Stereospecific pharmacodynamics and pharmacokinetics of carprofen in the dog. *Journal of Veterinary Pharmacology and Therapeutics*, **17**, 447–454.

Mauleon, D., Mis, R., Ginesta, J. *et al.* (1994) Pharmacokinetics of ketoprofen enantiomers in monkeys following single and multiple oral administration. *Chirality*, **6**, 537–542.

Meade, E., Smith, W. & DeWitt, D. (1993) Differential inhibition of prostaglandin endoperoxide synthase (cyclooxygenase) isoenzymes by aspirin and other non-steroidal anti-inflammatory drugs. *Journal of Biological Chemistry*, **268**, 6610–6614.

Mehvar, R., Gross, M.F. & Kreamer, R.N. (1990) Pharmacokinetics of atenolol enantiomers in humans and rats. *Journal of Pharmaceutical Sciences*, **79**, 881–885.

Mikus, G., Eichelbaum, M., Fischer, C., Gumulka, S. & Klotz, U. (1990) Interaction of verapamil and cimetidine: stereochemical aspects of drug metabolism, drug disposition and drug action. *Journal of Pharmacology and Experimental Therapeutics*, **253**, 1042–1048.

Muir, W.W. & Hubbell, J.A. (1988) Cardiopulmonary and anesthetic effects of ketamine and its enantiomers in dogs. *American Journal of Veterinary Research*, **49**, 530–534.

Papich, M.G., Davis, L.E. & Davis, C.A. (1986) Procainamide in the dog: anti-arrhythmic plasma concentrations after intravenous administration. *Journal of Veterinary Pharmacology and Therapeutics*, **9**, 359–369.

Parraga, M.E., Kittleson, M.D. & Drake, C.M. (1995) Quinidine administration increases steady state serum digoxin concentrations in horses. *Equine Veterinary Journal*, Suppl. **19**, 114–119.

Pasutto, F.M. (1992) Mirror images: the analysis of pharmaceutical enantiomers. *Journal of Clinical Pharmacology*, **32**, 917–924.

Peters, R.A. Wakelin, R.W., Rivett, D.E.A. & Thomas, L.C. (1953) Fluoracetate poisoning: comparison of synthetic fluorocitric acid with enzymically synthesized fluorotricarboxylic acid. *Nature*, **171**, 1111–1112.

Prescott, J.F. & Baggot, J.D. (1993) *Antimicrobial Therapy in Veterinary Medicine*, 2nd edn, pp. 300–307. Iowa State University Press, Ames.

Rubin, A., Knadler, M.P., Ho, P.P.K., Bechtol, L.D. & Wolen, R.L. (1985) Stereoselective inversion of (R)-fenoprofen to (S)-fenoprofen in humans. *Journal of Pharmaceutical Sciences*, **74**, 82–84.

Rudy, A.C., Liu, Y., Brater, D.C. & Hall, S.D. (1998) Stereoselective pharmacokinetics and inversion of (R)-ketoprofen in healthy volunteers. *Journal of Clinical Pharmacology*, **38**, 3S–10S.

Satoh, K., Yanagisawa, T. & Taira, N. (1980) Coronary vasodilator and cardiac effects of verapamil in the dog. *Journal of Cardiovascular Pharmacology*, **2**, 309–318.

Schroff, C.D. (1852) Uber belladonna, atropin und datura. *Z. Gez. Arzte* (Wien), **3**, 211.

Sedgwick, A.D. & Lees, P. (1986) Studies of eicosanoid production in the air pouch model of synovial inflammation. *Agents and Actions*, **18**, 429–438.

Skadhauge, E., Warui, C.N., Kamau, J.M.Z. & Maloiy, G.M.D. (1984). Function of the lower intestine and osmoregulation in the ostrich, *Struthio camelus*: preliminary anatomical and physiological considerations. *Quarterly Journal of Experimental Physiology*, **69**, 809–18.

Shen, T.Y. (1981) Non-steroidal anti-inflammatory agents. In: *Burger's Medicinal Chemistry*, Vol. III, (ed. M.E. Wolff) 4th edn. pp. 1205–1271. Wiley Interscience, New York.

Silber, B. & Riegelman, S. (1980) Stereospecific assay for (−)- and (+)-propranolol in human and dog plasma. *Journal of Pharmacology and Experimental Therapeutics*, **215**, 643–648.

Soraci, A.L. & Benoit, E. (1996) *In vitro* fenoprophenyl–coenzyme A thioester formation: interspecies variations. *Chirality*, **7**, 534–540.

Soraci, A.L., Benoit, E., Olivier, L. & Delatour, P. (1995) Comparative metabolism of R(−)-fenoprofen in rats and sheep. *Journal of Veterinary Pharmacology and Therapeutics*, **18**, 167–171.

Souhali El Amri, H., Mothe, O., Totis, M. *et al.* (1988) Albendazole sulfonation by rat liver cytochrome P450c. *Journal of Pharmacology and Experimental Therapeutics*, **246**, 758–764.

Stoltenberg, J.K., Puglisi, C.V., Rubio, F. & Vane, F.M. (1981) High-performance liquid chromatographic determination of stereoselective disposition of carprofen in humans. *Journal of Pharmaceutical Sciences*, **70**, 1207–1212.

Swart, D., Mackie, R.I. & Hayes, J.P. (1993). Influence of liver mass, rate of passage and site of digestion on energy metabolism and fibre digestion in the ostrich (*Struthio camelus var domesticus*). *South African Journal of Animal Science*, **23**, 119–126.

Taylor, P. & Insel, P.A. (1990) Molecular basis of pharmacologic selectivity. In: *Principles of Drug Action: The Basis of Pharmacology*, (eds W.B. Pratt & P. Taylor), *3rd* edn. pp. 1–102. Churchill Livingstone, New York.

Taylor, P.M., Delatour, P., Landoni, M.F., Deal, C., Pickett, C., Shojaee Aliabadi, F., Foot, R. & Lees, P. (1996) Pharmacodynamics and enantioselective pharmacokinetics of carprofen in the cat. *Research in Veterinary Science*, **60**, 144–151.

Tomaszewski, J. & Rumore, M.M. (1994) Stereoisomeric drugs: FDA's policy statement and the impact on drug development. *Drug Development and Industrial Pharmacy*, **20**, 119–139.

Tucker, G.I. & Lennard, M.S. (1990) Enantiomer specific pharmacokinetics. *Pharmacology and Therapeutics*, **45**, 309–329.

Twomey, B. & Dale, M. (1992) Cyclooxygenase-independent effects of nonsteroidal anti-inflammatory drugs on the neutrophil respiratory burst. *Biochemical Pharmacology*, **43**, 413–418.

Vane, J.R. (1971) Inhibition of prostaglandin synthesis as a mechanism of action for aspirin-like drugs. *Nature (New Biology)*, **231**, 232–235.

Vane, J.R. & Botting, R.M. (1995) New insights into the mode of action of anti-inflammatory drugs. *Inflammation Research*, **44**, 1–10.

Walle, T. & Walle, U.K. (1986) Pharmacokinetic parameters obtained with racemates. *Trends in Pharmacological Sciences*, **7**, 155–158.

White, P.F., Ham, J., Way, W.L. & Trevor, A.J. (1980) Pharmacology of ketamine isomers in surgical patients. *Anesthesiology*, **52**, 231–239.

Wilkinson, G.R. & Shand, D.G. (1975) A physiological approach to hepatic drug clearance. *Clinical Pharmacology and Therapeutics*, **18**, 377–390.

Chapter 5
Drug Permeation Through the Skin and Topical Preparations

Introduction

There are a wide variety of veterinary drug preparations available for topical application to the skin. While most of these preparations are intended to produce local effects, some are formulated to distribute via the systemic circulation to skin covering all regions of the body or to produce systemic effects. Percutaneous absorption of topically applied drugs entails diffusive penetration and permeation of a drug substance into and through the *stratum corneum*, other strata ('living' layers) of the epidermis and some portion of the dermis (Elias *et al.*, 1981; Schalla *et al.*, 1989). The skin, with its appendages and vasculature, is an organized, heterogenous, multilayer organ that contains a complex series of diffusion barriers which retard water loss and limit access of drugs and foreign chemical substances (xenobiotics) to the systemic circulation. Skin is one of the most water-impermeable biological barriers found in nature (Idsen, 1975). The skin accounts for approximately 10% of live body weight in cattle, goats and dogs, 7.5% in horses and 3.7% in man. While skin receives approximately 6% of cardiac output, cutaneous blood flow rate to various regions differs between species (Monteiro-Riviere *et al.*, 1990). In humans and pigs the cutaneous circulation supplies blood (in musculocutaneous arteries) to both the skin and underlying musculature, whereas in dogs and cats (loose-skin species) blood is supplied directly to the skin.

The epidermis is composed mainly of stratified squamous keratinized epithelial cells arranged in layers according to their stage of differentiation. Epidermal cells originate in the *stratum basale* and become progressively more keratinized as they move towards the surface of the skin. The outermost layer (*stratum corneum*) of the epidermis constitutes the major barrier to transdermal penetration of drugs and xenobiotics, especially hydrophilic substances. Beneath the epidermal layers lies the dermis, which is composed of connective tissue and contains blood vessels, lymphatics, hair follicles, and exocrine (sweat and sebaceous) glands. Although located deep in the dermis, sebaceous glands are appendages of the epidermis that secrete sebum into the follicular canals leading to the skin surface. Analysis of skin surface lipids has shown wide variation in sebum composition among animal species. A poorly vascularized layer of areolar connective tissue (hypodermis) that permits deposition of a layer of fat of variable depth underlies the dermis. Highly lipophilic substances, whether applied topically or administered systemically, can accumulate and persist (reservoir effect) in the epidermis or subcutaneous fat.

The intact epidermis behaves qualitatively as do cellular membranes in general (Scheuplein & Blank, 1971). Topically applied chemical substances diffuse through the functional barrier provided by the epidermis at rates determined largely by their lipid/water partition coefficients but more slowly than through cellular barriers elsewhere in the body (Scheuplein, 1965). Percutaneous absorption *in vivo* is a summation of ten steps that have been enumerated by Wester & Maibach (1983).

Absorption process

The absorption process for a topically applied drug essentially involves the following stages: dissolution of the drug in and release from the vehicle, drug penetration (by diffusion) through the *stratum corneum* and permeation through the 'living' layers of the epidermis to the underlying dermis where absorption into the systemic circulation takes place. While the initial stage is formulation-dependent in that it relates to the form of the drug and the nature of the vehicle, the translocation stages are largely governed by the molecular structure and physicochemical properties of the drug. Penetration of the *stratum corneum* is generally the rate-limiting step in the absorption process (Riegelman, 1974). Only lipid-soluble drugs can diffuse through the dead compacted keratinized cells (corneocytes) of the *stratum corneum*. However, passive diffusion through the epidermis, including the *stratum corneum*, can take place by one or more of the following routes: transcellular through the corneocytes, intercellular through the lipid matrix (a tortuous path), or along the sweat gland ducts and hair follicles (appendageal path). Even though lipophilic substances may penetrate the *stratum corneum* by transcellular diffusion, some degree of water solubility is required for passage through the 'living' layers of the epidermis. Polar drugs have a low capacity to penetrate the *stratum corneum* but may gain access to the 'living' epidermal layer by shunt diffusion along the appendageal path. Additional factors that influence percutaneous absorption include the nature of the vehicle, the state of hydration of the *stratum corneum*, drug persistence in the *stratum corneum* or other strata of the epidermis, biotransformation in the epidermis, and species differences in histological structure of skin. In aquatic mammals, the *stratum corneum* is very thick and the corneocytes are solidly apposed, while the epidermis is devoid of a *stratum granulosum* regardless of whether the skin is glabrous (as in whales) or hairy (as in seals) (Montagna, 1967).

The average thickness of the *stratum corneum* in laboratory and domestic animals and humans is in the range of 10–35 μm. The thickness of this epidermal layer might not influence the penetration of chemical substances, whereas the density of appendages per unit surface area, which differs among animal species, does influence passage through the epidermis. Human skin contains an average of 40–70 hair follicles and 200–250 sweat glands per cm^2, whereas cattle skin contains approximately 2000 hair follicles, with associated sweat and sebaceous glands, per cm^2 (Pitman & Rostas, 1981). The mean follicle density in ten British breeds of sheep varies from 1000 to 2000 per cm^2 of skin, with a secondary to primary follicle ratio of 2.4:1 to 5.9:1 (Ryder, 1957). The ratio of secondary to primary follicles appears to be higher in wool-growing regions of Merino sheep skin. The sebaceous glands of cattle and sheep exude large quantities of lipoid material (lanolin in the case of sheep) that serve to protect their skin. The emulsifying properties of exocrine secretions may enhance dissolution and thus facilitate percutaneous absorption of topically applied compounds in cattle and sheep. Seasonal changes in the composition of secretions may cause variations in absorption of moderately lipid-soluble drugs (e.g. levamisole applied by 'pour-on') at different times of the year (Forsyth *et al.*, 1983). Because of the larger number of skin appendages per unit surface area, the appendageal path will probably contribute more to percutaneous absorption of hydrophilic substances in cattle and sheep than in other species. Horses and humans have highly effective sweat glands, whereas cattle, sheep, pigs, dogs and cats are unable to sweat profusely; elephants and koalas do not have sweat glands. In horses, sweat glands are under adrenergic control (β$_2$-adrenoceptors), while in humans sweat glands are innervated by postganglionic sympathetic axons that release acetylcholine rather than noradrenaline (norepinephrine). Changes in ambient temperature appear to affect animal skin temperature to a larger degree than human skin temperature, which suggests that skin plays a greater role in thermoregulation in humans than in animals.

The state of hydration of the *stratum corneum*, which is normally maintained at 10–15%, affects the rate of penetration of chemical substances. By increasing the state of hydration to 50%, the rate of permeation of some chemical substances through the epidermis can be increased up to tenfold (Idson, 1983). Occlusion has been shown to enhance the pharmacological effect of topically applied hydrocortisone and fluocinolone acetonide (McKenzie, 1962), but percutaneous absorption of drugs is not necessarily increased. The degree of occlusion-induced absorption enhancement appears to increase with increasing lipophilicity of drug substances.

Formulations containing an absorption promoting substance, such as propylene glycol or sodium lauryl sulphate, may increase the permeability of the *stratum corneum* to water-soluble drugs. Propylene glycol is a commonly used vehicle in topical corticosteroid preparations for veterinary use. Various aprotic solvents, which include dimethylacetamide, dimethylformamide, dimethylsulphoxide, tetrahydrofurfuryl alcohol, and 2-pyrrolidone, serve as penetration enhancers of polar drugs (Barry, 1983). Dimethylsulphoxide

(DMSO) is used in formulating some topical veterinary preparations. The penetration-enhancing property of DMSO is markedly concentration-dependent. At concentrations below 50% DMSO in water, the penetration rate of many drugs differs little than from aqueous solutions. The penetration rate of levamisole through skin of cattle and sheep was somewhat slower from a formulation containing DMSO (concentration not specified) than from an aqueous solution of the drug (Pitman & Rostas, 1981). Plasma and gastro-intestinal fluid concentrations of levamisole were lower following 'pour-on' application to cattle than following oral administration or subcutaneous injection of the drug (Forsyth *et al.*, 1983). Parathion penetrated the skin of pigs more rapidly when formulated in DMSO than in other vehicles (glycerol–for-mal/isopropranol mixture, octanol, macrogol 400) (Table 5.1) (Gyrd-Hansen *et al.*, 1991). The formation of a stable 2:1 water hydrate at a concentration of 67% v/v DMSO may explain its dehydrating and penetration-enhancing effects when present at high concentration (Scheuplein, 1978). These effects are accompanied by, or perhaps attributable to, epidermal tissue damage. Mineral oil may be used in formulating long-acting, water-based topical preparations of synthetic pyrethroids (permethrin, cypermethrin) for application to ruminant animals. This type of preparation would not be washed off by rain and could provide protection against flies for an extended period. Water-insoluble substances can be formulated as emulsifiable concentrates. The emulsifiable concentrate contains one or more surfactant and produces an emulsion or micellar solution with the water-insoluble drug in the non-aqueous phase, when mixed with water (Pitman & Rostas, 1981).

Species variations

The barrier properties of skin vary with the species of animal, and within a species may differ between regions of the body. Based on limited data obtained

Table 5.1 Pharmackinetic parameters for parathion (50 mg/kg) applied topically in various vehicles to pigs.

Pharmacokinetic parameter	Vehicle			
	GFI[a]	DMSO	Octanol	Macrogol 400
AUC (μg · h/L)	1460–1795	1630–3050	2010–3310	595–600
MRT (h)	57–106	9.7–14.5	22–31	54–60
MAT (h)	55–104	7.5–12.5	20–29	52–58
Bioavailability[b] (%)	16–20	19–28	15–29	3.9–54

[a] Glycerol–formal/isopropanol mixture.
[b] Bioavailability (absolute) was based on $AUC_{topical}/AUC_{i.v.}$, with correction for dose.
Source: Gyrd-Hansen *et al.* (1991).

from *in vitro* studies of skin permeability, it could be speculated that species can, in general, be ranked in the following order: rabbits > rats > guinea pigs > cats > dogs > pigs and Rhesus monkeys ≥ humans (least permeable skin). Because of a lack of data, horses, cattle, sheep and goats are not included in the comparison of skin permeability. The emulsifying property and occlusive effect of sebum and the high density of appendages per unit surface area would be expected to facilitate percutaneous absorption of substances in ruminant species.

The maximal rate of penetration of an organophosphorus compound through skin sections excised from the dorsal thorax of various species largely supports the skin permeability ranking of species (*vide supra*) (Table 5.2) (McCreesh, 1965). The compound rapidly penetrated skin of rabbits and rats, while penetration through pig skin occurred more slowly than through skin of the other species. Even though pig skin and human skin are similar in many respects (Monteiro-Riviere & Stromberg, 1985; Carver & Riviere, 1989), percutaneous absorption of a variety of compounds in the pig was found to range from zero to four times that in humans *in vivo* (Bartek *et al.*, 1972; Reifenrath & Hawkins, 1986). Advantage can be taken of the often similar permeability characteristics of pig and human skins with avoidance of the systemic and/or fat distribution difference *in vivo* by using the isolated perfused porcine skin flap *in vitro* model (Riviere & Monteiro-Riviere, 1991; Riviere *et al.*, 1995). The diffusion of chemical substances through skin and metabolism within the skin can be determined by assay of the perfusate. The sum of the amount of compound that diffused into the perfusate and the residual amount in the skin preparation at the end of the exposure period to the drug provides an estimation of percutaneous absorption.

Regional variations in percutaneous absorption contribute to differences in the systemic availability of a drug depending on the site of topical application.

Table 5.2   Maximal penetration of radiolabelled organophosphorus compound through excised skin from dorsal thorax of various species.

Species	Rate ($\mu g/cm^2/min$)
Pig	0.3
Dog	2.7
Monkey	4.2
Goat	4.4
Cat	4.4
Guinea pig	6.0
Rabbit	9.3
Rat	9.3

Source: McCreesh (1965).

The Rhesus monkey (*Macaca mulatta*) could probably serve as an animal model for human skin regional variation (Wester & Maibach, 1999).

The absolute bioavailability of a topically applied drug can be determined only by measurement of plasma concentrations and comparing total areas under the curves (AUCS) or, less reliably, the amounts excreted in urine over a period of at least six half-lives following topical application and intravenous injection of the drug. An appropriate washout period must be allowed to elapse between the phases of a crossover study, which is the experimental design that should be used whenever feasible. Because of species variations in ultrastructure of skin, cutaneous blood supply, density of appendages per unit surface area, and activity of biotransformation pathways, the percutaneous absorption (rate and extent) of a drug is best determined by performing the study in the species of interest.

Cutaneous biotransformation

As biotransformation of drugs and xenobiotics takes place to a variable extent in skin, topically applied substances may be incompletely available systemically, even though they penetrate the *stratum corneum*. Cytochrome P450-mediated oxidative reactions, hydrolytic reactions, formation of glucuronide, sulphate and glutathione conjugates, and acetylation of primary aromatic amines take place in the skin (Krishna & Klotz, 1994; Bashir & Maibach, 1999). While the activity of cytochrome P450 enzymes in skin may be only 1–5% of that in the liver, the activity of transferases, which are involved in various conjugation reactions, in skin could approach 10% of that in liver (Merk *et al.*, 1996).

Epidermal cytochrome P450 and hydrolytic enzymes in the lipid matrix of the *stratum corneum* as well as in the *stratum granulosum* may be involved in conversion reactions of topically applied steroids (Behrendt *et al.*, 1989). In pigs, epidermal cytochrome P450 has been shown to convert parathion to paraoxon by oxidative desulphuration (Riviere & Chang, 1992). The oxygen analogue formed is rapidly hydrolysed to inactive metabolites. The large difference between mammals and insects in the rate at which the hydrolytic reaction takes place accounts for the selective toxicity of thiophosphate insecticides. The extent to which the ultrastructural difference in the epidermis of aquatic and terrestrial mammals affects the activity of drug-metabolizing enzymes in skin is not known. Fish appear to be unable to detoxify thiophosphate insecticides.

Benzoyl peroxide, the active ingredient in some shampoos for dogs, is almost completely metabolized to benzoic acid in the epidermis. Benzoic acid undergoes conjugation with glycine, mainly in the liver, and is excreted in urine as hippuric acid. Methylation of noradrenaline (norepinephrine) to adrenaline (epinephrine), an *N*-transferase-mediated conjugation reaction, in human and animal skin preparations has been reported (Kao & Carver, 1990).

Biotransformation of propranolol, which involves microsomal-mediated oxidative reactions and glucuronide conjugation, is stereoselective both in the liver and the skin. Based on *in vitro* studies, using intact human skin and microsomal preparations, of percutaneous absorption and metabolism of racemic propranolol, it was concluded that the S(−)-enantiomer (eutomer) is metabolized more efficiently by skin than the R(+)-enantiomer (Ademola *et al.*, 1991). The converse applies to hepatocytes, which metabolize the R(+)-enantiomer more efficiently (Ward *et al.*, 1989). The cytochrome P450 mono-oxygenase enzymes in skin, like in the liver, can be induced (by dex-amethasone, for example) or inhibited (chloramphenicol, imidazole antifungal agents). The clinical significance of altered microsomal enzyme activity in the epidermis has not been established. Metronidazole, which is available as a topical gel, inhibits acetaldehyde dehydrogenase (a non-microsomal enzyme), but whether the enzyme is present in skin does not appear to be known.

Susceptibility of cats

Because of the fastidious grooming behaviour of cats some topical, especially 'spot-on', preparations must be applied to the skin at a location that is inaccessible to the tongue, such as the back of the neck. Certain insecticidal drugs which are available as topical preparations for application to other species (e.g. amitraz liquid concentrate in shampoo for dogs, benzyl benzoate lotion for application to horses) are toxic to cats. Disinfectants, especially those containing phenolic compounds, commonly used in kennels and considered to be safe could produce toxicity in cats following licking (ingestion) of the chemical residue adhered to their paws (Spinelli & Enos, 1978). Defective glucuronide synthesis, which is characteristic of Felidae, contributes to the toxicity of phenolic disinfectants. Crude citrus oil extract contains *d*-limonene and linalool, substances with insecticidal properties. Topical application of these substances, which are formulated as sprays and shampoos for control of fleas, can cause toxicity in cats (Hooser, 1990). Because organophosphorus compounds inhibit plasma pseudocholinesterase activity and reduce micro-somal cytochrome P450-mediated oxidative reactions, the rate of metabolism of a wide variety of drugs is considerably decreased in cats and dogs wearing flea collars containing an organophosphorus compound (dimpylate, dichlorvos). Flea collars containing a carbamate insecticide (carbaril, propoxur) could similarly decrease the rate of metabolism (hydrolytic and oxidative reactions) of various drugs. A prolonged duration of action is the invariable outcome of the interaction and a normally minor (alternative) metabolic pathway could become significant. Cats appear to be more prone than dogs to side-effects produced by griseofulvin (Helton *et al.*, 1986).

Topical veterinary preparations

The classes of drug for which topical veterinary preparations are commer-cially available include ectoparasiticides, antibacterial agents, antifungal agents, corticosteroids, and compound antimicrobial–corticosteroid preparations.

Ectoparasiticides

Selection of the type of ectoparasiticide preparation depends on the species of animal and the purpose to be served by applying an ectoparasiticide, the physiochemical properties and spectrum of activity of the drug against the major ectoparasites which affect the animal species, the margin of safety based on selectivity of action of the drug, and the susceptibility of the species (or breed) of interest to adverse effects that could be produced by the ectoparasiticide. When the objective is to treat an identified species of ectoparasite, selection of the drug of choice can be more specific.

Even though different classes of drug may have activity against the same range of ectoparasites, the drugs differ in their clinical effectiveness. Quantitative differences in clinical effectiveness could be due to the susceptibility of the parasite to the action of the drug, which would be decreased by the development of parasite resistance, or to the accessibility of the drug to the site where the parasite is located. The latter would be influenced by the formulation of the drug preparation and the method of application to the host animal (Table 5.3).

Because avermectins and milbemycins (macrolide endectocides) can be administered by various routes depending on the animal species, and cythioate

Table 5.3 Dosage forms and methods of application of topical ectoparasiticide preparations to individual species.

Species	Dosage form	Method of application
Cattle	Solution	Pour-on
	Liquid concentrate[a]	Spray
	Ear tag	Attach to ears
Sheep	Liquid concentrate[a]	Dip, spray
	Solution	Spot-on, pour-on
Pigs	Solution	Pour-on, spot-on
	Liquid concentrate[a]	Spray
Horses	Solution	Pour-on
	Liquid concentrate[a]	Spray, shampoo
	Lotion	Dab-on
Dogs and cats	Solution	Spot-on, spray (dogs)
	Collar	Surrounding neck
	Dusting power	Apply to coat
	Liquid concentrate[a]	Sponge-on (dogs)
	Shampoo	Wash (dogs)

[a] Liquid concentrates must be appropriately diluted before use on animals.

(an organophosphorus compound administered orally to dogs) produce ectoparasiticidal effects following absorption into the systemic circulation, they are classified as systemic ectoparasiticides. The classes of drugs used as ectoparasiticides, their spectrum of activity and the preparations available for application are presented on an animal species basis in Tables 5.4–5.8. When preparing these tables the intention was to provide examples of drugs in the various ectoparasiticide classes and of the available preparations: consequently the information presented is generally and not all inclusive.

'Pour-on' preparations of ectoparasiticides are available generally as prepared solutions or as liquid concentrates which, after dilution with water, form an emulsion. Diluted liquid concentrates are usually applied 'by spray'. The 'pour-on' method is most suitable for topical application of ectoparasiticides to cattle (Table 5.4). Drugs formulated as 'pour-on' preparations must be sufficiently lipid-soluble to penetrate and persist in the *stratum corneum* and *stratum germinativum* to provide clinical effectiveness and protection against reinfestation for a reasonable length of time, and have adequate water solubility to pass into the deeper layers of the epidermis and the dermis for absorption to take place. Ivermectin, doramectin and moxidectin (macrolide endectocides) and phosmet (an organophosphorus compound) meet these requirements. Specified withdrawal periods are associated with 'pour-on' preparations of individual drugs. In addition to effectively treating the biting louse (*Bovicola bovis*) and sucking lice (*Haematopinus eurysternus* and *Linognathus vituli*), infestation with mites and warble-fly (*Hypoderma bovis*) larvae, and providing protection against warble flies and horn flies (*Haematobia irritans*), the 'pour-on' preparation of ivermectin is 99–100% effective against gastrointestinal and pulmonary nematodes in cattle (Alva-Valdes *et al.*, 1986). Ivermectin or moxidectin could alternatively be administered to cattle by subcutaneous injection (200 µg/kg) of a parenteral solution, or for long-term (up to 135 days) endectocidal activity, ivermectin could be administered as the modified-release ruminal bolus.

Cypermethrin or permethrin (synthetic pyrethroids) could be applied by 'pour-on' of a prepared solution or by attaching ear tags to both ears of cattle. Insecticidal ear tags provide protection against flies, with the notable exception of the warble-fly, for up to 5 months. Deltamethrin is available as a prepared solution for 'spot-on' application and fenvalerate as a liquid concentrate which, after dilution, can be applied by spray. Synthetic pyrethroids possess the rapid knock-down property of natural pyrethrins, but are more stable and have longer residual activity. Amitraz, a liquid concentrate to be diluted before application by spray, has activity against ticks (*Ixodes, Dermacentor, Haemaphysalis*) as well as against mites (*Chorioptes bovis, C. ovis* var *bovis, Sarcoptes scabiei* var *bovis*), sucking lice (*Haematopinus eurysternus, Linognathus vituli*), and the biting louse (*Bovicola bovis*). Amitraz causes detachment of ticks from the skin of the host animal rather than producing an acaricidal effect (Stone & Knowles, 1974). Fluazuron, a chitin synthesis inhibitor, is formulated as a 'pour-on' for application to beef cattle for control of the one-host tick (*Boophilis*

Table 5.4 Representative ectoparasiticides for application to cattle.[a]

Ectoparasiticide class & representative drugs	Spectrum of activity	Preparation	Method of application
Avermectin	Mites, lice, horn fly		
Ivermectin		Solution	Pour on
		Parenteral solution	Subcutaneous
		Controlled-release ruminal bolus (p.o.)	injection
Doramectin		Solution	Pour on
		Parenteral solution	Subcutaneous injection
Milbemycin	Warble fly larvae		
Moxidectin		Solution	Pour on
		Parenteral solution	Subcutaneous injection
Organophosphate	Mites, lice, warble fly larvae		
Phosmet		Solution	Pour on
Pyrethroid	Lice, flies		
Cypermethrin		Solution	Pour on
		Ear tag	
Permethrin		Solution	Pour on
		Ear tag	
Deltamethrin		Solution	Spot on
Fenvalerate		Liquid concentrate	Spray diluted solution
Amidine	Lice, mites, ticks		
Amitraz		Liquid concentrate	Spray diluted solution

[a] Ectoparasites that affect cattle:

Mites	*Chorioptes bovis, Psoroptes ovis* var *bovis, Sarcoptes scabiei* var *bovis*
Lice	*Bovicola bosi, Haematopinus eurysternus, Linognathus vituli*
Warble-fly	*Hypoderma bovis*
Horn fly	*Haemotobia irritans*
Other flies	*Stomoxys calcitrans, Hydrotaea irritans, Musca autumnalis, Musca domestica*
Ticks	*Ixodes, Dermacentor, Haemaphysalis*

microplus). Cattle, goats and sheep are distinct ruminant species, and, from a pharmacological point of view, goats more closely resemble cattle than sheep. Unlike cattle and sheep, goats do not develop an effective immunity against nematode infections.

Dipping is the usual method of ectoparasiticide application to sheep. The drug must be stable in the dip (emulsifiable) concentrate and in the diluted form in the dipping bath. Dimpylate (diazinon) and propetamphos (organophosphorus compounds), cypermethrin and flumethrin (synthetic pyrethroids) and amitraz (an amidine) are available as dip concentrates. While the spectrum of activity of organophosphates and synthetic pyrethroids against ectoparasites that affect sheep is, in general, similar (Table 5.5), dips containing an organophosphorus compound or flumethrin will treat and, for a limited time, prevent infestation with the sheep scab mite (*Psoroptes ovis*) whereas cypermethrin-containing dip is effective only for treatment. Psoroptes mite infestation can be treated systemically, by subcutaneous injection of a parenteral solution of an

Table 5.5 Representative ectoparasiticides for application to sheep.[a]

Ectoparasiticide class & representative drugs	Spectrum of activity	Preparation	Method of application
Organophosphate Dimpylate (diazinon)	Mites, lice, sheep ked, ticks, blowfly larvae	Dip concentrate	Dip
Pyrethroid Cypermethrin Flumethrin Deltamethrin	Mites, lice, sheep ked, ticks, blowfly larvae, flies	Dip concentrate Solution Dip concentrate Solution Solution Dip concentrate	Dip Spot on Dip Spot on Spot on Dip
Amidine Amitraz	Lice, ticks, sheep ked	Dip concentrate	Dip
Avermectin Ivermectin	Mites, nasal bot	Parenteral solution Oral solution Controlled-release ruminal capsule (p.o.)	Subcutaneous injection Drench
Doramectin		Parenteral solution Oral solution	Subcutaneous injection Drench
Cyromazine	Blowfly larvae	Solution	Pour-on

[a] Ectoparasites that affect sheep:

Mites	*Psoroptes ovis*
Lice	*Haematopinus, Linognathus*
Sheep ked	*Melophagus ovinus*
Ticks	*Ixodes ricinus*
Blowfly	*Calliphora, Lucilia cuprina*
Nasal bot	*Oestrus ovis*
Flies	*Hydrotaea irritans* (head fly)

avermectin. Either ivermectin, two doses (each 200 µg/kg) administered 7 days apart, or doramectin, a single subcutaneous dose (200 µg/kg) may be used. Avermectins provide no residual protection against *Psoroptes* reinfestation. Subcutaneously administered ivermectin or doramectin is effective in treating nasal bots (*Oestrus ovis*) in sheep. As ivermectin is available as an oral solution, this preparation could be administered as a drench at the same dose (200 µg/kg) as the parenteral solution (s.c. injection). Based on comparison of AUCs following administration of the oral solution and subcutaneous injection of the parenteral solution of ivermectin to sheep, the relative bioavailability of the drug administered orally was 36% (Marriner *et al.*, 1987). This suggests that subcutaneous injection would be the preferred route of ivermectin administration for systemic treatment of sheep infested with *P. ovis* or *O. ovis*.

When choosing between an organophosphorus compound (dimpylate, propetamphos) and a synthetic pyrethroid (flumethrin, cypermethrin) for dipping sheep, a consideration (in addition to residual protection) which could be of practical relevance is that there is no withdrawal period associated with the use of synthetic pyrethroids. The selective toxicity of synthetic pyrethroids for insects (mammalian-to-insect toxic dose ratio of more than 1000:1, compared with 33:1 for organophosphorous compounds) makes this class of ectoparasiticide the safest available. The low toxicity of pyrethroids in mammals is largely due to their rapid biotransformation by ester hydrolysis and/or hydroxylation. Unlike mammals, fish are extremely sensitive to pyrethroid toxicity. Because of the large quantities of drug required for dipping sheep and the difficulty of dip disposal, application of diluted dip concentrate, but at a higher concentration than used in the dip bath, as a spray is becoming a more popular method of ectoparasiticide application by sheep farmers. The relative effectiveness of spraying versus dipping sheep for the treatment and prevention of ectoparasite infestation is open to question. The ultimate assessment of clinical efficacy of an ectoparasiticide requires determination of the effectiveness of the drug in killing the parasite of interest. An indication of the relative effectiveness of different methods of application of a diluted dip concentrate of an organophosphorus compound can be obtained by comparing the plasma concentration profiles and AUCs following application of the drug by the different methods as well as monitoring both plasma and blood cholinesterase activity over an extended period. Interpretation of the effect on cholinesterase activity requires that untreated sheep (control group) be studied for each method of drug application. Organophosphorus compounds 'irreversibly' inhibit cholinesterase activity by phosphorylating the esteratic site of the enzyme and also inhibit microsomal cytochrome P450 oxidative activity.

Deltamethrin (synthetic pyrethroid) is available as a prepared solution for 'spot-on' application to sheep and is effective against lice, keds, ticks and blowfly (*Calliphora, Lucilia*) larvae. Cyromazine, a prepared solution for 'pour-on' application to sheep, is effective against blowfly larvae; because of the persistence of the drug, it is particularly indicated for the prevention of blowfly strike. Cyromazine protects sheep against blowfly strike (*Lucilia cuprina*) for up to 14 weeks after application. This chemical substance is an insect growth regulator with activity against ova and larvae of manure-breeding flies. Because insect growth regulators (cyromazine, methoprene, fenoxycarb) affect pre-adult stages of insects, effective control is generally not achieved for some weeks following their use.

As the sucking louse (*Haematopinus suis*) and the burrowing mange mite (*Sarcoptes scabiei* var *suis*) are the major ectoparasites that affect pigs, the use of a drug with activity against lice and mites could be an advantage. Such drugs include amitraz for topical application and avermectins (ivermectin, dor-amectin) for systemic administration (Table 5.6). Amitraz is available as a prepared solution for 'pour-on' application and as a liquid concentrate which, following appropriate dilution, can be applied to pigs by spray or 'pour-on'. Ivermectin can be administered in the form of a pre-mix for addition to the daily feed for 7 days, or the parenteral solution can be given by subcutaneous injection. Doramectin (parenteral solution) can be administered by intramus-cular injection in the lateral aspect of the neck. The parenteral dose of aver-mectins for pigs is 300 μg/kg, which is higher than that for ruminant animals (200 μg/kg). Deltamethrin is available as a prepared solution for 'spot-on' application to pigs but has activity only against lice. Specified withdrawal periods are associated with the use of all of these drugs in pigs.

Synthetic pyrethroids (cypermethrin, permethrin) and natural pyrethrins (pyrethrum extract) combined with piperonyl butoxide constitute the most important class of insecticide applied topically to horses (Table 5.7). The liquid concentrate containing cypermethrin which, after dilution, is applied to horses by spray contains a mixture of the isomers in equal proportion (*cis: trans* 50:50).

Table 5.6   Representative ectoparasticides for application to pigs.[a]

Ectoparasticide class & representative drugs	Spectrum of activity	Preparation	Method of application
Pyrethroid	Lice		
Deltamethrin		Solution	Spot on
Amidine	Lice, mites		
Amitraz		Solution	Pour on
		Liquid concentrate	Pour on or spray
Avermectin	Lice, mites		
Ivermectin		Parenteral solution	Subcutaneous injection
		Premix	Add to feed
Doramectin		Parenteral solution	Intramuscular injection

[a] Ectoparasites that affect pigs:
Lice   *Haematopinus suis* (sucking louse)
Mites   *Sarccoptes scabiei* var *suis* (burrowing mange mite).

Table 5.7 Representative ectoparasiticides for application to horses.[a]

Ectoparasiticide class & representative drugs	Spectrum of activity	Preparation	Method of application
Pyrethroid			
Cypermethrin	Flies, lice	Liquid concentrate	Spray
Permethrin	Lice, *Culicoides* midges	Solution	Pour on
Pyrethrins–piperonyl butoxide	Lice, *Culicoides* midges	Liquid concentrate Lotion	Shampoo
Avermectin			
Ivermectin	Mites, horse bots	Oral paste	
Organophosphate	Horse bots		
Haloxon		Oral powder (horses)	
Dichlorvos		Oral gel (foals)	
Benzyl benzoate	*Culicoides* midges	Lotion	

[a] Ectoparasites that affect horses:

Flies	*Haematobia irritans, Hydrotaea irritans, Stomoxys calcitrans, Musca domestica, M. autumnalis*
Biting midges	*Culicoides* spp. (insect saliva induces hypersensitivity)
Lice	*Bovicola equi* (biting louse), *Haematopinus* spp. (sucking louse)
Mites	*Sarcoptes, Psoroptes, Chorioptes*
Horse bots	*Gasterophilus intestinalis, G. nasalis*

It is effective against nuisance non-biting flies (*Hydrotaea irritans, Musca* spp.), blood-sucking flies (*Stomoxys calcitrans*, the 'stable fly', and *Haematobia irritans*) and lice (*Bovicola equi*, the biting louse, and *Haematopinus* spp.). The prepared solution of permethrin for 'pour-on' application (maximum volume of 40 ml) contains the isomers in unequal proportions (*cis: trans* 80:20). Permethrin has activity against *Culicoides* midges and lice. The spectrum of activity of the combination preparations containing natural pyrethrins and piperonyl butoxide (liquid concentrate and lotion) is similar to that of permethrin. Because piperonyl butoxide inhibits the inherently inefficient microsomal enzyme system of some arthropods, a synergistic action is produced by combining piperonyl butoxide with pyrethrins. Lotions containing a combination of pyrethrins and piperonyl butoxide or benzyl benzoate may be applied to horses for the control of sweet itch caused by hypersensitivity to *Culicoides* midges. The mechanism of action of benzyl benzoate is not known. Benzyl benzoate is toxic to cats. Lotions are usually aqueous solutions or suspensions of an active ingredient for application without friction to inflamed unbroken skin.

Ivermectin, an endectocide, has activity against endoparasites (gastro-intestinal roundworms and lungworms) and ectoparasites (mites and bots) of horses. The oral paste formulation of ivermectin (200 µg/kg) provides clinical efficacy against large strongyles (*Strongylus vulgaris, S. equinus, S. edentatus*), adult and most fourth stage larvae of the pathogenically important small strongyles (cyathostomes), ascarids (*Paracaris equorum*), stomach worms (*Draschia megastoma, Habronema* spp.), intestinal worms (*Trichostrongylus axei, Strongyloides westeri*), pinworms (*Oxyuris equi*) and lungworms (*Dictyocaulus arnfieldi*). In addition, the drug is effective against the migrating or stomach-attached stages of the three species of *Gasterophilus* bot (the most important of which is *G. intestinalis*) and in resolving skin lesions caused by *Onchocerca* microfilariae. The usual oral dose of ivermectin is effective against burrowing mites (*Sarcoptes* spp.) and non-burrowing mites (*Psoroptes* spp., *Chorioptes* spp.).

Even though haloxon and dichlorvos (organophosphorus compounds) have activity against some gastrointestinal nematodes of horses, the clinical indication for their use rests largely on their effectiveness against bots (*Gasterophilus* spp.). Haloxon is available as an oral powder for addition to the feed of adult horses, while an oral gel formulation of dichlorvos is specifically for use in foals over 5 weeks of age. Dichlorvos is clinically effective against ascarids (*Parascaris equorum*), pinworms (*Oxyuris equi, Probstmayria vivipara*) and *Strongylus vulgaris*, and against both migrating and sessile bots (*Gasterophilus intestinalis, G. nasalis*).

Dichlorvos, in liquid form for addition to bath water, is indicated for the treatment of salmon infested with sea lice (*Lepeophtheirus salmonis, Caligus elongatus*) before the stage at which serious skin damage is evident. As the organophosphate affects only mature lice, treatment should be repeated twice at intervals of 14 days. It is important that vigorous aeration of the bath water be provided at the time of medication. Teflubenzuron, a chitin synthesis inhibitor, may be an alternative to dichlorvos for the control of sea lice that infest farmed salmon. The drug, mixed with pelleted feed, is administered daily for 1 week.

There are several ectoparasitical preparations available for topical application to dogs and somewhat less for cats because of their characteristic behaviour and susceptibility to toxicity of certain drugs. Most of the ectoparasiticides have activity against fleas and application by 'spot-on' of a prepared solution or the wearing of an insecticidal collar, which provides continuous release of the drug, are the most popular methods of application, partly because of convenience for the pet owner (Table 5.8). Permethrin is indicated for the control of fleas (*Ctenocephalides felis, C. canis*) and lice (*Felicola, Trichodectes* – the biting louse) that infest dogs and cats, and may be effective against ticks (*Dermacentor, Rhipicephalus*). This synthetic pyrethroid is available as a variety of topical preparations which include prepared solution for 'spot-on' application (to dogs), collars, dusting powder, spray and shampoo (for dogs). The content of permethrin in these preparations is expressed in terms of the drug isomers (*cis:trans*), which may be present in varying proportions that range from 25:75 to 80:20, but most preparations contain the isomers in the proportion *cis:trans*, 40:60. The significance of the isomeric ratio with regard to the insecticidal activity of the drug is unclear. Pyrethrins and piperonyl butoxide, combined for their synergistic action, are present in various preparations for

Table 5.8 Representative ectoparasiticides for application to dogs and cats[a]

Ectoparasiticide class & representative drugs	Spectrum of activity	Preparation
Pyrethroid Permethrin Flumethrin Fenvalerate	Fleas, lice, (ticks)	Solution[b] (spot on); collars; spray; dusting powder; shampoo[b]; wash
Pyrethrins–piperonyl butoxide	Fleas, lice	Solution; dusting powder; spray; shampoo; wash
Organophosphate Dimpylate (diazinon) Dichlorvos Fenitrothion Fenthion Phosmet (dogs)	Fleas, ticks	Solution (spot on); collars; aerosol spray; liquid concentrate (sponge on)
Carbamate Propoxur Carbaril	Fleas, ticks	Collars; aerosol spray Solution
Fipronil	Fleas, ticks	Solution (spot on); spray
Amitraz[b]	*Sarcoptes, Demodex*	Liquid concentrate (sponge on)
Avermectin Ivermectin	Mites, ticks, fleas	Parenteral solution (s.c. injection); tablet (p.o.)
Milbemycin oxime Selamectin	*Otodectes cynotis*	Solution (spot on)

[a] Ectoparasites that affect dogs and cats:

Fleas	*Ctenocephalides felis, C. canis*
Lice	*Felicola, Trichodectes* (biting louse)
Mites	*Cheyletiella yasguri, Demoex canis, Sarcoptes scabiei* var *canis, Notoedres cati, Otodectes cynotis, Trombicula autumnalis, Pneumonyssus caninum*
Ticks (dogs)	*Rhipicephalus sanguineus. Dermacentor variabilis,* D. *reticulatus, Ixodes*

[b] For dogs.

the control of fleas mainly and lice on dogs and cats. *Ctenocephalides felis* resistance to various classes of insecticide, which include synthetic pyrethroids and organophosphorus compounds has been reported (Ross *et al.*, 1998).

Preparations for 'spot-on' application contain concentrated solutions of ectoparasiticides and should be applied directly to the skin at one (cats) or two (dogs) locations where the animal is unable to ingest the drug by licking it off.

The back of the neck is one such site. The total dose of a drug to apply will vary with the animal species (lower dose for cats) and the body weight range of dogs. Fenthion and fipronil are available for 'spot-on' application to dogs and cats, and permethrin for application to dogs. The prolonged insecticidal effect (for up to 2 months) of topically applied fipronil has been attributed to its slow release from sebaceous glands and skin surface migration by passive diffusion in sebum. There are insecticidal collars containing permethrin, dimpylate (diazinon), dichlorvos, carbaril or propoxur for dogs and cats, and a collar containing both flumethrin and propoxur for dogs. Insecticidal collars should be continuously worn by the animal, and most collars provide protection against fleas and ticks. The insecticide is slowly released from the collar during the period specified and is said to spread over the surface of the animal, similar to ear tags (contain permethrin or cypermethrin) for cattle. Carbaril and pro-poxur (carbamate insecticides) have very high lipid solubility. This property partly accounts for their effectiveness against fleas and ticks, but facilitates percutaneous absorption in the host animal and ultimately penetration of the blood–brain barrier. The mammalian-to-insect toxic dose ratio for carbamates (16:1) is approximately one-half of that for organophosphorus compounds (33:1) which explains the less selective toxicity of carbamates. The mammalian-to-insect toxic dose ratio is obtained from the rat oral LD_{50} to insect topical LD_{50} ratio.

Aerosol sprays containing propoxur (carbamate), combinations of pyrethrins and piperonyl butoxide, dichlorvos and fenitrothion (organophosphorus compounds) or fenvalerate (synthetic pyrethroid) and diethyltoluamide are more suitable for application of insecticides to dogs than to cats because cats resent (fearful response) being sprayed and lick the applied preparation from their coat. The combination preparation containing fenvalerate (0.09%) and diethyltoluamide (9.5%) has been reported to cause acute toxicity in some dogs and especially cats (Dorman *et al.*, 1990; Mount *et al.*, 1991). Diethyltoluamide (DEET), a cutaneous penetration-enhancing substance, may increase the absorption of fenvalerate to an extent which exceeds the immediate capacity of the body to metabolize the drug. Even though topically applied synthetic pyrethroids have a very wide margin of safety in mammalian species, caution should be exercised with the amount of compound applied to cats. There are non-aerosol sprays available that contain permethrin, fipronil, or a combination of pyrethrins and piperonyl butoxide. Fipronil (spray preparation) appears to be one of the few insecticides that may be applied to puppies and kittens under 12 weeks of age, which is the period during which the major pathways of drug metabolism develop. Liquid concentrates containing phosmet or amitraz, following dilution, can be applied by sponge to dogs for the treatment of sarcoptic (*Sarcopte scabiei* var *canis*) mange. Symptoms of amitraz toxicity, observed in a small proportion of dogs, resemble those produced by overdosing with α_2-adrenoceptor agonists and may be treated by administering tolazoline hydrochloride (5 mg/kg) slowly intravenously. Because idiosyncratic toxic reactions have been reported to occur in Chihuahuas and Miniature Poodles, amitraz should not be used on these breeds. Amitraz is toxic to cats, and the application of amitraz to horses is contra-indicated as the drug reduces intestinal motility which may result in impaction of the large colon.

Ivermectin, two doses (each 200 µg/kg) injected subcutaneously 14 days apart, appears to be effective in treating sarcoptic mange in dogs (Scheidt *et al.*, 1984), while a similar dosage regimen, apart from a higher dose (300 µg/kg), may be effective for the treatment of *Otodectes cynotis* and *Cheyletiella yasguri* infections. In cats, the subcutaneous injection of two doses (each 200 µg/kg) of the parenteral solution of ivermectin, 14 days apart, is clinically effective in treating *Notoedres cati* and *Otodectes cynotis* infections. The same dosage regimen can be used to treat *Pneumonyssus caninum* nasal mites in dogs and cats. The selective toxicity of ivermectin in based on the relative (mammal: insect) binding affinity of the drug for γ-aminobutyric acid (GABA) receptors, which are restricted to the central nervous system in mammalian species, and the impermeability of the blood–brain barrier of mammals to ivermectin. The idiosyncratic toxicity, manifested by neurological effects, to orally administered ivermectin at doses of 100 µg/kg or higher shown by a subpopulation of Collies could be attributed to a breed-related compromised blood–brain barrier, because the pharmacokinetic behaviour of the drug does not differ between 'ivermectin sensitive' and normal Collies (Tranquilli *et al.*, 1989). Adverse effects in Collies given ivermectin at the recommended oral dosage regimen for heartworm (*Dirofilaria immitis*) prevention (6–12 µg/kg given once a month) have not been reported. At this dose ivermectin is 100% effective in killing the developing third and fourth stage larvae of *D. immitis* acquired during the previous approximately 45 days. Two oral preparations (chewable tablets) are available for administration to dogs. One of these preparations contains ivermectin alone, while the other is a combination preparation containing ivermectin and pyrentel pamoate. Milbemycin oxime, chewable tablet administered orally to dogs at a dose of 500 µg/kg once a month, may be used as an alternative to ivermectin for the prevention of canine dirofilariasis and, in addition, provides clinical efficacy against mites and intestinal nematodes (*Toxocara canis*, *Trichuris vulpis*, *Ancylostoma caninum*, but unreliably *Unicinaria stenocephala*). Milbemycin oxime is moderately effective against *Demodex canis* when a prolonged course of treatment (1.5–3 mg/kg per day for 60 days) is applied. The animal owner should be advised of the cost of the treatment and the need for compliance with the dosage regimen. Commercially available oral formulations of ivermectin and milbemycin oxime have similar potential for producing toxicity in avermectin-sensitive Collies at 10–20 times the manufacturer's recommended dose for the prevention of heartworm infection; the recommended dose ranges are 6–12 µg/kg for ivermectin and 0.5–1 mg/kg for milbemycin oxime (Tranquilli *et al.*, 1991). Moxidectin, formulated as a tablet for administration to dogs, appears to have a wider margin of safety than ivermectin or milbemycin oxime, because signs of toxicity were not observed in avermectin-sensitive Collies at doses up to 30 times the manufacturer's recommended heartworm preventative dose, which is 3 µg/kg, of moxidectin (Paul *et al.*, 2000).

Selamectin is formulated as a topical preparation for 'spot-on' application at monthly intervals to dogs and cats. As selamectin, an avermectin endectocide, is percutaneously absorbed, the drug has clinical efficacy against both intestinal nematode and external (arthropod) parasites. It is indicated for the treatment, control and prevention of flea (*Ctenocephalides* spp.) infestation and of ear mites (*Otodectes cynotis*) in dogs and cats. Other indications in dogs include the treatment and control of sarcoptic mange mites (*Sarcoptes scabiei*), control of ticks (*Rhipicephalus sanguineus, Dermacentor variabilis*), prevention of heartworm (*Dirofilaria immitis*) infection, and the control of intestinal ascarid roundworms (*Toxocara canis*). It is indicated for the treatment and control of intestinal hookworms (*Ancylostoma tubaeforme*) and ascarid roundworms (*Toxocara cati*) in cats. The total dose for cats (2.5–7.5 kg body weight) is 45 mg, while the dose for dogs is related to the range of body weight: the total dose for dogs in the weight range of 10–20 kg is 120 mg. Following 'spot-on' application of the topical preparation of selamectin (Fig. 5.1), the systemic availability of the drug was substantially higher in cats (74%) (probably due to ingestion resulting from their grooming behaviour) than in dogs (4%). The apparent half-life of topically applied selamectin is approximately 8 days in cats and 11 days in dogs.

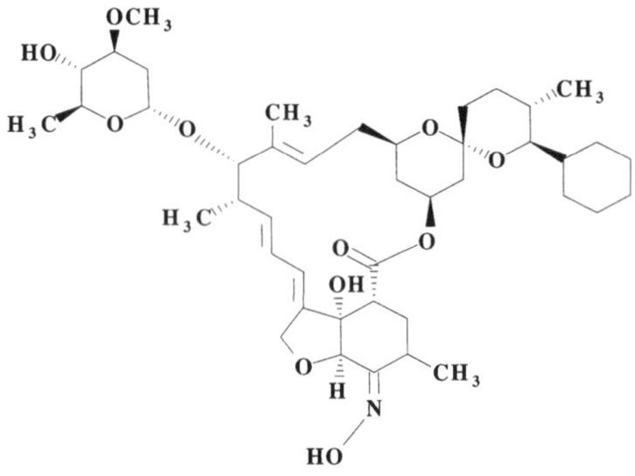

Fig. 5.1 Structural formula of selamectin (endectocide); $C_{43}H_{63}NO_{11}$, molecular weight 770 g/mol.

Antibacterial agents

When formulating dermatological preparations, an active ingredient should be incorporated in a vehicle that will facilitate application of the preparation, enhance delivery of the drug to the site of infection and cause little, ideally no, irritation. Depending on the vehicle used, dermatological preparations containing antibacterial agents include solutions, (aerosol) sprays, gels, creams, ointments and dusting powders. The type of preparation influences the stability and release of the active ingredient(s) and also evaporation from the surface of the skin. Release of the active ingredient is greatest from solutions, while evaporation from the site of application is most retarded from ointments. The application of an occlusive dressing will further decrease evaporation and may enhance penetration of the active ingredient, depending on its lipophilicity, to the site of infection.

Bacteria commonly isolated from primary skin infections in animals include *Staphylococcus* spp. (a large proportion of isolates show penicillinase activity), *Streptococcus* spp., *Proteus* spp. and *Escherichia coli*. Prolonged exposure to wet weather and muddy conditions under foot predispose horses and ruminant animals, respectively, to skin infection caused by *Dermatophilus congolensis*. Bacterial infections of the foot are generally caused by *Fusobacterium necrophorum* and *Bacteroides* spp.; footrot in sheep is caused by *Bacteroides (Dichelobacter) nodosus*.

The selection of an antibacterial agent should be based on the clinical diagnosis and, whenever feasible, *in vitro* culture and susceptibility testing of the microorganisms isolated. The microbiological results should be considered in conjunction with the pharmacological properties of the drugs that have activity against the causative pathogenic microorganism(s). In the treatment of superficial skin infections a topically applied antibacterial preparation may suffice, but in severe and deep-seated skin infections both local and systemic treatment should be applied. The selection of antibacterial agents for combined therapy requires consideration of potential interactions that would decrease clinical effectiveness (antagonistic action) or increase toxicity. Antibacterial agents that may be used for systemic treatment of skin infections and the route of administration will vary with the species of animal. In ruminant species, the intramuscular injection of enrofloxacin, trimethoprim–sulphadiazine combination or a long-acting preparation of oxytetracycline may be suitable. In addition to the antibacterial agents that may be administered to ruminant species, lincomycin hydrochloride (i.m. injection) could be considered for use in pigs. The choice of antibacterial preparations for use in horses is largely limited to procaine penicillin G (i.m. injection), cefadroxil (p.o.), or trimethoprim–sulphadiazine oral paste. The choice of antibacterial agent for use in dogs and cats is wide, and the oral route of administration is usual. The antibacterials include amoxycillin, alone or combined with clavulanic acid, cephalexin monohydrate, trimethoprim–sulphadiazine (or sulphamethoxazole) combination, marbofloxacin, clindamycin hydrochloride, and erythromycin (base or estolate).

Some antibacterial agents that are liable to produce systemic toxicity, especially kidney damage, when administered parenterally (neomycin, polymyxin B, bacitracin) can be applied topically because of poor percutaneous absorption. Neomycin has activity (bactericidal effect) against many opportunistic Gram-negative bacterial pathogens and *Staphylococcus aureus*, but its activity against other Gram-positive bacteria is generally low. Streptococci have a natural permeability barrier to aminoglycosides and, consequently, are inherently resistant. Cleansing the affected skin of exudate and cellular debris before the topical application of neomycin, either alone or combined with other antibacterial agents, will increase effectiveness. Neomycin sulphate is available as an aqueous solution and as a spray containing propylene glycol (vehicle) for topical application. Propylene glycol increases the permeability of the *stratum corneum* to water-soluble drugs (such as neomycin sulphate), and most of the small fraction which is percutaneously absorbed undergoes oxidation in the liver to lactic and pyruvic acids. Neomycin sulphate and zinc bacitracin are combined in a cream formulation to provide a broad spectrum of activity, and the combination may act synergistically against Gram-positive bacteria. Gels and creams are easier to apply than ointments, but are less occlusive. An ointment and an aerosol spray containing neomycin sulphate – zinc bacitracin–polymyxin B sulphate are available for the treatment of skin infections. Polymyxin B produces a rapid bactericidal effect on many Gram-negative aerobic bacteria including *E. coli* and *Pseudomonas aeruginosa*, but most strains of *Proteus* are resistant, as are all Gram-positive bacteria. A combination of polymyxin B sulphate and zinc bacitracin is formulated as an ointment to provide broad-spectrum activity.

Oxytetracycline hydrochloride, formulated as an aerosol spray for application to ruminant animals and pigs, may be effective for the treatment of superficial skin infections caused by streptococci *Clostridium* spp., *Actinomyces* spp., *Bacteroides nodosus* or *Fusobacterium necrophorum*. Because staphylococci, *E. coli* and *Proteus* spp., show variable susceptibility to tetracyclines, the determination of quantitative susceptibility, using the broth dilution method, of these microorganisms would indicate whether oxytetracycline would be effective. *Pseudomonas* spp. are resistant to tetracyclines. A dusting powder containing chlortetracycline hydrochloride and benzocaine is available for topical application to ruminant animals, pigs and horses. Nitrofurazone has activity (bactericidal effect) against *Streptococcus* spp., *Staphylococcus aureus* and *E. coli*, but *Proteus* spp. are often and *Pseudomonas* spp. are always resistant. For topical application, nitrofurazone is formulated as a solution and soluble dressing in polyethylene glycols, and as an ointment in polyglycol base. In contrast to propylene glycol, which enhances the skin permeability of certain substances (steroids and metronidazole), liquid polyethylene glycols appear ineffective in promoting percutaneous absorption. Nitrofurazone may be effective in the treatment of superficial skin infections caused by susceptible microorganisms. Silver sulphadiazine cream has been used to treat chronic otitis externa caused by multiply resistant *Pseudomonas aeruginosa*. It is effective in controlling bacteria that infect burn wounds in human patients. Fusidic acid is a lipophilic steroid antibiotic that is active mainly against Gram-positive bacteria. It is formulated as a cream and a gel, while sodium fusidate (soluble salt) is formulated as an ointment. These dermatological preparations are suitable for topical application in the treatment of skin infections caused by Gram-positive bacteria. The concurrent use of a penicillin, administered parenterally to horses and pigs, or orally to dogs and cats, prevents the emergence of resistant strains of *Staphylococcus aureus*.

Dermatophilosis can be treated systemically by administering intramuscularly a long-acting oxytetracyline preparation to ruminant animals. Infected horses should be groomed and bathed daily with either chlorhexidine gluconate solution or povidone–iodine solution and, if deemed necessary (severe or generalized infection), procaine penicillin G (two doses 24 h apart) can be administered intramuscularly. Chlorhexidine gluconate is used in water-based formulations as an antiseptic. At pH 5.5–7.0, chlorhexidine is active against vegetative bacteria and mycobacteria, and has moderate activity against fungi and viruses. It strongly adsorbs to bacterial membranes, causing leakage of small molecules and precipitation of cytoplasmic proteins. Chlorhexidine is most effective against Gram-positive cocci and somewhat less active against other bacteria. Because of its persistence, chlorhexidine has residual activity (bactericidal effect) when used repeatedly. The activity of chlorhexidine is relatively unaffected by the presence of blood, pus or necrotic tissue, but surfactants may neutralize its action. It is non-irritating to skin, and oral toxicity is low because of poor absorption. Povidone–iodine is an iodophore, i.e. a complex of iodine and a surface-active agent (polyvinylpyrrolidone). Solutions of povidone–iodine gradually release elemental iodine which exerts an antiseptic effect on vegetative bacteria, mycobacteria, fungi and lipid-containing viruses. In the 10% aqueous solution of povidone–iodine, the content of available iodine is low (1%) but, in contrast to tincture of iodine, the solution is non-irritating when applied to the skin. Tincture of iodine contains 2% iodine and 2.4% sodium iodide in 47% alcohol. It is the most active antiseptic for application to intact skin, producing an effect which is bactericidal, sporicidal, fungicidal, viricidal and protozoacidal.

Antifungal agents

Cutaneous mycotic infections caused by dermatophytic fungi can be treated either topically or systemically, depending on the location and severity of the skin lesions. Topical antifungal preparations should be formulated to promote penetration and persistence of the drug at the site of infection. Drugs that may be applied topically include various imidazole derivatives (clotrimazole, miconazole, enilconazole, ketoconazole), natamycin, nystatin and tolnaftate, while drugs administered orally include ketoconazole, fluconazole, itraconazole, nystatin and griseofulvin. Superficial infections caused by *Candida* spp. may be treated locally by applying an imidazole derivative or nystatin. Chronic generalized mucucutaneous candidiasis could be expected to respond to long-term oral therapy with ketoconazole.

In domestic animals and humans, the common fungal organisms that cause skin infections are *Trichophyton mentagrophytes* (the usual cause of ringworm in calves between 2 and 7 months of age), *Microsporum gypseum*, and *Trichophyton verrucosum* (in species other than dogs and cats). Superficial mycotic infections of the skin are also caused by *Trichophyton equinum* (horses, cattle, humans), *Microsporum nanum* (pigs, cattle, humans), and *Microsporum canis* (dogs and cats). Filamentous fungal keratitis in horses is usually caused by *Fusarium* spp. Yeasts, mainly *Candida* spp. can cause mastitis in cows, metritis in mares and occasionally inhabit the skin, mainly at mucocutaneous junctions, in dogs. *Malassezia pachydermatis* (*Pityrosporum canis*) causes pruritic skin disease in dogs, particularly in seborrhoeic conditions and in otitis externa. Although ringworm is generally a self-limiting disease, treatment with an antifungal drug can often shorten the duration of the infection. The success of treatment is greatly assisted by implementing management practices which reduce spread of this contagious mycotic disease.

The azole antifungal agents (e.g. ketoconazole) are generally fungistatic against a wide range of filamentous fungi, which include *Aspergillus* spp. and dermatrophytes (*Microsporum* and *Trichopyton* spp.), yeasts (*Cryptococcus neoformans*, *Candida* and *Malassezia* spp.) and dimorphic fungi (*Blastomyces dermatitidis*, *Histoplasma capsulatum*). The antifungal activity of azole drugs results from the reduction of ergosterol synthesis, the principal sterol incorporated in the cell membranes of fungi and yeasts, by causing inhibition of fungal cytochrome P450 enzymes (Grant & Clissold, 1989). The selectivity of antifungal azoles is due to their greater affinity for fungal than for mammalian cytochrome P450 enzymes. Because imidazoles (ketoconazole, miconazole, clotrimazole, enilconazole) are less selective in action than triazoles (itraconazole, fluconazole), the former subgroup would be expected to interfere to a greater extent with the biosynthesis of endogenous steroid hormones and to show a higher incidence of pharmacokinetic interactions with other drugs that undergo microsomal-mediated biotransformation. Itraconazole has the most selective action. In contrast to the other antifungal azoles, fluconazole is eliminated by renal excretion. For topical application, imidazoles are formulated as creams and lotions, and there appears to be no clear preference for the use of one imidazole over others. Ketoconazole alone and miconazole nitrate combined with chlorhexidine gluconate are available as shampoos for dogs. Enilconazole is formulated as a liquid concentrate, which must be diluted before topical application (by wash) to horses and dogs, and by spray to cattle. Even though topically applied ketoconazole or enilconazole is generally effective in the treatment of *Malassezia pachydermatis* infection in dogs, the shampoo containing miconazole nitrate and chlorhexidine gluconate is the treatment of choice. Following topical application, imidazoles attain effective concentrations in the outer layers, including the *stratum corneum*, of the epidermis and percutaneous absorption appears to be minimal.

For systemic treatment of fungal infections in dogs and cats, ketoconazole and fluconazole are available as tablets and oral suspensions, itraconazole as capsules, while miconazole and fluconazole are available as parenteral solutions. Even though ketoconazole is often effective, itraconazole may be the preferred azole for the treatment of systemic disease caused by dimorphic fungi (*Blastomyces dermatitidis*, *Histoplasma capsulatum*, *Sporothrix schenckii*). The activity of fluconazole against dimorphic fungi is limited to coccidioidal disease (*Coccidioides immitis*), but this azole penetrates the blood–brain barrier.

Consequently, fluconazole is the azole of choice for the treatment of crypto-coccal meningitis.

There is wide variation in the oral bioavailability of ketoconazole in dogs: systemic availability may be increased by the presence of food in the stomach. The oral dosage of ketoconazole for the treatment of cutaneous mycotic infections in dogs is 10 mg/kg administered daily for 4–6 weeks. Because low gastric pH is required for absorption of ketoconazole, dissolution of the drug in 0.2 N hydrochloric acid before administration by nasogastric tube increases systemic availability of the drug in horses. As ketoconazole undergoes exten-sive hepatic metabolism (microsomal-mediated oxidative reactions), the first-pass effect influences systemic availability of the drug. Even though cimetidine (H$_2$-receptor antagonist) inhibits cytochrome P450-mediated metabolism of a wide variety of drugs, concomitantly used cimetidine may decrease the sys-temic availability of ketoconazole due to the lowering of gastric acidity.

Nystatin, a polyene macrolide structurally similar to amphotericin B, avidly binds to ergosterol in the cellular membranes of yeasts and dermatophytic fungi, causing pore formation which allows leakage of intracellular ions and macromolecules, eventually leading to cell death (fungicidal effect). Nystatin is used mainly to treat cutaneous yeast infections caused by *Candida* spp., although some *Candida* spp. other than *C. albicans* may be resistant. It is avail-able as a cream and as an ointment for topical application. A cream containing a combination of nystatin and chlorhexidine hydrochloride is also available. Nystatin is not absorbed to any significant extent from skin, mucous mem-branes or the gastrointestinal tract. The oral suspension of nystatin may be effective for the treatment of gastrointestinal candidiasis, caused by *C. albicans*, in dogs and cats.

Natamycin is a polyene antibiotic with fungicidal activity against a wide range of filamentous fungi, including dermatophytes (*Microsporum* spp., *Tri-chophyton* spp.) and against yeasts (*Candida* spp., *Cryptococcus neoformans*). It is available as a suspension, powder for reconstitution and dilution with water, for topical application. Natamycin, applied by spray or sponge using 1 L of 100 ppm (0.01%) aqueous solution/suspension on two occasions with a 4-day interval and applied again after 14 days if required, is effective in the treatment of ringworm in horses. It is important that all grooming utensils and tackle be thoroughly cleansed and immersed in the natamycin suspension, which should be prepared in plastic or galvanized containers (Oldenkamp, 1979). Natamycin has been used successfully to treat filamentous fungal keratitis, particularly when caused by *Fusarium* spp. in horses (Hodgson & Jacobs, 1982; Beech & Sweeney, 1983). A recommended treatment is to apply one drop of a 5% aqu-eous suspension every 1 or 2 h, decreasing to six or eight times daily after a few days. If *Aspergillus* is mycologically identified as the causative organism of a corneal infection, miconazole (10 mg/ml parenteral solution) may be the anti-fungal of choice. Locally applied natamycin suspension is generally effective in the treatment of nasal aspergillosis in horses. The drug has potential applica-tion in the local treatment of *Candida* metritis in mares and *Candida* mastitis in cows. In either condition, 20 ml of a 2.5% aqueous suspension of natamycin should be infused once daily for 3 days.

Tolnaftate is a synthetic antifungal agent with a narrow spectrum of activity which is limited to dermatophytes (*Epidermophyton, Microsporum* and *Trichophyton* spp.). It could be used to treat mild localized dermatophytic infection. For topical application to dogs, tolnaftate is formulated as a 1% cream containing both polyethylene glycol and propylene glycol. The powder aerosol preparation is less likely to be effective for treatment, but could be applied to prevent spread of the infection.

Griseofulvin is a very poorly soluble fungistatic antibiotic which is administered orally to treat cutaneous infection caused by dermatophytes (*Trichophyton, Epidermophyton* and *Microsporum* spp.). The selectivity of action of griseofulvin is due to an energy-dependent preferential uptake of the drug by susceptible dermatophytic fungi. Having entered fungal cells the drug acts by disrupting the mitotic spindle, causing mitotic arrest in metaphase. Griseofulvin is active only against growing cells. A prolonged duration of treatment (6–8 weeks) is invariably required. The drug is available as tablets for administration to dogs and cats, as an oral paste for horses, and as oral granules for addition to the feed for horses, donkeys and cattle. Griseofulvin should not be administered to pregnant animals. In dogs and cats, absorption of griseofulvin is increased when the drug is given in conjunction with a fatty meal. Decreasing particle size from micronized to ultramicronized griseolfulvin further increases oral bioavailability and would allow up to 50% reduction in the daily dose. The systemically available drug distributes to the various layers of the epidermis, including the *stratum corneum*. It is eliminated by hepatic biotransformation. Cats appear to be more prone than dogs to the development of side-effects during therapy (Helton *et al.*, 1986). Because diligently applied topical treatment of dermatophytic infection is often effective, systemic therapy with an orally administered antifungal agent (griseofulvin, ketoconazole, itraconazole) should be reserved for severe or refractory cases. Topical treatment would avoid side-effects and/or interaction (decreased rate of elimination) with concomitantly administered drugs that undergo hepatic cytochrome P450-mediated metabolism. Ringworm is highly contagious and even though *Trichophyton equinum, Microsporum canis, Microsporum nanum* and possibly *Trichophyton verrucosum* are primarily fungal pathogens of animals, infection can be transmitted to humans (zoonotic disease).

Topical corticosteroids

The therapeutic effectiveness of topically applied corticosteroids results primarily from their anti-inflammatory activity. The local action could be largely due to inhibition of phospholipase A_2, which is responsible for the release of arachidonic acid from epidermal cells and vascular endothelial cells. This action would result in decreased production of prostaglandins and leukotrienes (inflammatory mediators and/or modulators). Glucocorticoids are capable of stabilizing lysosomal membranes within neutrophils that infiltrate the dermis and/or epidermis in inflammatory skin diseases. The relative efficacy of the various topical glucocorticoids appears to be in the following order: hydrocortisone, prednisolone, betamethasone < hydrocortisone valerate or butyrate, betamethasone valerate, triamcinolone acetonide, flucinolone acetonide < betamethasone dipropionate, fluocinonide (which is the 21-acetate derivative of fluocinolone acetonide). In addition to the nature of the glucocorticoid, its solubility and, to a lesser extent, the concentration used, the formulation of the preparation influences clinical efficacy. Glucocorticoids tend to have greater efficacy when formulated in ointment bases than in cream or lotion vehicles. This could be attributed to the occlusive effect provided by ointments. When applied to normal skin, glucocorticoids slowly penetrate the *stratum corneum* where they tend to persist; absorption into the systemic circulation is minimal. The application of an occlusive (water impermeable) dressing enhances penetration, leading to increases in both the concentration and persistence of the steroid (reservoir effect) in the *stratum corneum* (Munro & Stoughton, 1965; Barry, 1983). When clinical remission of the inflammatory condition has been achieved, the once daily application of a lower efficacy glucocorticoid preparation should suffice.

In the treatment of secondarily infected dermatoses, which are usually colonized with streptococci, staphylococci, or both, compound anti-inflammatory and antibacterial preparations are indicated when the underlying disorder has been diagnosed. Corticosteroids do not appear to inhibit the activity of antibacterial agents in compound preparations for topical application. Examples of topical compound preparations include: betamethasone valerate–fusidic acid gel (for dogs), betamethasone sodium phosphate–neomycin sulphate cream (for dogs and cats), prednisolone–neomycin sulphate–nitrofurazone ointment (for horses, dogs and cats). The use of compound preparations is contra-indicated in pregnant animals.

There are various topical compound preparations available for the treatment of otitis externa in dogs and cats. The majority of these preparations are formulated as ear drops. Some compound preparations contain an antibacterial agent (neomycin sulphate or polymyxin B sulphate), an antifungal agent (nystatin, natamycin or miconazole nitrate) and a corticosteroid (hydrocortisone, betamethasone, prednisolone or triamcinolone acetonide). Other preparations contain an antibacterial agent and an ectoparasiticide (synthetic pyrethroid or pyrethrins and piperonyl butoxide). A local anaesthetic (tetracaine or benzocaine) is incorporated in a minority of topical compound preparations, e.g. ear drops containing neomycin sulphate, permethrin (*cis:trans* 25:75) and tetracaine hydrochloride for use in dogs and cats. Selection of the drug product should be based on clinical, supported by microbiological, diagnosis of the underlying cause of otitis externa infection. Whenever the infection is caused by a single type of organism, the product selected should contain a drug with activity against the causative organism either alone or combined with a topical corticosteroid. The collection of specimens for microbiological diagnosis must precede the initiation of therapy. Cleansing of the ear canal (generally using a solution containing propylene glycol) to remove wax and cellular debris before each application of the drug product will enhance the effectiveness of treatment. *Otodectes cynotis* infection in cats can be treated with an avermectin, either selamectin applied by 'spot-on' or ivermectin administered by subcutaneous injection.

Transdermal therapeutic systems

A transdermal therapeutic system is a rate-controlled drug delivery system which, applied to the surface of the skin, continuously releases the drug at a rate that will provide a desired steady-state plasma concentration for a specified duration. A candidate drug must possess high activity (i.e. be effective at low plasma concentrations) and efficiently penetrate the *stratum corneum*; percutaneous absorption must be reliably consistent. Based on technological design there are four types of rate-controlled transdermal drug delivery system (Chien, 1987):

- Membrane permeation-controlled
- Adhesive dispersion type
- Matrix diffusion-controlled
- Microreservoir dissolution-controlled.

Membrane permeation-controlled transdermal drug delivery (Fig. 5.2) has been successfully applied in therapeutic systems for scopolamine (prevention of motion sickness for a 3-day period), nitroglycerin (prophylaxis against attack of angina pectoris over a 24-h period), clonidine (control of hypertension for a 7-day period), and fentanyl (control of constant pain for 72 h).

Transdermal therapeutic systems of various types that will deliver nitro-

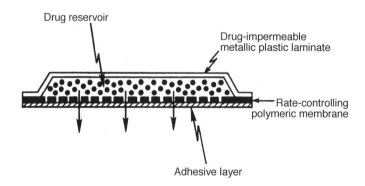

Fig. 5.2 Cross-sectional view of a membrane-moderated transdermal drug delivery system showing major structural components. (Reproduced with permission from Chien (1985).)

glycerin at a constant rate over a 24-h period are commercially available. Nitroglycerin (glyceryl trinitrate) is rapidly metabolized in the liver by reductive hydrolysis which is catalysed by the enzyme glutathione–organic nitrate reductase. This high-capacity hepatic enzyme converts lipid-soluble organic nitrate esters into more water-soluble denitrated metabolites that form glucuronide conjugates and inorganic nitrite. Avoidance of hepatic first-pass metabolism is a primary consideration with regard to the manner of administration of nitroglycerin. A comparative transdermal bioavailability study carried out in six normal volunteers showed that there was no statistically significant difference between the plasma concentration profiles of nitroglycerin delivered by the Transderm-Nitro (type 1), Nitro-Dur (type 3) and Nitrodisc (type 4) transdermal therapeutic systems (Shaw, 1984). In another study, the steady-state plasma concentration of nitroglycerin was found to be linearly proportional to the drug-releasing surface area of the transdermal therapeutic system (Transderm-Nitro) in contact with the skin (Good, 1983). For each unit area (cm^2) of the drug-releasing surface of the system in intimate contact with the skin, a plasma nitroglycerin concentration of 14 pg/mL was achieved.

Clonidine, a centrally acting α_2-adrenoceptor agonist causing a consequent decrease in plasma renin concentration, is a suitable drug for controlled-release transdermal delivery, both because of its effectiveness in controlling hypertension at very low plasma concentrations and its physicochemical properties, which include low molecular weight and high lipid solubility. Percutaneous absorption avoids first-pass hepatic metabolism, although metabolism may occur in the epidermis, while constant-rate entry into the systemic circulation avoids the variability associated with gastrointestinal absorption and the fluctuation in plasma concentrations that occurs during the intervals between successive oral doses, particularly of conventional dosage forms. The membrane permeation-controlled transdermal delivery system designed to release clonidine at a constant rate for 7 days can maintain steady-state plasma concentrations within the narrow therapeutic concentration range for this drug (0.2–2 ng/mL). As the average half-life of clonidine in humans is 12 h, the attainment of steady-state plasma concentration will be slow (Shaw, 1984). This is not a major drawback because the indication for clonidine is the control of hypertension and a prolonged effect is more important than an immediate effect.

The transdermal therapeutic system containing fentanyl [μ (mainly)-opioid agonist] which was designed to release the drug at a constant rate for 72 h, may have application in dogs for the control of post-operative (surgical) pain. Secure placement of the transdermal system that releases 50 μg/h of fentanyl on the dorsal aspect of the thorax of Beagle dogs (11.4–16.5 kg body weight) provided an average steady-state plasma fentanyl concentration of 1.6 ng/mL, which is within the range of plasma concentrations (1–2 ng/mL) considered to provide analgesia without producing other significant effects (Holley & Van Steennis, 1988; Kyles *et al.*, 1996). A steady-state concentration of fentanyl in plasma was reached at approximately 24 h after placement of the transdermal system, as would be expected because the half-life of fentanyl in Beagles is 6 h, and was maintained until removal of the system at 72 h. As the dosing rate (3.7 µg/h·kg) exceeded the amount of drug cleared systemically (2.7 µg/h·kg) and the transdermal bioavailability of fentanyl is 64%, a fraction of the released drug either persists in the *stratum corneum* or is metabolized in the epidermis preceding absorption into the systemic circulation, or both may contribute to incomplete systemic availability of the drug. Because of the 24 h delay in achieving plasma concentrations within the analgesia-producing range, either an intravenous dose (approximately 30 µg/kg) could be administered at the time of placement of the transdermal system or the system could be securely placed on the animal 12 h before performing the surgery.

When the transdermal penetration of a drug is inadequate to achieve and maintain a plasma concentration above the minimum therapeutic concentration required to produce the desired effect, a lipophilic prodrug that will be metabolized in the epidermis to the active drug could be used in the development of a controlled-release transdermal delivery system. This approach has been applied to estradiol esters (diacetate and valerate) which are rapidly converted by esterases in the skin tissue to estradiol (Chien *et al.*, 1985). The prodrug serves to increase the transdermal bioavailability of the active drug to which it is converted by metabolism (generally ester hydrolysis) during the percutaneous absorption process.

Whenever a drug delivery device, such as an insecticidal collar or a transdermal system, is securely placed on an animal, the increased potential for drug interaction must be borne in mind at the time of selecting another drug for administration by any route and throughout the course of therapy.

References

Ademola, J.I., Chow, C.A., Wester, R.C. & Maibach, H.I. (1991) Metabolism of propranolol during percutaneous absorption in human skin. *Journal of Pharmaceutical Sciences*, **82**, 767–770.

Alva-Valdes, R., Wallace, D.H., Holste, J.E., Egerton, J.C., Cox, J.L., Woodes, J.W. & Barrick, R.A. (1986) Efficacy of ivermectin in a topical formulation against induced gastrointestinal and pulmonary nematode infections and naturally acquired grubs and lice in cattle. *American Journal of Veterinary Research*, **47**, 2389–2392.

Barry, B.W. (1983) Properties that influence percutaneous absorption. In: *Dermatological Formulations: Percutaneous Absorption*, pp. 127–233. Marcel Dekker, New York.

Bartek, M.J., LaBuddle, J.A. & Maibach, H.I. (1972) Skin permeability in vivo: comparison in rat, rabbit, pig and man. *Journal of Investigative Dermatology*, **58**, 114–123.

Bashir, S.J. & Maibach, H.I. (1999) Cutaneous metabolism of xenobiotics. In: *Percutaneous Absorption*, (eds R.L. Bronaugh & HI Maibach), pp. 65–80. Marcel Dekker, New York.

Beech, J. & Sweeney, C.R. (1983) Keratomycoses in 11 horses. *Equine Veterinary Journal* (Suppl. 2: Equine ophthalmology), 123–124.

Behrendt, H., Korting, H. Ch. & Braun-Falco, O. (1989) Zum metabolismus von pharmaka in der haut. *Hautarzt*, **40**, 8–13.

Carver, M.P. & Riviere, J.E. (1989) Percutaneous absorption and excretion of xenobiotics after topical and intravenous administration to pigs. *Fundamental and Applied Toxicology*, **13**, 714–722.

Chien, Y.W. (1985) The use of biocompatible polymers in rate-controlled drug delivery systems. *Pharmaceutical Technology*, **9**, 50–66.

Chien, Y.W. (1987) Developmental concepts and practice in transdermal therapeutic systems. In: *Transdermal Controlled Systemic Medications*, (ed. Y.W. Chien), pp. 25–81. Marcel Dekker, New York.

Chien, Y.W., Valia, K.H. & Doshi, U.B. (1985) Long-term permeation kinetics of estradiol. V. Development and evaluation of transdermal bioactivated hormone delivery system. *Drug Development and Industrial Pharmacy*, **11**, 1195–1212.

Dorman, D.C., Buck, W.B., Trammel, H.L., Jones, R.D. & Beasley, V.R. (1990) Fenvalerate/N, N-diethyl-*m*-toluamide (DEET) toxicosis in two cats. *Journal of the American Veterinary Medical Association*, **196**, 100–102.

Elias, P.M., Cooper, E.R., Korc, A. & Brown, B.E. (1981) Percutaneous transport in relation to stratum corneum structure and lipid composition. *Journal of Investigative Dermatology*, **76**, 297–301.

Forsyth, B.A., Gibbon, A.J. & Pryor, D.E. (1983) Seasonal variations in anthelmintic response by cattle to dermally applied levamisole. *Australian Veterinary Journal*, **60**, 141–146.

Good, W.R. (1983) Transderm-Nitro: controlled delivery of nitroglycerin via the transdermal route. *Drug Development and Industrial Pharmacy*, **9**, 647–670.

Grant, S.M. & Clissold, S.P. (1989) Itraconazole: a review of its pharmacodynamic and pharmacokinetic properties, and therapeutic use in superficial and systemic mycoses. *Drugs*, **37**, 310–344.

Gyrd-Hansen, N., Brimer, L. & Rasmussen, R. (1991) Percutaneous absorption and recovery of parathion in pigs. *Acta Veterinaria Scandinavica*, **87** [Suppl. (Proceedings of the 5th Congress of EAVPT)], 410–412.

Helton, K.A., Nesbitt, G.H. & Caciolo, P.L. (1986) Griseofulvin toxicity in cats: literature review and report of seven cases. *Journal of the American Animal Hospital Association*, **22**, 453–458.

Hodgson, D.R. & Jacobs, K.A. (1982) Two cases of *Fusarium* keratomycosis in the horse. *Veterinary Record*, **110**, 520–522.

Holley, F.O. & van Steennis, C. (1988) Postoperative analgesia with fentanyl: pharmacokinetics and pharmacodynamics of constant-rate IV and transdermal delivery. *British Journal of Anaesthesia*, **60**, 608–613.

Hooser, S.B. (1990). D-Limonene, linalool, and crude citrus oil extracts. *Veterinary Clinics of North America: Small Animal Practice*, **20**(2), 383–385.

Idsen, I. (1975) Percutaneous absorption. *Journal of Pharmaceutical Sciences*, **64**, 901–924.

Idson, B. (1983) Vehicle effects on percutaneous absorption. *Drug Metabolism Reviews*, **14**, 207–222.

Kao, J. & Carver, M.P. (1990) Cutaneous metabolism of xenobiotics. *Drug Metabolism Reviews*, **22**, 363–410.

Krishna, D.R. & Klotz, U. (1994) Extrahepatic metabolism of drugs in humans. *Clinical Pharmacokinetics*, **26**, 144–160.

Kyles, A.E., Papich, M. & Hardie, E.M. (1996) Disposition of transdermally administered fentanyl in dogs. *American Journal of Veterinary Research*, **57**, 715–719.

McCreesh, A.H. (1965) Percutaneous toxicity. *Toxicology and Applied Pharmacology*, **7** (Suppl. 2), 20–26.

McKenzie, A.W. (1962) Percutaneous absorption of steroids. *Archives of Dermatology*, **86**, 91–94.

Marriner, S.E., McKinnon, I. & Bogan, J.A. (1987) The pharmacokinetics of ivermection after oral and subcutaneous administration to sheep and horses. *Journal of Veterinary Pharmacology and Therapeutics*, **10**, 175–179.

Merk, H.F., Jergert, F.K. & Frankenberg, S. (1996) Biotransformations in the skin. In: *Dermatotoxicology*, (eds F.N. Marzulli & H.I. Maibach), 5th edn. pp. 61–74. Marcel Dekker, New York.

Montagna, W. (1967) Comparative anatomy and physiology of the skin. *Archives of Dermatology*, **96**, 357–363.

Monteiro-Riviere, N.A. & Stromberg, M.W. (1985) Ultrastructure of the integument of the domestic pig (*Sus scrofa*) from one through fourteen weeks of age. *Zentralblatt für Veterinarmedizin*, [*Reihe C: Anatomia, Histologia, Embryologia*], **14**, 97–115.

Monterio-Riviere, N.A., Bristol, D.G., Manning, T.O., Rogers, R.A. & Riviere, J.E. (1990) Interspecies and interregional analysis of the comparative histologic thickness and laser doppler blood flow measurements at five cutaneous sites in nine species. *Journal of Investigative Dermatology*, **95**, 582–586.

Mount, M.E., Moller, G., Cook, J., Holstege, D.M., Richardson, E.R. & Ardans, A. (1991) Clinical illness associated with a commercial tick and flea product in dogs and cats. *Veterinary and Human Toxiocology*, **33**, 19–27.

Munro, D.D. & Stoughton, R.B. (1965) Dimethylacetamide (DMAC) and dimethylformamide (DMFA): effect on percutaneous absorption. *Archives of Dermatology*, **92**, 585–586.

Oldenkamp, E.P. (1979) Treatment of ringworm in horses with natamycin. *Equine Veterinary Journal*, **11**, 36–38.

Paul, A.J., Tranquilli, W.J. & Hutchens, D.E. (2000) Safety of moxidectin in avermectin-sensitive collies. *American Journal of Veterinary Research*, **61**, 482–483.

Pitman, I.H. & Rostas, S.J. (1981) Topical drug delivery to cattle and sheep. *Journal of Pharmaceutical Sciences*, **70**, 1181–1194.

Reifenrath, W.G. & Hawkins, G.S. (1986) The weanling Yorkshire pig as an animal model for measuring percutaneous penetration. In: *Swine in Biomedical Research*, (ed. M.E. Tumbleson), pp. 673–680. Plenum Press, New York.

Reigelman, S. (1974) Pharmacokinetics: pharmacokinetic factors affecting epidermal penetration and percutaneous absorption. *Clinical Pharmacology and Therapeutics*, **16**, 873–883.

Riviere, J.E. & Chang, S.K. (1992) Transdermal penetration and metabolism of organophosphate insecticides. In: *Organophosphates: Chemistry, Fate and Effects*. Academic Press, New York.

Riviere, J.E. & Monteiro-Riviere, N.A. (1991) The isolated perfused porcine skin flap as an *in vitro* model for percutaneous absorption and cutaneous toxicology. *Critical Reviews in Toxicology*, **21**, 329–344.

Riviere, J.E., Monteiro-Riviere, N.A. & Williams, P.L. (1995) The isolated perfused porcine skin flap as an *in vitro* model for predicting transdermal pharmacokinetics. *European Journal of Pharmaceutics and Biopharmaceutics*, **41**, 152–162.

Ross, D.H., Young, D.R., Young, R. & Pennington, R.G. (1998) Topical pyriproxyfen for control of the cat flea and management of insecticide resistance. *Feline Practice*, **26**, 18–22.

Ryder, M.L. (1957) A survey of the follicle populations in a range of British breeds of sheep. *Journal of Agricultural Science*, **49**, 275–282.

Schalla, W., Jamoulle, J. & Schaefer, H. (1989) Localization of compounds in different skin layers and its use as an indicator of percutaneous absorption. In: *Percutaneous Absorption*, (eds R.L. Bronaugh & H.I. Maibach), pp. 283–312. Marcel Dekker, New York.

Scheidt, V.J., Medleau, L., Seward, R.L. & Schwartzman, R.W. (1984) An evaluation of ivermectin in the treatment of sarcoptic mange in dogs. *American Journal of Veterinary Research*, **45**, 1201–1202.

Scheuplein, R.J. (1965) Mechanisms of percutaneous absorption. I. Routes of penetration and influence of solubility. *Journal of Investigative Dermatology*, **45**, 334–346.

Scheuplein, R.J. (1978) Site variations in diffusion and permeability. In: *The Physiology and Pathophysiology of the Skin*, Vol. 5, (ed A. Jarrett), pp. 1731–1752. Academic Press, New York.

Scheuplein, R.J. & Blank, I.H. (1971) Permeability of the skin. *Physiological Reviews*, **51**, 702–746.

Shaw, J.E. (1984) Pharmacokinetics of nitroglycerin and clonidine delivered by the transdermal route. *American Heart Journal*, **108**, 217–222.

Spinelli, J.S. & Enos, J.R. (1978) Veterinary therapeutics and drug interactions. In *Drugs in Veterinary Practice*, pp. 12–28. CV Mosby, St. Louis.

Stone, B.F. & Knowles, C.O. (1974) A laboratory method for evaluation of chemicals causing detachment of the cattle tick *Boophilus microplus*. *Journal of the Australian Entomological Society*, **12**, 163–172.

Tranquilli, W.J., Paul, A.J. & Seward, R.L. (1989) Ivermectin plasma concentrations in Collies sensitive to ivermectin-induced toxicosis. *American Journal of Veterinary Research*, **50**, 769–770.

Tranquilli, W.J., Paul, A.J. & Todd, K.S. (1991) Assessment of toxicosis induced by high-dose administration of milbemycin oxime in Collies. *American Journal of Veterinary Research*, **52**, 1170–1172.

Ward, S., Walle, T., Walle, K., Wilkinson, G.R. & Branch, R.A. (1989) Propranolol's metabolism is determined by both mephenytoin and debrisoquin hydroxylase. *Clinical Pharmacology and Therapeutics*, **45**, 72–78.

Wester, R.C. & Maibach, H.I. (1983) Cutaneous pharmacokinetics: 10 steps to percutaneous absorption. *Drug Metabolism Reviews*, **14**, 169–205.

Wester, R.C. & Maibach, H.I. (1999) Regional variation in percutaneous absorption. In: *Percutaneous Absorption*, (eds R.L. Bronaugh & H.I. Maibach), 3rd edn. pp. 107–116. Marcel Dekker, New York.

Chapter 6
Antimicrobial Disposition, Selection, Administration and Dosage

Introduction

In the treatment of a bacterial infection, the antimicrobial agent selected must have activity against the causative pathogenic microorganism and must attain effective concentrations at the site of infection. The ultimate criterion of successful therapy is a favourable clinical response to the treatment. Such a response depends on the interrelations between the causative pathogenic microorganism, the animal receiving treatment, and the antimicrobial drug selected and dosage used. Inadequacy of host defence mechanisms, particularly in neonatal foals and in immunocompromized animals, could contribute to a discrepancy between the expected and actual response to antimicrobial therapy. In these animals, it is preferable to use antimicrobial agents, alone or combined, that produce a bactericidal effect.

Antimicrobial classification

Antimicrobial agents are classified on the basis of molecular structure, which determines their chemical nature and related physicochemical properties (pK_a/pH-dependent degree of ionization, lipid solubility). The drugs within each class generally have the same mechanism of action, a broadly similar spectrum of antimicrobial activity (Table 6.1) and reasonably similar disposition (i.e. extent of distribution and elimination processes) (Table 6.2). Individual drugs within a class differ quantitatively in antimicrobial activity and, when mainly eliminated by hepatic metabolism, in the rate of elimination (usually expressed as half-life). Bioavailability, which refers to the rate and extent of absorption, and the withdrawal period vary with the dosage form of a drug and may differ between animal species. Selective tissue binding (e.g. aminoglycosides) is a cause for concern in terms of the pathological lesion that may be produced in the particular tissue and the persistence of drug residues (a long withdrawal period is required).

Table 6.1 Spectrum of antimicrobial activity (semi-quantitative).[a]

Antimicrobial class	Usual effect	Gram-positive	Gram-negative	Anaerobic bacteria	Other microorganisms	Protozoa
Penicillins	C					
Penicillin G[b]		+++	(+)	+(+)	—	
Aminobenzyl penicillins[c]		++	+(+)	+	—	
Carboxypenicillins[d]		+	+(+)	+	—	
Isoxazolyl penicillins[e]		++	—	—	—	
Cephalosporins	C					
First-generation[f]		++	+	+	—	
Second-generation[g]		+	++	++ [cefoxitin]	—	
Third-generation[h]		+	++(+)	+ [ceftizoxime]	—	
Aminoglycosides	C	(+)	+++	—	(*Mycoplasma* spp.)	
Fluoroquinolones	C	+(+)	+++	(+) [difloxacin]	*Mycoplasma* spp. *Chlamydia* spp.	
Trimethoprim–sulphonamide	C	++	++	+	*Chlamydia* spp.	*Toxoplasma* spp.
Tetracyclines	S	++	++	+	*Mycoplasma* spp. *Chlamydia* spp. *Rickettsia* spp.	*Theileria* spp. *Eperythrozoon* spp. *Anaplasma* spp.
Chloramphenicol	S	++	+(+)	++	(*Mycoplasma* spp.) (*Chlamydia* spp.) *Rickettsia* spp.	

Contd.

Table 6.1 *Contd.*

Antimicrobial class	Usual effect	Gram-positive	Gram-negative	Anaerobic bacteria	Other microorganisms	Protozoa
Macrolides	S	++	(+)	(+)	Mycoplasma spp. [Tylosin]	
Lincosamides	S	++	–	++ (clindamycin)	(Mycoplasma spp.)	
Rifampin	C	++	–/(+)	+(+)	Chlamydia spp. Rickettsia spp.	
Metronidazole	C	–	–	+++	–	Trichomonas foetus Giardia lamblia Histomonas meleagridis
Sulphonamides	S	+	(+)	+	Chlamydia spp.	

[a] C, bactericidal; S, bacteriostatic; +++, most active; (+), some activity; (+(+) is greater than + and less than ++; –, no activity; the drug of choice (most active) within a class is shown in square brackets.
[b] Phenoxymethyl penicillin (penicillin V) – acid stable.
[c] Ampicillin, amoxycillin and prodrugs.
[d] Ticarcillin, carbenicillin – anti-pseudomonal (*P. aeruginosa*).
[e] Cloxacillin, oxacillin, nafcillin, methicillin – relatively resistant to staphylococcal β-lactamase; acid stable.
[f] Cefadroxil, cephalexin (both oral); cafezolin, cephalothin (both parenteral).
[g] Cefuroxime (oral); cefoxitin (i.v.).
[h] Cefixime (oral); cefotaxime, ceftizoxime, cefoperazone, ceftriaxone, ceftazidime (all i.v.).

Table 6.2 Extent of distribution and processes of elimination of antimicrobial agents.

Antimicrobial agent	Extent of distribution (comment)	Elimination process(es)[a]
β-Lactams	Limited – low intracellular concns	E(r), except nafcillin, cefoperazone and ceftriaxone, E(r + h)
Aminoglycosides	Limited – mainly extracellular fluid (selective binding to renal cortex; inner ear)	E(r)
Fluoroquinolones	Wide (developing cartilage)	M(h) + E(r + h)
Trimethoprim	Wide	M(h) + E(r)
Sulphonamides	Moderate	M(h) + E(r), except sulfisoxazole, E(r) + M(h)
Tetracyclines	Wide (sites of ossification; developing teeth)	E(r + h), except doxycycline, E(f) and minocycline M(h)
Chloramphenicol[b]	Wide	M(h) + E(r)
Metronidazole[c]	Wide	M(h) + E(r)
Erythromycin[b]	Wide – high intracellular concn	M(h) + E(h)
Clinidamycin	Wide	M(h) + E(r)
Rifampin**[d]	Wide – high intracellular concn, including phagocytes	M(h) + E(h + r)

[a] E(r), excretion (renal); M(h), metabolism (hepatic); E(r + h), excretion (renal and hepatic); E(f), excretion (faecal).
[b] Inhibits hepatic microsomal enzymes.
[c] Inhibits aldehyde dehydrogenase (non-microsomal enzyme).
[d] Induces hepatic microsomal enzymes.

Mechanisms of action

Antimicrobial action usually depends on the inhibition of biochemical events that exist in or are essential to the bacterial pathogen but not the host animal. Unfortunately, the action of antimicrobial agents is not selective for pathogenic microorganisms and the balance between the commensal flora can be seriously disturbed, particularly in the colon of horses (macrolides, lincosamides and, parenterally administered doxycycline).

The actions of antimicrobial agents can be adequately distinguished by the following general mechanisms:

- Selective inhibition of bacterial cell wall synthesis (penicillins, cephalosporins, bacitracin, vancomycin). Following attachment to receptors (penicillin-binding proteins), β-lactam antibiotics inhibit transpeptidation enzymes and thereby block the final stage of peptidoglycan sysnthesis. This action is followed by inactivation of an inhibitor of autolytic enzymes in the bacterial cell wall. Bacitracin and vancomycin inhibit early stages of peptidoglycan synthesis.
- Inhibition of cell membrane function by disrupting functional integrity of the bacterial (polymyxins) or fungal (antifungal azoles and polyenes) cytoplasmic membrane. Antifungal azoles (e.g. ketoconazole, miconazole, fluconazole) act by inhibiting the biosynthesis of fungal membrane lipids, especially ergosterol. Polyenes (e.g. amphotericin B, natamycin) require ergosterol as a receptor in the fungal cell membrane to exert their effect; this sterol is absent from the bacterial cell membrane. Polyene antibiotics and the synthetic antifungal azoles act on fungi, whereas the polymyxins act on Gram-negative bacteria.
- Inhibition of protein synthesis through an action on certain subunits of microbial ribosomes (aminoglycosides, tetracyclines, chlorampenicol and its derivatives, macrolides and lincosamides). Each class of antimicrobial agent attaches to a different receptor site apart from macrolides and lincosamides, which bind to the same site on the 50S subunit of the microbial ribosome.
- Inhibition of nucleic acid synthesis. Fluoroquinolones block the action of DNA gyrase; rifampin binds strongly to DNA-dependent RNA polymerase; metronidazole, following chemical reduction of the nitro group of the molecule within anaerobic bacteria or sensitive protozoal cells, produces a bactericidal effect by reacting with various intracellular macromolecules.
- Inhibition of folic acid synthesis in susceptible microorganisms and ultimately the synthesis of nucleic acids. By competing with *para*-aminobenzoic acid (PABA) for the enzyme dihydropteroate synthetase, sulphonamides prevent the incorporation of PABA into dihydrofolate, while trimethoprin, by selectively inhibiting dihydrofolate reductase, prevents the reduction of dihydrofolate to tetrahydrofolate (folic acid). Animal cells, unlike bacteria, utilize exogenous sources of folic acid. Pyrimethamine inhibits protozoal dihydrofolate reductase, but is less selective for the microbial enzyme and therefore more toxic than trimethoprim to mammalian species.

Knowledge of the mechanisms of action of antimicrobial agents is required for understanding resistance acquired through chromosomal mutation and selection, and forms the basis of selecting antimicrobials for concurrent use, either as combination preparations or separately.

Antimicrobial resistance

There are many different mechanisms by which micro-organisms might exhibit resistance to antimicrobial drugs. Inherent and acquired resistance to an antimicrobial agent are clearly distinguishable and due to different mechanisms, although the lack of a favourable clinical response (therapeutic failure) is the invariable outcome.

Inherent resistance

Inherent resistance largely limits the spectrum of activity of an antimicrobial agent, while acquired resistance invariably decreases the quantitative susceptibility of pathogenic microorganisms.

In order to reach receptors (penicillin-binding proteins), β-lactam antibiotics must penetrate the outer layers of the bacterial cell envelope. Inherent resistance of many Gram-negative bacteria to penicillin G (benzylpenicillin) is due to low bacterial permeability, lack of penicillin-binding proteins and/or a wide variety of β-lactamase enzymes. Gram-negative bacteria have an outer phospholipid membrane that may hinder passage of β-lactam antibiotics. Some (such as ampicillin and amoxicillin) pass through pore molecules in this outer barrier more readily than penicillin G. Due to their higher penetrative capacity of cell membranes, third-generation cephalosporins (except cefoperazone) have activity against an expanded range of Gram-negative aerobic bacteria and reach infection sites in the central nervous system. Streptococci have a natural permeability barrier to aminoglycosides. Their penetrative capacity can be enhanced by the simultaneous presence of a cell wall-active drug, such as a penicillin.

Most Gram-negative aerobic bacteria, with the notable exception of *Brucella* ssp., are relatively impermeable and therefore inherently resistant to rifampin; the site of action of rifampin is intracellular. Microbial susceptibility to tetracyclines depends on the attainment of high intracellular drug concentrations. Individual tetracyclines differ in lipid solubility. A distinction must be made between microorganisms that have low penetrative capacity for tetracyclines (inherently resistant) and those that acquire resistance through defective active transport of these drugs across the inner cytoplasmic membrane. As mycoplasmas are bounded by a triple layered 'unit membrane' and lack a rigid cell wall, these microorganisms are inherently resistant to β-lactam antibiotics. The inherent resistance of aerobic bacteria to metronidazole may be attributed to the absence of an anaerobic environment for activation (chemical reduction of the nitro group) of the drug to take place.

Acquired resistance

The potential for genetic exchange between bacteria, combined with their short generation time, can rapidly lead to resistant bacterial populations. Acquired, genetically based resistance may be due to chromosomal mutation (altered structural target or metabolic pathway essential for antimicrobial action) or, more importantly, the acquisition, by bacterial conjugation, of resistance (R) plasmids (Prescott & Baggot, 1993). Resistance plasmids (transferable genetic material) may be present in bacteria as extrachromosomal circular DNA molecules that replicate independently of, but synchronously with, chromosomal DNA. Plasmid genes for antimicrobial resistance often control the formation of bacterial enzymes that are capable of either inactivating antimicrobial agents or decreasing bacterial membrane permeability to antimicrobials (Jacoby & Archer, 1991).

Plasmid-mediated resistance to penicillins and cephalosporins (β-lactam antibiotics) is due to the formation of β-lactamase enzymes by *Staphylococcus aureus* or enteric Gram-negative rods. Some β-lactamases can be firmly bound by compounds such as clavulanic acid (combined with amoxycillin or ticarcillin) and sulbactam (combined with ampicillin) and can thus be prevented from attacking hydrolysable penicillins. Gram-positive bacteria, apart from staphylococci, generally lack the ability to acquire R plasmids.

Gram-negative bacteria that are resistant to aminoglycosides produce enzymes that inactivate drugs in this class, apart from amikacin, by adenylation, acetylation or phosphorylation. This type of resistance is usually plasmid-mediated. Plasmids code for the enzyme acetyltransferase that inactivates chloramphenicol. Florfenicol, an analogue of thiamphenicol, is less susceptible than chloramphenicol to inactivation by bacterial acetyltransferase. Defective active transport of tetracyclines across the inner cytoplasmic membrane of microorganisms that have acquired resistance may be plasmid-mediated. As the plasmid genes that code for tetracycline resistance are closely associated with those for chloramphenicol and aminoglycosides (especially streptomycin), multiple drug resistance may result. Multiple drug resistance plasmids, which commonly occur in Enterobacteriaceae such as *Salmonella, E. coli* and *Proteus*, will be maintained in a population by the use of any antibiotic to which resistance is encoded by the plasmid genes.

The spread of multiple drug resistance has serious implications because of its persistence. Plasmid-mediated resistance to lincosamides and macrolides is the result of methylation of the shared receptor site on the 50S subunit of the bacterial ribosome. Plasmid transferable resistance has recently been reported for fluoroquinolones (Martinez-Martinez *et al.*, 1998).

Chromosomal mutants are commonly resistant by virtue of a change in a structural receptor for an antimicrobial agent. Resistance to β-lactam antibiotics (penicillins and cephalosporins) may be attributed to the loss (or alteration) of penicillin-binding proteins. Chromosomal resistance to aminoglycosides (including amikacin) is associated with the deletion (or alteration) of a specific receptor (protein) on the 30S ribosomal subunit. Resistance to fluoroquinolones (especially in coagulase-positive staphylococci and *Pseudomonas* spp.) may be due to mutation of the target enzyme, DNA gyrase. The rapid development of high-level resistance to rifampin, associated with its use as the sole antimicrobial agent, results from chromosomal mutation of bacterial RNA polymerase. In sulphonamide-resistant mutants, the affinity of dihydropteroate synthetase for *para*-aminobenzoic acid may exceed that for sulphonamide, which is a reversal of the situation in sulphonamide-sensitive microorganisms.

At least some sulphonamide-resistant bacteria can, like mammalian cells, utilize preformed folic acid for nucleic acid synthesis.

Significance of transferable drug resistance

Acquired resistance to several antibiotics is of particular concern in Enterobacteriaceae and is increasingly found in non-enteric Gram-negative bacterial pathogens, as well as in the commensal flora. A causal relationship has been shown between the use of antimicrobials and the development of resistance. The use of antimicrobials does not induce resistance but rather provides an intense selection pressure which, by destroying the susceptible bacteria in the host animal, allows the resistant bacteria to proliferate (Hinton, 1986). The gravity of this adverse situation lies in the fact that, once developed, multi-resistant organisms can persist in the individual or exposed animal population and in the environment. The control of antimicrobial resistance, in so far as is possible, depends on the judicious selection and appropriate use of anti-microbial agents.

Cross-resistance

Microorganisms that are resistant to a certain antimicrobial agent may also be resistant to other antimicrobials with the same mechanism of action, or share the same receptor-binding site. Cross-resistance mainly applies to anti-microbial agents that are closely related structurally, i.e. are within the same class (e.g. aminoglycosides, fluoroquinolones, lincosamides, sulphonamides, chloramphenicol and its derivatives). As all tetracyclines have the same basic structure, cross-resistance between tetracyclines is to be expected. Although lincosamides and macrolides are structurally unrelated, they share the same receptor-binding site, have the same mechanism of plasmid-mediated resistance, and cross-resistance among drugs in these two classes is common. Because of its unique action (inhibition of RNA polymerase), cross-resistance between rifampin and other antimicrobial agents is unlikely to occur.

Distribution and elimination

The chemical nature and related physicochemical properties largely govern the distribution and elimination, which refers to biotransformation (metabolism) and excretion, of antimicrobial agents. The majority of antimicrobial agents are weak organic electrolytes, either weak acids (penicillins, cephalosporins, sulphonamides) or weak bases (aminoglycosides, lincosamides, macrolides, diaminopyrimidines, metronidazole), while fluoroquinolones, tetracyclines and rifampin are amphoteric compounds, and chloramphenicol and its derivatives (thiamphenicol, florfenicol) are neutral molecules. Lipid solubility and, for antimicrobial agents that are weak organic electrolytes, the pK_a/pH-dependent degree of ionization in the blood and body fluids influence the extent of distribution and the rate of elimination. Both molecular structure and lipid solubility determine the process(es) by which a drug is eliminated from the body.

Following entry into the systemic circulation, antimicrobial agents undergo reversible binding to plasma proteins. While most classes of antimicrobial agents bind to plasma albumin, some classes (which include macrolides, lincosamides and diaminopyrimidines) bind to α_1-acid glycoprotein (globulin). The extent of protein binding varies with the individual drug, may be concentration-dependent (ceftriaxone, cefoperazone), and differs somewhat between animal species. Extensive (>80%) binding to plasma proteins limits extravascular distribution and the concentration that could be attained at sites of infection, and may either hinder (which is generally the case) or facilitate elimination depending on the mechanism of the principal elimination process. When glomerular filtration is the principal mechanism of elimination, extensive binding delays elimination. Antimicrobial agents that bind extensively to plasma proteins include cloxacillin, ceftriaxone, erythromycin (estolate), clindamycin, doxycycline and sulphadimethoxine. Decreased protein binding, whether due to the presence of a disease state (such as hypoalbuminaemia, uraemia) or competitive displacement by a concomitantly administered therapeutic agent with higher affinity for protein-binding sites, increases the fraction of unbound (free) drug in the blood. Gram-negative bacterial infections may cause an elevated free fatty acid concentration in plasma, resulting in decreased binding of acidic drugs to albumin. A relatively small decrease in the extent of protein binding of a drug that is normally more than 92% bound would cause a large increase, which could be of clinical significance, in the unbound (free) fraction of the drug in the plasma. For example, a decrease in protein binding from 98% to 92% represents a fourfold increase in the unbound fraction in the plasma which is available for extravascular distribution and elimination by passive processes. While decreased protein binding increases the apparent volume of distribution of the drug, the change in drug elimination that might ensue is difficult to predict. It largely depends on whether clearance of the drug by the organ of elimination is restricted by plasma protein binding (the half-life would be decreased) or non-restricted by protein binding (the half-life could be increased).

The unbound drug in the systemic circulation is available to distribute extravascularly. The extent of distribution is mainly determined by lipid solubility and, for weak organic acids and bases, is influenced by the pK_a/pH-dependent degree of ionization because only the more lipid-soluble non-ionized form can passively diffuse through cell membranes and penetrate cellular barriers such as those which separate blood from transcellular fluids (cerebrospinal and synovial fluids and aqueous humour). The milk-to-plasma equilibrium concentration ratio of an antimicrobial agent provides a reasonably good indication of its distribution capacity. In normal lactating cows (milk pH range 6.5–6.8), weak organic acids (penicillins, cephalosporins, sulphonamides) attain milk ultrafiltrate-to-plasma ultrafiltrate equilibrium concentration ratios less than unity; oxytetracycline and rifampin, amphoteric drug molecules with moderate and high lipid solubility, attain equilibrium concentration ratios of 0.75 and about unity, respectively; weak organic bases, apart from aminoglycosides, spectinomycin and polymyxin B (polar drugs with low solubility in lipid), attain milk ultrafiltrate-to-plasma ultrafiltrate equilibrium concentration ratios greater than unity (Prescott & Baggot, 1993). The high concentration ratios attained by lipophilic organic bases (macrolides, lincosamides, trimethoprim) can be partly attributed to the ion-trapping effect in the milk, which is acidic relative to blood (pH 7.4). An undesirable feature of the distribution of lipophilic organic bases is their diffusion from the systemic circulation into ruminal fluid (pH 5.5–6.5) where the ion-trapping effect applies to an even greater extent than in milk. Enrofloxacin and its active metabolite ciprofloxacin, formed by N-deethylation (a microsomal-mediated oxidative reaction) in the liver, would be expected to attain concentrations in milk that would be effective against susceptible Gram-negative aerobic bacteria. Selective binding of spiramycin and aminoglycoside antibiotics to certain tissue components is a feature of their distribution which limits their clinical use in food-producing animals because of the persistence of tissue residues.

Apparent volume of distribution is the pharmacokinetic parameter that indicates the extent of distribution of a drug. Based on this parameter, macrolides, lincosamides, fluoroquinolones, tetracyclines and trimethroprim are widely distributed ($V_d > 0.7$ L/kg); sulphonamides, rifampin and metronidazole are moderately well distributed (V_d, 0.3–0.7 L/kg); while β-lactam and aminoglycoside antibiotics have limited distribution (V_d, 0.15–0.3 L/kg). Volume of distribution does not reveal the pattern of distribution of a drug in the various organs and tissues of the body or provide evidence of selective tissue binding. However, an exceedingly large volume of distribution is suggestive of a high degree of tissue sequestration; further evidence for sequestration would be provided by a prolonged terminal elimination half-life.

Antimicrobial agents, other than β-lactam, aminoglycoside and tetracycline antibiotics, are eliminated mainly by the liver and to a much lesser extent by the kidney (Table 6.2). This is because the majority of antimicrobials are at least moderately lipid-soluble and have in their molecular structure a functional group which is suitable to undergo biotransformation. The role of biotransformation is to convert lipid-soluble drugs to less lipid-soluble (ultimately water-soluble) polar metabolites which can be rapidly removed from the body by renal or biliary excretion, or both excretion routes. In general, the more rapidly a drug is metabolized the smaller the contribution of excretion to overall elimination. This is shown by considering the half-life of intravenously administered trimethoprim and the fraction of dose excreted unchanged (parent drug) in the urine of various species (Table 6.3). The types of biotransformation reaction that antimicrobial agents may undergo depend on

Table 6.3   Half-life and urinary excretion of trimethoprim.

Species	Half-life (h)	Fraction of dose excreted unchanged (%)
Goat	0.7	2
Cow	1.25	3
Pig	2.0	16
Horse	3.2	10
Dog	4.6	20
Human	10.6	69 ± 17

the functional groups present in or introduced (by microsomal-mediated oxidation) into their molecular structure. They include various types of oxidation, reduction, hydrolysis (phase I metabolic reactions) and formation of conjugates, principally glucuronides and ethereal sulphates (phase II synthetic reactions). Glucuronide conjugates, being highly ionized and water-soluble, are rapidly removed from the body by biliary excretion and renal tubular secretion. Those excreted in the bile may be reactivated by intestinal microflora β-glucuronidase (hydrolytic reaction) and the liberated parent drug may be at least partly reabsorbed from the intestine, thereby establishing a form of enterohepatic circulation. Cats (and other Felidae) have a low capacity compared with other mammalian species to synthesize glucuronide conjugates. The slow rate of glucuronide synthesis in cats can be attributed to a relative deficiency of the transferring enzyme, microsomal glucuronyl transferase, required for glucuronide synthesis. The half-lives of antimicrobial agents that form predominantly glucuronide conjugates, e.g. chloramphenicol (5.1 h), tinidazone (8.4 h) and enrofloxacin/ciprofloxacin (6.7 h), are longer in cats (values shown) than in dogs and horses. The relatively low capacity of pigs to synthesize ethereal sulphates is due to a limited source of sulphate for conjugation, but is generally compensated for by increased glucuronide synthesis. Fish appear to have a limited capacity to synthesize glucuronide and sulphate conjugates. This deficiency could partly account for the slow elimination of drugs for which conjugation constitutes a major metabolic pathway. Conjugation increases water solubility of drugs with the notable exception of the acetyl derivatives of most sulphonamides. Dogs, foxes (and presumably other Canidae) are unable to acetylate the aromatic amino group ($Ar-NH_2$) of sulphonamides and other drugs. This conjugation defect could be due to the absence in Canidae of a specific N-acetyltransferase. However, dogs, like other species, do acetylate the sulphamoyl group ($Ar-SO_2NH_2$) of sulphanalamide (Fig. 6.1) (Williams, 1967). The lower solubility of acetylated sulphonamides, particularly under acidic urinary conditions, formed in several species including human beings, increases the risk of renal tubular damage (crytalluria). Aromatic hydroxylation (microsomal oxidative reaction) followed by glucuronide and sulphate conjugation of the phase I metabolite is a major

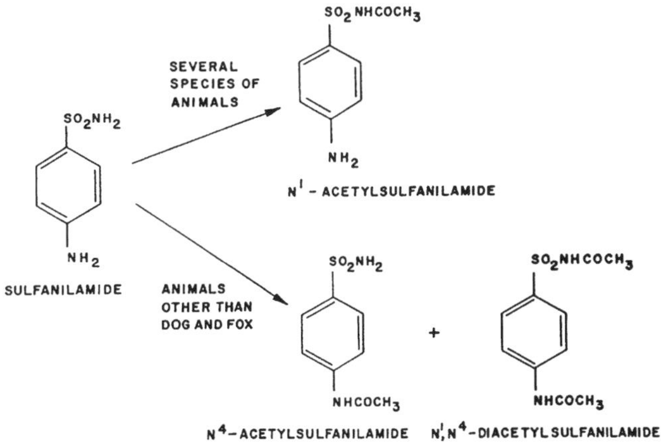

Fig. 6.1 Acetylation reactions of sulphanilamide in several species of animals. The dog and fox are unable to form the N^4-acetyl derivative.

alternative metabolic pathway to acetylation of sulphonamides in herbivorous species (ruminant animals and horses). Because of wide variation between species in the rate at which various biotransformation reactions take place, species differences in the half-lives of antimicrobial agents that are mainly eliminated by hepatic metabolism are usual (Table 6.4). The half-lives of most antimicrobials that undergo extensive metabolism are shorter in cattle (and other ruminant animals) than in monogastric species, particularly human beings. As well as showing interspecies variations, the half-lives of individual drugs in an antimicrobial class differ within each species (intraspecies variation). The half-lives of fluoroquinolones in the dog, for example, are: ciprofloxacin, 2.2 h; enrofloxacin, 3.4 h; norfloxacin, 3.6 h; difloxacin, 8.2 h; and marbofloxacin, 12.4 h.

The high degree of lipid solubility of macrolides and lincosamides enables these antibiotics to penetrate cell membranes and distribute widely in tissues. Extensive binding to plasma proteins (α_1-acid glycoprotein) coupled with rapid elimination by the liver, limit the concentrations that are attained in cerebrospinal fluid. Under steady-state conditions these antibiotics attain high concentrations in the milk (pH 6.5–6.8) of lactating cows. The membrane penetrative capacity of erythromycin and ion-trapping effect in acidic prostatic fluid (pH 6.4) of dogs would allow relatively high concentrations to be attained. However, because *E. coli* is the most common causative organism of bacterial protatitis, a fluoroquinolone (in particular difloxacin because of its higher activity in the acidic environment) or trimethoprim–sulphamethoxazole combination may be the treatment of choice. Clindamycin is one of the few antimicrobials that can attain effective concentrations in bone. The half-life of clindamycin in dogs is 3.25 h. Macrolides and lincosamides are mainly eliminated by the liver, either unchanged in bile (erythromycin, azithromycin, lincomycin) or by metabolism (clarithromycin, clindamycin). Because they

Table 6.4 Average half-lives of antimicrobial agents in various species.

Drug	Process(es) of elimination[a]	Half-life (h)			
		Cattle	Horses	Dogs	Humans
Trimethoprim	M + E(r)	1.25	3.2	4.6	10.6
Sulphadiazine	M + E(r)	2.5	3.6	5.6	9.9
Sulphamethoxazole	M + E(r)	2.3	4.8	–	10.1
Sulphamethazine	M + E(r)	8.2	9.8	16.8	–
Sulphadimethoxime	M + E(r)	12.5	11.3	13.2	40
Sulphadoxine	M + E(r)	10.8	14.2	–	150
Norfloxacin	M + E(r)	2.4	6.4	3.6	5.0
Enrofloxacin	M + E(r)	1.7	5.0	3.4	–
Chloramphenicol	M + E(r)	3.6	0.9	4.2	4.6
Metronidazole	M + E(r)	2.8	3.9	4.5	8.5
Tinidazole	M + E(r)	2.4	5.2	4.4	14.0
Erythromycin	E(h) + M	3.2	1.0	1.7	1.6
Oxytetracycline	E(r ± h)	4.0	9.6	6.0	9.2
Penicillin G	E(r)	0.7	0.9	0.5	1.0
Ampicillin	E(r)	0.95	1.2	0.8	1.3
Cefazolin	E(r)	–	0.65	0.8	1.8
Ceftriaxone	E(r)	–	1.62	0.85	7.3[b]
Gentamicin	E(r)	1.8	2.2–2.8	1.25	2.75
Amikacin	E(r)	–	1.7	1.1	2.3

[a] See footnote a in Table 6.2.
[b] Eliminated by the liver (biliary excretion) in human beings

cause severe disturbance of the balance between the commensal microbial flora in the colon, which is essential for meeting nutrient requirements and maintaining health, of the horse, macrolides (erythromycin, azithromycin, clarithromycin, spiramycin, tylosin, tilmicosin), lincosamides (lincomycin, clindamycin) or tiamulin should not be administered by any route to horses. A notable exceptional indication is the concurrent oral administration of erythromycin estolate (20 mg/kg at 8-h intervals) and rifampin (5 mg/kg at 12-h intervals) for the treatment of *Rhodococcus equi* pneumonia in 6–16-week-old foals. This antimicrobial combination attains effective intracellular concentrations at the site of infection and acts synergistically against *R. equi*. Diagnosis at an early stage of the infection and prompt initiation of therapy largely influence the required duration of treatment. Improvement in clinical symptoms, return of white blood cell count and plasma fibrinogen concentration to within normal ranges and radiographic resolution of pulmonary lesions serve as a useful guide to the duration of antimicrobial therapy.

As the ostrich, like the horse and the koala, is a hindgut fermenter that relies on microbial digestion of dietary fibrous material, various antimicrobial agents can severely disturb the balance of the commensal microbial flora. The large intestine, which has twin caeca, comprises 60% of the intestinal tract of the ostrich, whereas in chickens it accounts for 6% of the length of the tract.

Variations in clinical efficacy of individual tetracyclines are attributable to differences in their pharmacokinetic properties (absorption, distribution and elimination) rather than to differences in quantitative susceptibility of microorganisms. This is because equal concentrations of individual tetracyclines in body fluids or tissues have approximately equal antimicrobial activity. The factor that underlies the pharmacokinetic properties of tetracyclines (amphoteric compounds) is lipid solubility; the degree of lipid solubility differs between individual tetracyclines (minocycline and doxycycline are more lipidsoluble than oxytetracycline, chlortetracycline and tetracycline). Because tetracyclines have moderate to high lipid solubility, these antibiotics distribute widely in the body in that they enter most tissues and body fluids with the exception of cerebrospinal fluid. Minocycline, the most lipid-soluble drug in this antimicrobial class, may attain effective concentrations at relatively inaccessible sites of infection. Extensive binding to plasma proteins limits the concentrations attained by doxycycline in extravascular fluids and tissues. Tetracyclines undergo enterohepatic circulation and, apart from the small (although variable) fraction of the amount excreted in bile that is not reabsorbed from the intestine, are slowly eliminated by renal excretion (glomerular filtration). The half-life of oxytetracycline differs widely between domestic animal species: goats (3.4 h), cattle (4.0 h), sheep (5.2 h), pigs (6.0 h), dogs (6.0 h), donkeys (6.5 h), horses (9.6 h). For comparative purposes, the half-life of oxytetracycline in rabbits is 1.3 h, in human beings is 9.2 h and in red-necked wallabies is 11.4 h, while in rainbow trout (*Oncorhynchus gairdneri*) acclimatized at 12°C it is 80.3 h. Unlike other tetracyclines, minocycline is mainly eliminated by hepatic metabolism, while doxycycline is eliminated by excretion in bile and by diffusion from the systemic circulation into the intestine for excretion in the faeces. The half-life of doxycycline is short in cats (4.6 h) and not related to the unbound fraction of the drug in plasma, which is lower in cats and dogs than in humans (an unusual situation). As doxycycline elimination does not involve renal excretion, it can be administered orally to dogs and cats with renal impairment for the treatment of systemic infections caused by susceptible microorganisms.

The penicillins and cephalosporins (β-lactam antibiotics) are weak organic acids that, due to their low pK_a values, are predominantly ionized in the blood plasma. Binding of β-lactam antibiotics to plasma proteins (albumin) differs between individual penicillins (from 16–22% for ampicillin to over 80% for cloxacillin and nafcillin) and individual cephalosporins (from 15–20% for cephalexin and cefadroxil to over 80% for cefazolin, cefoperazone and ceftriaxone). The consequence of extensive protein binding on clinical efficacy of β-lactam antibiotics is incompletely understood, apart from decreasing the availability of the drug (unbound fraction) for extravascular distribution. Because of their high degree of ionization in the plasma and consequently relatively low solubility in lipid, the extravascular distribution of β-lactam antibiotics is limited in that they attain low intracellular concentrations and, apart from cefuroxime, cefotaxime and ceftriaxone (even though this drug binds extensively to plasma proteins), penetrate poorly into transcellular fluids (cerebrospinal and synovial fluids, aqueous humour). The presence of fever and inflammation increases the penetration, at least of penicillins, through cellular barriers. The β-lactam antibiotics are rapidly eliminated almost entirely by renal excretion as unchanged (parent drug) in the urine. Because of the renal mechanisms involved in their elimination (glomerular filtration and carrier-mediated proximal tubular secretion), their half-lives (related to intravenous administration) are short (0.5–1.5 h) in domestic animal species. The extent of protein binding does not influence the half-life but individual drugs that are relatively more widely distributed have somewhat longer half-lives (ampicillin and amoxycillin compared with penicillin G in several species). The concurrent administration of probenecid and a penicillin (usually penicillin G) prolongs the duration of effective penicillin concentrations by delaying penicillin excretion and does not interfere with antimicrobial activity of the penicillin. Probenecid competitively inhibits proximal tubular secretion of penicillin by combining with the carrier that actively transports organic anions into proximal renal tubular fluid. β-Lactamase inhibitors combined with penicillins (amoxycillin–clavulanate, ticarcillin–clavulanate, ampicillin–sulbactam) enhance the activity of the penicillin against β-lactamase producing bacteria that would otherwise be resistant and do not alter the disposition (distribution and elimination) of the penicillin. Nafcillin, cefoperazone and ceftriaxone bind extensively to plasma proteins and, unlike other β-lactam antibiotics, are mainly eliminated by biliary excretion. The half-life of ceftriaxone is unusually long in human beings (7.3 h) compared with dogs (0.85 h), horses (1.62 h) and sheep (1.73 h).

The aminoglycoside antibiotics are polar organic bases that have restricted extravascular distribution with limited capacity to enter cells and penetrate cellular barriers. Their polarity largely accounts for the pharmacokinetic properties that are shared by all the drugs in this antimicrobial class. Aminoglycosides bind to a low extent (<25%) to plasma proteins, their distribution is largely limited to extracellular fluid and they do not readily attain effective concentrations in transcellular fluids, particularly cerebrospinal fluid. Restricted access to a site of infection could account for a discrepancy between *in vitro* susceptibility of a bacterial pathogen and clinical efficacy of the drug. Aminoglycosides are eliminated entirely by renal excretion (glomerular filtration). The half-lives associated with clinically effective plasma concentrations are short and reflect the relative (not actual) rates of glomerular filtration in domestic animal species. While the range of half-lives of gentamicin and amikacin is similar (1–3 h, when several mammalian species are considered collectively, the half-life of amikacin is consistently somewhat shorter than that of gentamicin on an individual species basis. This could be due to a lower extent of distribution of amikacin than gentamicin. Based on comparison of minimum inhibitory concentrations (MIC_{90}), the antimicrobial activity of amikacin is lower than that of gentamicin against susceptible Gram-negative aerobic bacteria. This underlies the requirement for higher plasma concentrations of amikacin which should be administered at double the dose level (mg/kg) used for gentamicin while the same dosage interval is appropriate for both drugs. Acquired (plasmid-mediated) resistance of Gram-negative aerobes to aminoglycoside antibiotics may be due to inactivation of these drugs, with the exception of amikacin, by bacterial enzymes. It would appear that the use of amikacin should probably be reserved for the treatment of bacterial infections caused by microorganisms that have become resistant to gentamicin (and other aminoglycosides) but remain susceptible to amikacin. The widespread use of aminoglycosides promotes the emergence of resistant bacterial strains and thereby ultimately limits their effectiveness. Because aminoglycosides have a narrow margin of safety, being potentially both ototoxic and nephrotoxic, and gradually accumulate when administered at therapeutic dosage for an extended period, adjustment of the dosage rate is important when their use in an animal with renal impairment is considered necessary. Increasing the dosage interval, based on the decrease in renal function (glomerular filtration rate), is the preferred adjustment to reducing the size of the dose. The usual dose should be administered at a longer dosage interval and the serum/plasma concentrations of the aminoglycoside monitored; for gentamicin the trough serum concentration should not be allowed to exceed $2\,\mu g/ml$.

The selective binding of aminoglycosides to anionic membrane phospholipids of proximal renal tubular cells (kidney cortex) and cochlear tissue leads to a slow decline in subtherapeutic plasma drug concentrations, causing delayed elimination of aminoglycosides from the body. The half-life of the prolonged terminal elimination phase of gentamicin disposition has been estimated to be 88.9 h in sheep (Brown *et al.*, 1986) and 142 h in horses (Bowman *et al.*, 1986). The terminal phase half-life is several-fold the half-life on which the dosage interval associated with multiple dosing is based. In the case of horses, for example, the usual dosage interval for gentamicin sulphate (2–4 mg/kg), administered by intramuscular injection, is 8–12 h which is based on an apparent half-life of gentamicin of 3 h. The relevant application of a particular half-life may be defined in terms of the fraction of the clearance and volume of distribution that is related to each half-life and whether plasma concentration or amounts of drug in the body are best related to measurements of response (Benet, 1984). With reference to gentamicin elimination, the relevance of a particular half-life depends on the intended application, whether it be selection of the dosage interval (use the half-life associated with clinical efficacy) or prediction of the withdrawal period (use the terminal phase half-life) for a food-producing animal species. The preferential accumulation with selective binding of aminoglycosides to phospholipid (phosphatidylinositol)-rich tissues of particularly the kidney cortex and inner ear substantially contributes to their toxicity and necessitates the application of a long withdrawal period in food-producing animals. The risk of producing toxicity is reduced when an aminoglycoside is administered at appropriate dosage and the duration of treatment is not prolonged. Aminoglycoside toxicity in domestic and laboratory animal species was reviewed by Riviere (1985).

Average values of the major pharmacokinetic parameters describing the disposition of antimicrobial agents in adult horses are presented in Table 6.5. The half-lives of the majority of antimicrobials are short (between 0.8 and 5.0 h, apart from rifampin (6.0 h), oxtetracycline (9.6 h) and sulphadoxine (14.2 h). This implies that multiple doses would have to be administered at short dosage intervals when the intravenous route of injection is used. Oxytetracycline hydrochloride (conventional parenteral preparation) can be administered by slow intravenous injection to horses when specifically indicated. Erythromycin should not be administered by any route to horses, but may be administered orally to foals less than 4 months of age. With the notable exception of procaine benzylpenicillin (aqueous suspension), long-acting parenteral preparations are unsuitable for administration to horses because they cause tissue irritation at the injection site. Antimicrobial agents that do not adversely affect commensal microbial flora in the colon may be administered orally, provided systemic availability is adequate and an oral dosage form that is convenient to administer to horses is commercially available. Volumes of distribution vary widely between antimicrobials due mainly to differences in lipid solubility. Values of

Table 6.5 Disposition kinetics of antimicrobial agents in horses.

Drug	Half-life (h)	$V_{d\ (area)}$ (mL/kg)	Cl_B (mL/min·kg)
Penicillin G	0.90	195	2.50
Ampicillin	1.20	300	2.89
Amoxycillin	1.43	556	4.55
Ticarcillin	0.94	250	3.10
Cefazolin	0.65	291	5.27
Cefadroxil	0.77	462	6.95
Cefoxitin	0.82	125	1.72
Ceftriaxone	1.62	650	5.22
Gentamicin	2.50	254	1.20
Amikacin	1.70	180	1.23
Enrofloxacin	4.96	2495	5.75
Ciprofloxacin	4.71	3900	9.70
Trimethoprim	3.16	1378	5.03
Sulphadiazine	3.64	465	1.45
Sulphamethoxazole	4.80	500	1.20
Sulphadoxine	14.20	390	0.32
Chloramphenicol	0.92	700	8.80
Metronidazole	3.92	660	1.97
Rifampin	6.00	635	1.34
Erythromycin	1.00	2300	26.6
Oxytetracycline	9.60	1500	1.25

systemic clearance exceed 1 mL/min·kg for the various antimicrobials apart from sulphadoxine, which reflects the efficiency of the renal and hepatic elimination processes in the horse.

Active metabolites

High-performance liquid chromatographic (HPLC) methods measure separately the concentrations of parent drug and metabolites in biological fluid samples, whereas microbiological assay measures the combined antimicrobial activity of parent drug and active metabolite(s). The phase I metabolites of some antimicrobial agents possess activity (Table 6.6). The antimicrobial activity of desfuroylceftiofur, which is very rapidly formed from ceftiofur, and of ciprofloxacin, which is formed by *N*-deethylation of enrofloxacin, is at least equal to that of the parent drug.

Table 6.6 Antimicrobial agents that form active metabolites.

Drug	Active metabolite
Cefotaxime	Desacetylcefotaxime
Ceftiofur	Desfuroylceftiofur
Clarithromycin	14-Hydroxyclarithromycin
Difloxacin	Sarafloxacin
Enrofloxacin	Ciprofloxacin
Metronidazole	Hydroxymethyl metabolite
Rifampin	Desacetylrifampin

Potential pharmacokinetic interactions

Certain antimicrobial agents inhibit hepatic microsomal cytochrome P450 activity and can thereby decrease the rate of elimination of drugs that are mainly metabolized by microsomal-mediated oxidative reactions. Examples include chloramphenicol, macrolide antibiotics and imidazole antifungal drugs (ketoconazole). Metronidazole inhibits aldehyde dehydrogenase, which catalyses some non-microsomal oxidative reactions. Rifampin, which should always be used in conjunction with another antimicrobial agent to reduce the rapid emergence of resistant strains, is a potent inducer of cytochrome P450 isoenzymes of the subfamily CYP3A (Park & Kitteringham, 1988, 1990).

Norfloxacin and ciprofloxacin decrease the systemic clearance of theophylline to an extent that could be of clinical significance (Prince *et al.*, 1989). The effect of the interaction can be avoided by adjusting the dosage rate of theophylline in accordance with the decreased clearance so that steady-state plasma theophylline concentrations remain within the therapeutic range (6–16 µg/mL).

The concomitant administration of enrofloxacin, which is converted to ciprofloxacin, and theophylline (sustained-release oral dosage form) to Beagle dogs progressively and significantly increased the trough (12 h) plasma concentration of theophylline by decreasing systemic clearance of the drug. The effect of enrofloxacin on the plasma concentration profile of theophylline under steady-state conditions is shown in Fig. 6.2 (Intorre *et al.*, 1995). The basis of the interaction could be selective inhibition by fluoroquinolone antimicrobials of cytochrome P450 isoenzymes that metabolize theophylline. The lower clearance of theophylline may be attributed to a decreased rate of hepatic microsomal oxidative metabolism (*N*-demethylation) of the drug (Rogge *et al.*, 1988).

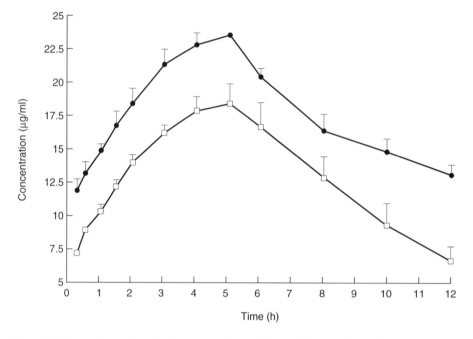

Fig. 6.2   Mean plasma theophylline concentration–time profiles on days 9 (□; theophylline alone) and 14 (●; theophylline + enrofloxacin); $n = 6$.

Relationship between plasma concentrations and clinical effectiveness

Penicillins and cephalosporins act by causing selective inhibition of bacterial cell wall synthesis; they interfere with the final stage of peptidoglycan synthesis. β-Lactam antibiotics produce a time-dependent bactericidal effect on susceptible bacteria. The overall effectiveness of therapy with penicillins (and cephalosporins) is largely influenced by the aggregate time, though not necessarily continuous, during which effective plasma concentrations (greater than MIC for pathogenic microorganism) are maintained; peak height determines the rate of penicillin penetration to the site of infection. The clinical effectiveness of discontinous dosage regimens for penicillins could be attributed to the post-antibiotic sub-MIC effect they exert on Gram-positive bacteria. The post-antibiotic sub-MIC effect (PASME) refers to a temporally limited suppression of bacterial growth that occurs at subinhibitory concentrations following exposure of susceptible bacteria to drug concentrations above the MIC.

Aminoglycosides inhibit ribosomal protein synthesis in susceptible bacteria by inducing misreading of the genetic code on the messenger RNA template (30S ribosomal subunit). Fluoroquinolones block nucleic acid synthesis in susceptible bacteria by selectively inhibiting DNA gyrase, an intracellular enzyme. Both classes of antimicrobial agent produce a concentration-dependent bactericidal effect.

The clinical effectiveness of aminoglycosides and fluoroquinolones is influenced both by the height of the peak plasma concentration relative to the minimum inhibitory concentration (C_{max}:MIC ratio) and the area under the plasma concentration–time curve that is above the MIC during the dosage interval (AUIC = AUC/MIC). The former is relatively more important for fluoroquinolones; maximum activity is achieved when C_{max} is in the range 5–10 times the MIC.

Clinical effectiveness of the aminoglycosides is mainly determined by the area under the inhibitory plasma concentration–time curve (AUIC). The AUIC indicates the degree of exposure of a microorganism to the drug. Aminoglycosides and fluoroquinolones induce a PASME on some species of Gram-negative aerobic bacteria. Because of its variable duration, generally 1–6 h, the post-antibiotic effect is not taken into account when calculating dosage regimens. For the treatment of systemic bacterial infections caused by susceptible microorganisms, the usual dosage intervals are 8–12 h for aminoglycosides, injected intramuscularly or subcutaneously, and 12 h for fluoroquinolones (with the exception of marbofloxacin, 24 h), administered orally, in dogs. Some authors contend, from both a safety and clinical efficacy standpoint, that the dosage interval for aminoglycosides could be 24 h (Zhanel, 1993; Swan *et al.*, 1995). As aminoglycosides are potentially ototoxic and nephrotoxic, and can accumulate due to their prolonged terminal elimination, the monitoring of trough serum/plasma concentrations (C_{min}), which for gentamicin should not be allowed to exceed 2 µg/mL, is important, particularly in the presence of renal impairment.

Antimicrobial agents, unlike pharmacological agents, do not have a defined range of therapeutic plasma concentrations. When designing a dosage regimen for an antimicrobial agent the objective is to calculate the dose that, when administered at a constant dosage interval, will maintain plasma concentrations above the MIC (generally a small multiple of the MIC) throughout the dosage interval. This applies especially to antimicrobial agents that produce a bacteriostatic effect (e.g. tetracyclines, macrolides and lincosamides, sulphonamides, chloramphenicol and its derivatives). Whether maintaining plasma concentrations above the MIC for most of the dosage interval would suffice remains controversial for antimicrobials that produce a bactericidal effect (penicillins and cephalosporins, aminoglycosides and fluoroquinolones). The terms bacteriostatic and bactericidal are relative, not absolute, and are influenced by antimicrobial concentration and local conditions.

Approach to therapy

The approach to antimicrobial therapy involves both microbiological and pharmacological considerations as well as assessment of the severity of the infectious disease. Having diagnosed the presence of a bacterial infection, appropriate specimens should be properly collected to identify the causative pathogenic microorganism(s) and, when considered necessary, to determine its susceptibility to antimicrobial agents that could be effective in treatment of the infection. Immediate examination of a specimen including, whenever feasible, a Gram-stained direct smear greatly assists with the selection of a drug for initial therapy which, although empirical, should commence at this stage. The value of immediate examination of clinical specimens in the initial selection of an antimicrobial agent cannot be overemphasized. Blood culture is a useful, although not invariably certain, technique for making a microbiological diagnosis of septicaemia in neonatal foals.

Antimicrobial therapy involves the following stages:

- Initial (tentative) diagnosis and informed empirical treatment
- Bacterial culture, identification of the causative pathogenic microorganism, susceptibility testing, definitive diagnosis, selection of the antimicrobial agent of choice, and
- Provision of maintenance therapy for an adequate duration.

A favourable clinical response is the ultimate criterion of successful therapy. However, recovery from an infection may not be entirely attributable to the treatment applied.

Initial (empirical) treatment

As there will be some delay in obtaining laboratory results, antimicrobial therapy should be initiated on an informed empirical basis. The choice of drug for initial therapy is largely based on clinical experience, the nature (and site) of the infectious disease process and epidemiological pattern in the herd or geographical region, but should be supported by the findings of specimen examination. A suggested choice of drug for initial therapy based on knowledge (although tentative at this stage) of the pathogenic microorganism is presented in Table 6.7. While the drug of choice presented in this table is generally applicable, selection of the antimicrobial agent must be related to the site of the

Table 6.7 Empiric antimicrobial drug selection based on knowledge of pathogenic microorganisms.

Microorganism	Drug of choice	Alternatives
Gram-positive aerobic bacteria		
Streptococcus spp.	Penicillin G	First-generation cephalosporin; trimethoprim–sulphonamide
Staphylococcus		
Non-penicillinase-producing	Penicillin G	First-generation cephalosporin
Penicillinase-producing	Isoxazoyl penicillin	First-generation cephalosporin; fluoroquinolone; amoxycillin–clavulanate
Methicillin-resistant	Fluoroquinolone	Trimethoprim–sulphonamide
Bacillus spp.	Penicillin G	Erythromycin
Erysipelothrix rhusiopathiae	Penicillin G	Erythromycin
Corynebacterium spp.	Penicillin G	Erythromycin
Listeria monocytogenes	Aminobenzyl penicillin	Chloramphenicol; trimethoprim–sulphonamide
Nocardia spp.	Trimethoprim–sulphonamide	Minocycline ($\pm$ sulphonamide)
Mycobacterium tuberculosis	Rifampin + isoniazid	Streptomycin
Gram-negative aerobic bacteria		
Coliforms (*E. coli*, *Klebsiella* spp., *Proteus* spp., *Enterobacter* spp.)	Gentamicin (or amikacin); amoxycillin–clavulanate for urinary tract infections	Fluoroquinolone; third-generation cephalosporin
Salmonella spp.	Trimethoprim–sulphonamide	Fluoroquinolone; aminobenzyl penicillin
Pasteurella multocida	Aminobenzyl penicillin	Aminoglycoside; fluoroquinolone
Actinobacillus spp.	Trimethoprim–sulphonamide	Fluoroquinolone; amoxicillin–clavulanate; tetracycline
Leptospira spp.	Aminobenzyl penicillin	Erythromycin; streptomycin
Helicobacter spp.	Erythromycin	Fluoroquinolone
Bordetella bronchiseptica	Tetracycline	Trimethoprim–sulphonamide; chloramphenicol; gentamicin
Pseudomonas aeruginosa	Gentamicin $\pm$ ticarcillin (or carbenicillin)	Ciprofloxacin; third-generation cephalosporin

Contd.

Table 6.7   *Contd.*

Moraxella bovis	Oxytetracycline	Cephalothin; chloramphenicol; aminoglycoside
Anaerobic bacteria *Clostridium* spp.	Penicillin G	First-generation cephalosporin; (clindamycin)
Actinomyces spp.	Penicillin G	Erythromycin; Trimethoprim– Sulphonamide
Fusobacterium spp.	Metronidazole	Penicillin G; clindamycin; first-generation cephalosporin
Bacteroides spp. (other than *B. fragilis*)	Metronidazole	Penicillin G; clindamycin; cefoxitin
Bacteroides fragilis	Metronidazole or clindamycin	Chloramphenicol; ampicillin– Sulbactam; cefoxitin
Other micro-organisms *Mycoplasma* spp.	Tylosin or tiamulin	Fluoroquinolone; tetracycline
Chlamydia spp.	Tetracycline	Trimethoprim–sulphonamide
Rickettsia spp.	Tetracycline	Chloramphenicol

infection, the animal species and the readily available dosage forms. When treating food-producing animals, the farmer should be informed of the specified withdrawal period for the drug preparation selected. The withdrawal period for a drug may vary with the preparation (dosage form) as well as between food-producing animal species. It is stated on the label (and package insert) of authorized drug preparations.

Supportive measures that would complement antimicrobial effectiveness and assist recovery of the animal from the infection should be provided. In neonatal animals, care must be taken to avoid a too-rapid rate of intravenous fluid administration. Fever may serve a useful purpose in infectious diseases, and the change in body temperature may be used to assess the progress of the infection. In the presence of an infectious diseased, the only indication for an antipyretic drug, e.g. aspirin or paracetamol (acetaminophen) in dogs but not in cats; metamizole (dipyrone) or sodium salicylate administered intravenously to horses, is to decrease body temperature to below a dangerous level, 41°C (105.8°F). Concurrent therapy with a NSAID and an aminoglycoside antibiotic increases the risk of nephrotoxicity. If the infection is suspected to be contagious, the diseased and in-contact animals should be isolated.

When an appreciable quantity of pus or a foreign body is present, the appropriate surgical intervention is indicated.

Bacterial culture and susceptibility testing

After the pathogenic microorganism has been isolated by bacterial culture (performed under various incubation conditions) and identified, the decision can be made as to whether susceptibility testing (particularly the determination of MIC) is necessary. The susceptibility of certain commonly isolated bacteria is generally predictable. For example, β-haemolytic streptococci isolated from horses are susceptible to penicillin G, as are anaerobes, except *Bacteroides* spp. In mixed infections and abscesses, the presence of anaerobic bacteria should always be considered. The fostering of a close working relationship with the clinical microbiology laboratory is important with regard to the relevance of the techniques performed to the clinical situation and the interpretation of the laboratory results.

Concerning susceptibility testing, the disk (agar)-diffusion method is satisfactory only when a microorganism is either very susceptible or very resistant. It should be understood that the method relates antimicrobial drug concentrations achieved in the serum of human beings given usual dosages to the susceptibility pattern of populations of fast-growing aerobic bacteria (Prescott & Baggot, 1985). The MIC of an organism can be extrapolated from inhibitory zone diameters, and these MIC values have been used to define breakpoints to describe bacteria as susceptible or resistant. The disk-diffusion method provides a qualitative or, at best, semi-quantitative indication of susceptibility, because some antimicrobials become concentrated while others penetrate poorly into certain body fluids and tissues; furthermore, the disposition of many antimicrobial agents differs between human beings and animal species. Because of the aforementioned limitations of the disk-diffusion method, it is necessary to determine quantitative susceptibility, using the broth dilution method (which measures MIC), of pathogenic microorganisms of frequently unpredictable susceptibility. They include coagulase-positive staphylococci (*S. aureus* and *S. intermedius*) and enteric microorganisms (*E. coli*, *Klebsiella*, *Proteus* and *Salmonella* spp.). The determination of quantitative susceptibility could be considered essential for bacteria that have developed multiple drug resistance.

Quantitative susceptibility varies between bacterial genera and species, as well as between strains of a particular species. Moreover, individual drugs within a class differ quantitatively in antimicrobial activity. Tetracyclines might constitute an exception, in that differences in clinical efficacy between tetracyclines are largely attributable to features of bioavailability, distribution and excretion. Suggested interpretative guidelines for MIC breakpoint values are presented (Table 6.8). The choice of antimicrobial agent for systemic therapy is almost invariably limited to drugs to which the bacterial pathogen is susceptible. For treatment of canine urinary tract infections, the range of antimicrobial agents can be extended to include drugs to which the bacterial pathogen is moderately susceptible, provided urinary concentrations exceeding four times the MIC could be maintained during therapy.

Table 6.8 Suggested guideline for the interpretation of MIC (µg/mL) of various antimicrobial agents based on bacterial isolates of equine origin, apart from fluoroquinolones which relate to isolates of canine origin.

Antimicrobial agent	Susceptible	Moderately susceptible	Resistant
Penicillin G	≤ 0.125	0.25–16	> 16
Ampicillin	≤ 1	2–16	> 16
Amoxycillin	≤ 1	2–16	> 16
Gentamicin	≤ 2	4–8	> 8
Amikacin	≤ 4	8–16	> 16
Fluoroquinolones[a]	≤ 1	2–4	> 4
Erythromycin	≤ 0.5	1–4	> 4
Tetracycline	≤ 1	2–4	> 4
Chloramphenicol	≤ 4	8–16	> 16
Trimethoprim– sulphamethoxazole	≤ 0.5/10	1/20–2.5/50	> 3/75

[a] Quantitative susceptibility of bacterial pathogens varies between individual fluoroquinolones, e.g. the minimum inhibitory concentration of enrofloxacin for the majority of susceptible *E. coli* strains isolated from calves is 0.25 µg/mL.

Knowledge of the susceptibility of a pathogenic microorganism is most useful for selecting the antimicrobial agent of choice and can be applied in tailoring dosage of the drug for an individual animal but, even though *in vitro* susceptibility (particularly MIC) generally correlates well with clinical efficacy, it cannot be relied upon to predict the response to therapy. Accumulated data on MIC_{90}, which is the MIC breakpoint value for 90% of isolates tested, compared over different time periods (e.g. on an annual basis), would reveal the pattern of resistance to a drug.

Maintenance therapy

The choice of drug for maintenance therapy rests with the clinician, and is based on the severity, site and nature of the infection, knowledge of the susceptibility of the causative pathogenic microorganism, the pharmacokinetic properties of the drug in the animal species, and on clinical experience (Fig. 6.3). Consideration must be given to the toxic potential of the antimicrobial agent of choice, the dosage forms that would be suitable for administration to the individual animal, the ease of repeated administration (which often determines owner compliance), and the overall cost of the likely course of therapy. Due account should be taken of the value, placed by the owner, of the animal in making the final choice of antimicrobial agent and the dosage form. The antimicrobial agent can usually be administered at the usual dosage regimen for the preparation selected or a dosage regimen tailored to the individual animal may be applied. The latter approach to dosage (specific therapy)

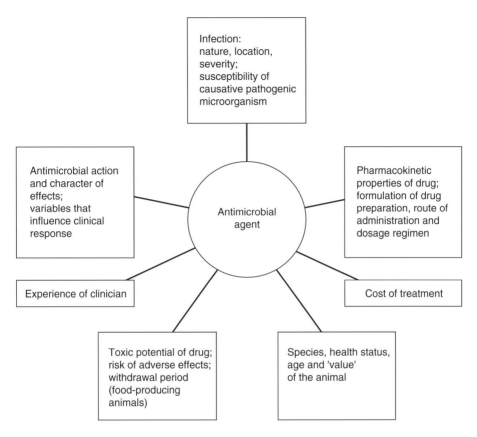

Fig. 6.3 Factors to consider in the selection of an antimicrobial agent for administration to an animal with a diagnosed infection.

assumes greater importance in the treatment of severe systemic infections, such as septicaemia.

Drug administration and dosage

The route of administration of an antimicrobial drug depends on the site and severity of the infection as well as on the animal species, but is often governed by the dosage forms that are available. It is because bacterial susceptibility (MIC) can be determined *in vitro* and drug disposition processes are quantifiable (in pharmacokinetic terms) that dosage rates for antimicrobial drugs can be calculated. However, various formulations may significantly differ from a standard (reference) formulation in bioavailability of the drug substance (active moiety). Only drug preparations that are bioequivalent in the target animal species would be expected to have similar clinical efficacy. Selected features of the plasma concentration–time profiles are used for bioequivalence assessment of formulations of an antimicrobial agent (Martinez & Berson, 1998).

Oral administration is used, particularly in dogs and cats, in the treatment of mild and moderate infections or when a prolonged duration of therapy is anticipated (Table 6.9). The oral bioavailability of many antimicrobial agents is affected by the temporal relationship between feeding and dosing (Table 6.10). Depending on this relationship, food should either be given 1 h before dosing (e.g. with doxycycline, erythromycin estolate, ketoconazole) or be withheld for

Table 6.9 Usual dosage regimens for antimicrobial preparations used in dogs and cats.

Drug preparation	Route of administration	Dosage regimen	
		Dose (mg/kg)	Interval (h)
Penicillin G, sodium	i.v. i.m., s.c.	20000–40000 IU/kg	4–6
Penicillin G, procaine	i.m. s.c.	25000 IU/kg	24
Penicillin V, calcium	p.o.	10–20	8
Ampicillin sodium	i.v. i.m. s.c.	10–20	8
Ampicillin	p.o.	25	8
Hetacillin or pivampicillin	p.o.	20–30	8
Amoxycillin trihydrate	p.o.	12.5–25	8–12
Amoxycillin trihydrate– clavulanate potassium	p.o.	12.5–25	8–12
Cloxacillin sodium	p.o.	25–35	8
Cefadroxil	p.o.	20–30	8–12
Cephalexin monohydrate	p.o.	20–30	8–12
Cefazolin sodium	i.v.	10–20	8
Gentamicin sulphate	i.m. s.c.	3–5	8–12 (dogs) 12–24 (cats)
Amikacin sulphate	i.m. s.c.	6–10	8–12
Enrofloxacin	p.o.	5–10	12
Marbofloxacin	p.o.	2–4	12–24
Trimethoprim–sulphadiazine	p.o.	5/25	12
Trimethoprim–sulphamethoxazole	p.o.	5/25	12
Tetracycline hydrochloride	p.o.	20	8
Oxytetracycline hydrochloride	p.o.	20	12
Oxytetracycline dihydrate	p.o.	40	12
Doxycycline hydrochloride	p.o.	5	12
Chloramphenicol	p.o.	25	8 (dogs) 12 (cats)
Chloramphenicol palmitate	p.o.	25	8 (dogs)
Metronidazole	p.o.	10–20	8–12
Erythromycin	p.o.	10–20	8–12
Erythromycin estolate	p.o.	10–20	8–12
Clindamycin hydrochloride	p.o.	5–10	8–12
Sulfisoxazole	p.o.	50	8
Sulfasalazine	p.o.	25	8 (dogs)
Ketoconazole	p.o.	5–10	12–24
Griseofulvin (micronized)	p.o.	25–50	12–24

Table 6.10 Influence of food on the oral bioavailability of antimicrobial agents in dogs and cats.

Antimicrobial class/preparation	Effect on oral bioavailability[a]
Most penicillins, apart from	↓
amoxycillin and	–
ampicillin pro-drugs	–
Cephalosporins	↓
Fluoroquinolones	–
Trimethoprim–sulphonamide	↓
Most tetracyclines, apart from	↓
doxycycline	↑
Chloramphenicol	–
Chloramphenicol palmitate	↑ (cats)
Metronidazole	↑ (dogs)
Erythromycin base	↓
Erythromycin stearate	↓
Erythromycin estolate	↑
Erythromycin ethylsuccinate	↑
Erythromycin enteric-coated formulations	–
Clarithromycin	–
Nitrofurantoin	↑ (dogs)
Ketoconazole	↑
Griseofulvin (micronized)	↑

[a] The oral bioavailability of an antimicrobial agent may vary with formulation of the oral dosage form.

up to 2h after dosing (e.g. with most penicillins, cephalosporins, tetracyclines, erythromycin base or stearate). The oral bioavailability of some antimicrobial agents (e.g. amoxycillin, fluoroquinolones) is indifferent to the time of feeding relative to dosing.

Many of the antimicrobial agents that are given orally to dogs are administered by intramuscular injection, depending on the availability of parenteral preparations, to ruminant animals (Table 6.11). The systemic availability (extent of absorption) of an antimicrobial agent from a parenteral formulation injected intramuscularly is generally higher when the site of injection is the lateral neck compared with the buttock (*m. semitendineus*) (Rutgers *et al.*, 1980; Nouws & Vree, 1983). Better antimicrobial absorption from the former injection site could be attributed to wider spread of the parenteral preparation (aqueous suspension or non-aqueous solution) providing greater access to a larger absorptive surface area and possibly to higher blood flow to tissues in this region. At least a portion of the volume injected is more likely to be deposited between muscles (intermuscular), which would facilitate spread of the preparation along fascial planes, in the neck than in the buttock. Even though the usual dosage interval for oxytetracycline dihydrate (a long-acting parenteral formulation) is 48h, the intramuscular injection of two doses

Table 6.11 Usual dosage regimens for antimicrobial preparations used in cattle, sheep and goats.

Drug preparation	Route of administration	Dosage regimen	
		Dose (mg/kg)	Interval (h)
Penicillin G, sodium	i.v., i.m.	25 000 IU/kg	6–8
Penicillin G, procaine	i.m.	25 000 IU/kg	24
Ampicillin sodium	i.v., i.m.	10–20	8
Ampicillin–sulbactam	i.m.	10	8–12
Amoxycillin trihydrate	i.m.	10	12
Trimethoprim–sulphonamide	i.m.	4/20	12
Enrofloxacin	i.m.	2.5–5	12
Oxytetracycline hydrochloride	i.v., i.m.	10	12
Oxytetracycline dihydrate (long-acting)	i.m.	20	48
Erythromycin lactobionate	i.v., i.m.	5	8–12
Lincomycin hydrochloride	i.m.	10	12
Tylosin	i.m.	20	12
Sulphamethazine (10% oral solution)	p.o.	50	12

(20 mg/kg, 72 h apart) can be recommended for the treatment of infectious bovine keratoconjunctivitis, caused by *Moraxella bovis* (George & Smith, 1985). Antimicrobial agents are administered to pigs either in the feed or drinking water, or by intramuscular injection (lateral neck) provided injection site damage is not produced (Table 6.12). Parenteral preparations should be formulated in a manner such that their intramuscular injection does not cause tissue damage with persistence of drug residues at the injection site. Antemortem methods for evaluating the extent of tissue irritation and rate of resolution at the injection site include the use of ultrasonography (Banting & Baggot, 1996) and determination of the kinetics of plasma creatine kinase (CK) activity (Aktas et al., 1995; Toutain et al., 1995).

The systemic availability of antimicrobial agents administered orally (pastes) or by nasogastric tube (aqueous suspensions) to horses is significantly decreased by feeding before dosing. Food should be withheld for up to 2 h after drug administration. Metronidazole, which is most useful for the treatment of anaerobic infections (e.g. pleuropneumonia, liver abscesses, peritonitis), is an exception in that the drug is well absorbed from the gastrointestinal tract (systemic availability, 60–90%) of fasted and fed horses. The addition of an antimicrobial agent to the feed (as a powder) is an unreliable method of dosing horses. Usual dosage regimens for antimicrobial preparations that may be used in horses are presented in Table 6.13. Parenteral (i.v. or i.m.) therapy with conventional (immediate-release) dosage forms is required in the treatment of severe infections. Procaine penicillin G occupies a unique position in the

Table 6.12 Usual dosage regimens for antimicrobial preparations used in pigs.

Drug preparation	Route of administration	Dosage regimen		Dose in	
		Dose (mg/kg)	Interval (h)	Feed (g/ton(US))	Water (mg/L)
Ampicillin sodium	i.m.	10–20	8	–	–
Penicillin G, procaine	i.m.	20 000–40 000 IU/kg	24	–	–
Amoxycillin trihydrate–clavulanate potassium	p.o.	10–15	12	–	–
Streptomycin sulphate	i.m.	10	8	–	–
Kanamycin sulphate	i.m.	10	8	–	–
Gentamicin sulphate	i.m.	2–4	8	–	12.5
Apramycin sulphate	p.o.	10–20	12	150	100
Neomycin sulphate	p.o.	10	8	140	100
Enrofloxacin	i.m.	2.5–5	12	–	–
Trimethoprim–sulphonamide	i.m.	4/20	12	–	–
Sulphamethazine (10% oral solution)	p.o.	50	12	–	80–120
Oxytetracycline hydrochloride	i.m.	10	12	200–800	–
Oxytetracycline dihydrate (long-acting)	i.m.	20	48	–	–
Lincomycin hydrochloride	i.m.	10	12	100–200	30
Tylosin[a]	i.m.	20–30	12	100	80
Tiamulin fumarate[b]	i.m.	10–15	24	200	60
Virginiamycin[a]	–	–	–	100	–
Bacitracin[a]	–	–	–	250	–
Monensin[b]	–	–	–	100	–

[a] Phased out as feed additive for pigs over a 6-month period commencing 1 January 1999 (EU Member States).
[b] The concurrent use of monensin and tiamulin must be avoided; otherwise toxicity will very probably occur.

Table 6.13 Usual dosage regimens for antimicrobial preparations used in horses.

Drug preparation	Route of administration	Dosage regimen	
		Dose (mg/kg)	Interval (h)
Penicillin G, sodium	i.v. i.m.	15000–30000 IU/kg	6
Penicillin G, procaine	i.m.	25000 IU/kg	12
Ampicillin sodium	i.v. i.m.	20	8
Ticarcillin sodium–clavulanate potassium	i.v. (slowly)	50	8
Cefadroxil	p.o.	25	8
Cephalexin monohydrate	p.o.	25	8
Cefazolin sodium	i.v.	20	8
Cefoxitin	i.v.	20	8
Gentamicin sulphate	i.m.	2–4	8–12
Amikacin sulphate	i.m.	4–8	8–12
Enrofloxacin	p.o.	5	12 (>4 years old)
Trimethoprim–sulphadiazine	p.o.	5/25	12
Chloramphenicol palmitate	p.o.	50	8
Chloramphenicol sodium succinate	i.v. i.m.	25	6
Metronidazole	p.o.	20	12
Oxytetracycline hydrochloride	i.v. (slowly)	3	12
Rifampin	p.o.	5	12
Erythromycin estolate	p.o.	20–25	8 (foals)
Ketoconazole	p.o.[a]	20	12–24

[a] Dissolve ketoconazole in 0.2 N hydrochloric acid and administer the solution by nasogastric tube.

treatment of equine bacterial infections. This long-acting parenteral dosage form (aqueous suspension) of penicillin G provides effective plasma concentrations of the antibiotic for at least 12 h, due to slow absorption from the intramuscular injection site, and has high activity against commonly isolated equine bacterial pathogens; however, care must be taken to avoid inadvertent intravenous administration. The intramuscular injection of procaine penicillin G in the neck region (*m. serratus ventralis cervicis*) produces a higher peak plasma concentration and higher systemic availability of penicillin G than injection of the long-acting product at other locations (Firth *et al.*, 1986) (Fig. 2.9). Oxytetracycline is the antimicrobial agent of choice for the treatment of tentatively diagnosed or confirmed cases of equine monocytic ehrlichiosis (Potomac horse fever) (Palmer *et al.*, 1988). Either a conventional preparation of oxytetracycline hydrochloride can be administered by slow intravenous injection, or a long-acting preparation containing oxytetracycline formulated in polyethylene glycol can be injected intramuscularly at a dosage rate of 6.6 mg/kg at 24-h intervals for 5–10 days (Dowling & Russell, 2000). Long-acting preparations of oxytetracycline formulated in other vehicles are unsuitable for administration to horses because of tissue irritation produced at injection sites. The prime site for intramuscular injection in the neck of the horse appears to be at the level of the fifth cervical vertebra, ventral to the funicular part of the *ligamentum nuchae* but dorsal to the brachiocephalic muscle (Boyd, 1987). The location of intramuscular injection site does not affect the bioavailability (refers to rate and extent of absorption) of gentamicin (50 mg/ml solution), nor does gentamicin bioavailability differ following intramuscular or subcutaneous injection (Gilman *et al.*, 1987; Wilson *et al.*, 1989).

Because of the slow elimination (long half-life) of antimicrobial agents in reptiles, dosage intervals are substantially longer in reptilian compared with mammalian species (Jacobson, 1993) (Table 6.14). To avoid significantly decreased systemic availability of drugs that are eliminated by renal excretion (e.g. β-lactam and aminoglycoside antibiotics), the site of intramuscular injection should be the anterior half of the body; most reptilian species have a well-developed renal portal system.

Fish, in common with reptiles, are poikilothermic (cold-blooded) animals, and ambient temperature may have a pronounced influence on the rate of drug elimination, particularly when biotransformation is the principal process of elimination. The half-life of trimethoprim, administered intravenously as trimethoprim–sulphadiazine combination, differs widely between carp (*Cyprinus carpio* L.) and mammalian species: carp (40.7 h at 10°C; 20 h at 24°C), cattle (1.25 h), horse (3.2 h), (dog 4.6 h) and human being (10.6 h). Sulphadiazine half-life similarly differs widely: carp (47 h at 10°C; 33 h at 24°C), cattle (2.5 h), horse (3.6 h), dog (5.6 h) and human being (9.9 h). Oxytetracycline is slowly eliminated by glomerular filtration because the drug undergoes enterohepatic circulation. The half-life of oxytetracycline is 89.5 h in rainbow trout (*Salmo gairdneri*) at 12°C and 80.3 h in African catfish (*Clarias gariepinus*) at 25°C (Grondel *et al.*, 1989), compared with half-lives in the range 3.4–9.6 h in domestic animals. In fish and reptiles, the elimination of antimicrobial agents increases with increase in ambient temperature. When developing drug products for use in farmed-fish (food-producing animals), studies of the relationship between pharmacokinetics of the drugs and ambient (water) temperature should be performed.

Antimicrobial combinations

When two antimicrobial agents act simultaneously on a homogenous microbial population, the resulting effect can be one of three types: additive (or indifferent), synergistic or antagonistic (Fig. 6.4) (Jawetz, 1975). The mechanisms of action of the drugs, their concentration ratio at the site of microbial action and bacterial (species and strain) susceptibility to the drugs determine the type of interaction that may occur when antimicrobial agents of different classes are used concurrently, either as combination preparations or administered

Table 6.14 Suggested dosage regimens for antimicrobial preparations that may be used in reptiles.

Drug preparation	Species	Route of administration	Dosage regimen	
			Dose (mg/kg)	Interval (h)
Ampicillin sodium	Tortoise	i.m.	50	12
Carbenicillin	Snakes	i.m.	400	24
	Tortoise	i.m.	400	48
Gentamicin sulphate	Alligator	i.m.	1.75	72–96
	Snakes	i.m.	2.5	72
Amikacin sulphate	Alligator	i.m.	2.5	96
	Snakes	i.m.	5.0	72
	Tortoise	i.m.	5.0	48
Enrofloxacin	Hermann's toirtoise	i.m.	10	24
	Gopher tortoise	i.m.	5	24
	Burmese python	i.m.	10	48
Ciprofloxacin	Snakes	p.o.	2.5	48–72
Trimethoprim–sulphadiazine	All species	i.m.	5/25	First 2 doses 24 h apart; thereafter 48
Tylosin	All species	i.m.	5–10	24
Ketoconazole	Tortoise	p.o.	15–30	24
Nystatin	All species	p.o.	100000 IU/kg	24

Adapted from Jacobson (1993), Table 29.4.

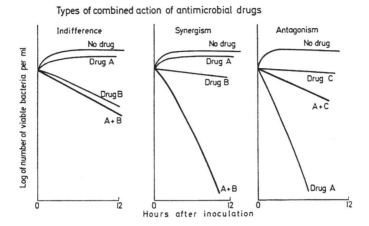

Fig. 6.4 Types of combined action of two antimicrobial drugs on a homogeneous microbial population. Schematic representation of bactericidal action *in vitro* showing the possible types of results seen when one drug, or two drugs, act on a homogeneous population of bacteria under conditions permitting growth.

separately. While the majority of interactions result in an additive effect, it is often little greater than that attributable to the more active drug in the combination.

Useful combination preparations include trimethoprim–sulphonamide which, through synergistic action, produces a bactericidal effect (at least *in vitro*), amoxycillin–clavulanate and ticarcillin–clavulanate (Table 6.15). The concurrent use of ampicillin (or amoxycillin) and gentamicin is likely to provide synergistic action at least against streptococci (have a natural permeability barrier to aminoglycosides), while ticarcillin (or carbenicillin) and gentamicin used concurrently act synergistically against some strains of *Pseudomonas, Proteus, Enterobacter* and *Klebsiella* spp. (i.e. Gram-negative rods). Note that penicillins and gentamicin should not be mixed *in vitro*, as activity of the aminoglycoside would be decreased (due to chemical interaction). The concurrent use of a bacteriostatic drug and a bactericidal drug, especially a β-lactam antibiotic, generally results in antagonism. Chloramphenicol and a fluoroquinolone are antagonistic. However, erythromycin and rifampin act synergistically against *Rhodococcus equi*, while tetracycline and rifampin (or streptomycin) used concurrently provide enhanced clinical efficacy against *Brucella* spp. in human beings, horses and dogs. While rifampin is particularly useful against macrophage-associated (intracellular) susceptible microorganisms, it should always be used concurrently with another antimicrobial drug to prevent the rapid emergence of strains resistant to rifampin. In mixed infections with anaerobic involvement, the concurrent use of clindamycin (or, in horses, metronidazole) and gentamicin is the treatment of choice.

Unless specifically indicated, which implies synergistic action and/or the prevention of acquired resistance, or there is circumstantial evidence to

Table 6.15 Activity of concurrently used antimicrobial drugs.

Antimicrobial agents	Activity
Combination preparations	
Trimethoprim–sulphonamide	Synergistic; bactericidal against susceptible microorganisms
Ampicillin–sulbactam	Enhanced (broader) activity of the penicillin
Amoxicillin–clavulanate	
Ticarcillin–clavulanate	
Administered separately	
Ampicillin (or amoxycillin) + gentamicin	May be synergistic, depending on the microorganism
Ticarcillin (or carbenicillin) + gentamicin	Synergistic against some strains of *Pseudomonas, Proteus, Enterobacter, Klebsiella* spp.
Erythromycin + rifampin	Synergistic; *Rhodococcus equi*
Isoniazid + rifampin	Prevents emergence of resistant strains *Mycobacterium tuberculosis*
Doxycycline + rifampin	*Brucella melitensis* (human beings)
Minocycline + rifampin (or streptomycin)	*Brucella canis* (dogs)
Oxytetracycline + rifampin (or streptomycin)	*Brucella abortus* (horses)
Clindamycin (or metronidazole)[a] + gentamicin	Additive; mixed Gram-negative + anaerobic infections
Lincomycin + spectinomycin	Additive; bacterial respiratory infections in cattle

[a] Use metronidazole in horses.

support the clinical effectiveness of antimicrobial combinations, the concurrent use of antimicrobial drugs should be avoided. When two antimicrobial agents are used concurrently, not as a combination preparation, they must be administered independently at usual dosage rates.

Duration of therapy

Antimicrobial therapy must be maintained for an adequate duration, which is based upon monitoring the response both by clinical assessment (resolution of fever, leukocytosis and other signs of inflammation) and bacterial culture. Definitive diagnosis at an early stage of infection and the application of specific therapy, based on knowledge of the causative pathogenic microorganism and its susceptibility, will decrease the overall duration of treatment and minimize residual sequelae. Therapy with an aminoglycoside should not be extended beyond the duration required to treat the infection. The speed of clinical response is generally inversely related to the length of time the infection was present before therapy was initiated.

There are certain infections which, due to the relative inaccessibility of the causative microorganisms to antimicrobial agents, invariably require a prolonged duration (3–5 weeks, rather than 5–8 days) of therapy. They include prostatitis, osteomyelitis and skin infections in dogs, and *Rhodococcus equi* pneumonia in foals (6–16 weeks of age). In the treatment of these infections, preference should be given to the use of orally effective antimicrobial agents.

Variables that influence clinical response

Even though the antimicrobial drug of choice is administered at the recommended dosage rate, the outcome of therapy is largely governed by the responsiveness of host defence mechanisms. This applies particularly to drugs that produce a bacteriostatic effect. The concentration attained by an antimicrobial agent at the site of infection may be influenced by disease-induced changes in the disposition of the drug as well as by local changes associated with tissue inflammation or abscess formation. Disease states that may alter the disposition of drugs include fever, dehydration, hypoalbuminaemia (associated with chronic liver disease) and uraemia (chronic renal failure). The bactericidal activity of aminoglycosides and fluoroquinolones (apart from difloxacin) against Gram-negative aerobic bacteria is greater in an alkaline than in an acidic environment. In the presence of impaired renal function, which may be detected by urinalysis (proteinuria and the presence of casts), dosage regimens for aminoglycosides should be adjusted (preferably by increasing the dosage interval in accordance with the decrease in glomerular filtration rate (GFR)) in order to avoid drug accumulation with attendant toxic effects (acute tubular necrosis and cochlear damage in dogs or vestibular damage in cats).

An indication of the extent of a decrease in the GFR may be obtained by measuring endogenous creatinine clearance. In dogs with decreased renal function (GFR < 3 mL/min·kg; in normal dogs, GFR = 4.07 ± 0.52 mL/min·kg), the reciprocal of serum creatinine concentration provides a clinically useful estimation of the glomerular filtration rate (Finco *et al.*, 1995) that could serve as a guide for dosage interval adjustment of aminoglycoside antibiotics. The monitoring of trough serum or plasma concentrations of an aminoglycoside is highly desirable in animals with severe infections or renal impairment, and is essential in animals with changing renal function.

After an infectious disease has been diagnosed in an animal, the decision has to be made as to whether an antimicrobial agent should be administered. When the answer is in the affirmative, and following proper collection of appropriate specimens, the treatment should be promptly initiated with an antimicrobial selected on an informed empirical basis. The microbiological and clinical chemistry results on the samples submitted for analysis, in conjunction with the response of the animal to the initial treatment, provide the requisite information for selecting the antimicrobial agent to use for the continuation of treatment. The usual dosage regimen for the particular antimicrobial preparation selected can generally be applied, while the duration of treatment should be based on monitoring the response both by clinical assessment of the animal and bacterial culture of properly collected specimens. By adopting the approach outlined in this chapter the success of antimicrobial therapy will probably be increased and the indiscriminate use of antimicrobial agents will be reduced. Moreover, the animal's owner will become increasingly aware of the fact that there is far more to antimicrobial therapy than the administration of an empirically selected antimicrobial preparation, and will ultimately appreciate the long-term benefits and cost-effectiveness of the scientific approach.

Therapy of bovine mastitis

Antimicrobial therapy is generally applied in the treatment of clinical mastitis during lactation and in treating subclinical mastitis at the end of lactation, while the implementation of preventive measures is essential for decreasing the incidence of mastitic infection in the dairy herd. Nutritional deficiencies, such as vitamin E and selenium deficiencies, predispose cows to mastitis and pro-long the duration of infection, probably due to decreased function of phago-cytes. The common causative pathogenic microorganisms of clinical mastitis are *Streptococcus uberis*, coliforms (*Escherichia coli*, *Klebsiella* spp.), *Staphylococcus aureus*, *Streptococcus dysgalactiae* and *Streptococcus agalactiae*. It is usual to treat clinical mastitis both systemically, using a parenteral antimicrobial prepara-tion, and locally with a quick-release intramammary preparation. The infusion via the teat canal of an intramammary preparation alone would be inadequate for the treatment of moderate-to-severe infection because of the decreased ability of an infused drug to ascend partially occluded milk ducts and the requirement, particularly in coliform mastitis, for frequent milkout (stripping) of the infected quarter of the mammary gland. In mild cases of mastitis that are diagnosed at an early stage of infection, the infusion of a quick-release intra-mammary preparation may suffice without concurrent systemic treatment. Slow-release intramammary preparations are used at the end of lactation (after the last milking) to treat subclinical mastitis, and to prevent the establishment of new infections, including summer mastitis commonly caused by *Actinomyces pyogenes* during the non-lactating (dry) period. Because *Staphylococcus aureus* is the principal causative microorganism of subclinical mastitis, the slow-release intramammary preparation selected for treatment should contain an anti-microbial that will be effective against all strains of the bacterium.

An 'ideal' antimicrobial agent for systemic therapy of bovine mastitis should possess the following properties (adapted from Ziv, 1980):

- Low MIC for the majority of mastitis-causing pathogenic microorganisms
- High systemic availability following intramuscular injection
- Be lipid-soluble and predominantly non-ionized in the blood and have a low degree of binding to plasma proteins

- Have a long apparent half-life to ensure that concentrations above (preferably several-fold) the MIC are maintained at the site of infection in the mammary gland throughout the recommended dosage interval (12 h is desirable)
- Cause minimal adverse effects in cows treated at effective dosage
- Short withdrawal periods (milk and slaughter).

Parenteral preparations with both antimicrobial activity, which depends on the causative pathogenic microorganism, and pharmacokinetic properties that meet most of these criteria include procaine penicillin G (aqueous suspension), amoxycillin trihydrate–clavulanate potassium combination (aqueous suspension), trimethoprim–sulphadiazine combination (for injection) and enrofloxacin (solution). Enrofloxacin is not approved for use in cows producing milk for human consumption. In order to attain effective concentrations in the mammary gland, oxytetracycline hydrochloride (conventional preparation) has to be administered by slow intravenous injection. Even though macrolide antibiotics attain high concentrations in milk, they also passively diffuse into ruminal fluid (pH 5.5–6.5) where the ion-trapping effect applies. This feature of their distribution may be undesirable. Moreover, slow intravenous injection is the preferred manner of administration, as the available parenteral preparations cause tissue irritation at intramuscular injection sites. Because spiramycin avidly binds to tissue components, long withdrawal periods would be associated with the use of this antimicrobial agent.

Intramammary preparations are formulated to provide either quick-release of the antimicrobial agent or slow-release of the antimicrobial over an extended period. A requirement of all intramammary preparations is that they be reasonably non-irritating to the parenchyma (epithelial tissue) of the udder. Quick-release preparations are used mainly in lactating cows for the treatment, often in conjunction with systemic therapy, of clinical mastitis. They should have short withdrawal periods. The vehicle used and viscosity of the formulation should allow rapid release of the antimicrobial agent while ensuring that effective concentrations will be maintained throughout the recommended dosage interval. Access of the released antimicrobial agent to the site of infection is determined by its uptake and distribution in mammary tissue, which are governed by the chemical nature and physiochemical properties (in particular lipid solubility) of the drug. Binding to milk proteins or components of mammary tissue limits distribution and extends the withdrawal periods. The transfer of an antimicrobial agent from a treated to untreated quarters of the udder takes place via the bloodstream and involves passive diffusion in both directions across the blood–milk barrier. Examples of intramammary preparations that are formulated as suspensions and have a recommended dosage interval of 12 h include cloxacillin sodium, ampicillin sodium–cloxacillin sodium combination, trimethoprim–sulphadiazine combination, and oxytetracycline hydrochloride (oily suspension), while erythromycin is formulated as an intramammary solution. Cefuroxime sodium and cefoperazone sodium (third-generation cephalosporins) are formulated as an oily paste and oily suspension, respectively. Quick-release intramammary preparations have short withdrawal periods, typically slaughter 7 days and milk withholding 3.5 days, either of which may be less depending on the preparation.

Slow-release intramammary preparations may be infused at the end of lactation (after the last milking) and into the teat canal of non-lactating cows to treat subclinical mastitis and to prevent the establishment of new infections during the non-lactating period. Either a poorly soluble salt of an antimicrobial agent may be used, or the formulation of the preparation be such that the rate of antimicrobial release is relatively constant, approaching zero-order. The antimicrobial agent must remain active (be stable) throughout the extended duration in the udder, and the preparation should not cause tissue irritation. Antimicrobial binding to mammary tissue components is not of particular concern, because slow-release preparations are not used in lactating cows. However, ability to penetrate cell membranes is important as, in chronic staphylococcal mastitis, the pathogenic bacteria often reside within epithelial cells, neutrophils and macrophages (Pyorala, 1995). Examples of slow-release intramammary preparations include cloxacillin (benzathine salt) with aluminium monostearate (suspension), ampicillin (trihydrate) and cloxacillin (benzathine) with aluminium monostearate (suspension) or formulated without aluminium monostearate as an oily suspension, procaine penicillin G (oily paste), dihydrostreptomycin sulphate and procaine penicillin G (oily paste). Penicillins and especially aminoglycosides have limited ability to penetrate cell membranes, whereas fluroquinolones, rifampin and macrolides have this capacity.

Compound preparations containing one or more antimicrobial agents and a corticosteroid (hydrocortisone or prednisolone) are available for intramammary infusion in lactating cows. The reduction in inflammation of the mammary gland is desirable, but the immunosuppressant effect and decrease in phagocyte function produced by glucocorticoids are undesirable. Amoxycillin trihydrate–clavulanate potassium combination and prednisolone is an example of a compound preparation (oily suspension) that can be administered by intramammary infusion at 12-h intervals and has short withdrawal periods (slaughter 7 days, milk 2 days). Unlike glucocorticoids, the NSAIDs do not cause immunosuppression. Flunixin meglumine (2.2 mg/kg), administered by intravenous injection at 24-h dosage intervals, may have a place in the treatment of acute *E. coli* (endotoxin) mastitis. The significance of the antipyretic, anti-inflammatory and analgesic effects produced by the drug is largely dependent on the stage of the inflammatory process at which treatment is commenced. Early diagnosis of coliform mastitis and prompt initiation of treatment with flunixin greatly increase the beneficial effect of the drug. The half-life of flunixin in cows is 8.1 h and the withdrawal periods are short (slaughter 7 days, milk 12 h). Flunixin does not interfere with the activity of concurrently administered antimicrobial agents should antimicrobial therapy be applied. There is no evidence to support the contention that systemic antimicrobial therapy causes a massive release of endotoxin in cows with coliform mastitis. Frequent stripping of the infected quarter(s) to remove bacteria and cellular debris is important, perhaps essential, in coliform mastitis (Sandholm & Pyorala, 1995). The slow intravenous injection of oxytocin, 5–10 units of diluted solution (10 units/mL), facilitates the completeness of stripping (milkout).

References

Aktas, M., Lefebvre, H.P., Toutain, P.L. & Braun, J.P. (1995) Disposition of creatine kinase activity in dog plasma following intravenous and intramuscular injection of skeletal muscle homogenates. *Journal of Veterinary Pharmacology and Therapeutics*, **18**, 1–6.

Banting, A.L. & Baggot, J.D. (1996) Comparison of the pharmacokinetics and local tolerance of three injectable oxytetracycline formulations in pigs. *Journal of Veterinary Pharmacology and Therapeutics*, **19**, 50–55.

Benet, L.Z. (1984) Pharmacokinetic parameters: which are necessary to define a drug substance? *European Journal of Respiratory Diseases*, **65**(Suppl. **134**), 45–61.

Bowman, K.F., Dix, L.P., Riond, J.-L. & Riviere, J.E. (1986) Prediction of pharmacokinetic profiles of ampicillin sodium, gentamicin sulfate, and combination ampicillin sodium–gentamicin sulfate in serum and synovia of healthy horses. *American Journal of Veterinary Research*, **47**, 1590–1596.

Boyd, J.S. (1987) Selection of sites for intramuscular injections in the neck of the horse. *Veterinary Record*, **121**, 197–200.

Brown, S.A., Coppoc, G.L., Riviere, J.E. & Anderson, V.L. (1986) Dose-dependent pharmacokinetics of gentamicin in sheep. *American Journal of Veterinary Research*, **47**, 789–794.

Dowling, P.M. & Russell, A.M. (2000) Pharmacokinetics of a long-acting oxytetracycline–polyethylene glycol formulation in horses. *Journal of Veterinary Pharmacology and Therapeutics*, **23**, 107–110.

Finco, D.R., Brown, S.A., Vaden, S.L. & Ferguson, D.C. (1995) Relationship between plasma creatinine concentration and glomerular filtration rate in dogs. *Journal of Veterinary Pharmacology and Therapeutics*, **18**, 418–421.

Firth, E.C., Nouws, J.F.M., Driessens, F., Schmaetz, P., Peperkamp, K. & Klein, W.R. (1986) Effect of the injection site on the pharmacokinetics of procaine penicillin G in horses. *American Journal of Veterinary Research*, **47**, 2380–2384.

George, L.W. & Smith, J.A. (1985) Treatment of *Moraxella bovis* infections in calves using a long acting oxytetracycline formulation. *Journal of Veterinary Pharmacology and Therapeutics*, **8**, 55–61.

Gilman, J.M., Davis, L.E., Neff-Davis, C.A., Koritz, G.D. & Baker, G.J. (1987) Plasma concentration of gentamicin after intramuscular or subcutaneous administration to horses. *Journal of Veterinary Pharmacology and Therapeutics*, **10**, 101–103.

Grondel, J.L., Nouws, J.F.M., Schutte, A.R. & Driessens, F. (1989) Comparative pharmacokinetics of oxytetracycline in rainbow trout (*Salmo gairdneri*) and African catfish (*Clarias gariepinus*). *Journal of Veterinary Pharmacology and Therapeutics*, **12**, 157–162.

Hinton, M. (1986) The ecology of *Escherichia coli* in animals including man with particular reference to drug resistance. *Veterinary Record*, **119**, 420–426.

Intorre, L., Mengozzi, G., Maccheroni, M., Bertini, S. & Soldani, G. (1995) Enrofloxacin–theophylline interaction: influence of enrofloxacin on theophylline steady-state pharmacokinetics in the Beagle dog. *Journal of Veterinary Pharmacology and Therapeutics*, **18**, 352–356.

Jacobson, E.R. (1993) Antimicrobial drug use in reptiles. In: *Antimicrobial Therapy in Veterinary Medicine*, (eds J.F. Prescott & J.D. Baggot), 2nd edn. Chapter 29, pp. 542–552. Iowa State University Press, Ames, Iowa.

Jacoby, G.A. & Archer, G.L. (1991) New mechanisms of bacterial resistance to antimicrobial agents. *New England Journal of Medicine*, **324**, 601–612.

Jawetz, E. (1975) Combined actions of antimicrobial drugs. In: *Concepts in Biochemical Pharmacology*, Part 3, (eds J.R. Gillette & J.R. Mitchell), pp. 343–358. Springer-Verlag, Berlin.

Martinez, M.N. & Berson, M.R. (1998) Bioavailability/bioequivalence assessments. In: *Development and Formulation of Veterinary Dosage Forms*, (eds G.E. Harde & J.D. Baggot), 2nd edn. Chapter 7, pp. 429–467. Marcel Dekker, New York.

Martinez-Martinez, L., Pascual, A. & Jacoby, G.A. (1998) Quinolone resistance from a transferable plasmid. *Lancet*, **351**, 797–799.

Nouws, J.F.M. & Vree, T.B. (1983) Effect of injection site on the bioavailability of an oxytetracycline formulation in ruminant calves. *Veterinary Quarterly*, **5**, 165–170.

Palmer, J.E., Whitlock, R.H. & Benson, C.E. (1988) Equine ehrlichial colitis: effect of oxytetracycline treatment during the incubation period of *Ehrlichia risticii* infection in ponies. *Journal of the American Veterinary Medical Association*, **192**, 343–345.

Park, B.K. & Kitteringham, N.R. (1988) Relevance of and means of assessing induction and inhibition of drug metabolism in man. In: *Progress in Drug Metabolism*, (ed G.G. Gibson), pp. 1–60. Taylor and Francis, London.

Park, B.K. & Kitteringham, N.R. (1990) Assessment of enzyme induction and enzyme inhibition in humans: toxicological implications. *Xenobiotica*, **20**, 1171–1185.

Prescott, J.F. & Baggot, J.D. (1985) Antimicrobial susceptibility testing and antimicrobial drug dosage. *Journal of the American Veterinary Medical Association*, **187**, 363–368.

Prescott, J.F. & Baggot, J.D. (1993) *Antimicrobial Therapy in Veterinary Medicine*, (eds J.F. Prescott & J.D. Baggot), 2nd edn. pp. 21–36. Iowa State University Press, Ames, Iowa.

Prince, R.A., Casabar, E., Adair, C.G., Wexler, D.B., Lettieri, J. & Kasik, J.E. (1989) Effect of quinolone antimicrobials on theophylline pharmacokinetics. *Journal of Clinical Pharmacology*, **29**, 650–654.

Pyorala, S. (1995) Staphylococcal and streptococcal mastitis. In: *The Bovine Udder and Mastitis*, (eds M. Sandholm, T. Honkanen-Buzalski, L. Kaartinen & S. Pyorala), pp. 143–148. Faculty of Veterinary Medicine, University of Helsinki, Helsinki.

Riviere, J.E. (1985) Aminoglycoside-induced toxic nephropathy. In: *CRC Handbook of Animal Models of Renal Failure*, (eds S.R. Ash & S.A. Thornhill), pp. 145–182. CRC Press, Boca Raton, Fla.

Rogge, M.C., Solomon, W.R., Sedman, A.J., Welling, P.G., Toothaker, R.D. & Wagner, J.C. (1988) The theophylline-enoxacin interaction: 1. Effect of enoxacin dose size on theophylline disposition. *Clinical Pharmacology and Therapeutics*, **44**, 579–587.

Rutgers, L.J.E., van Miert, A.S.J.P.A.M., Nouws, J.F.M. & van Ginneken, C.A.M. (1980)

Effect of the injection site on the bioavailability of amoxycillin trihydrate in dairy cows. *Journal of Veterinary Pharmacology and Therapeutics*, **3**, 125–132.

Sandholm, M. & Pyorala, S. (1995) Coliform mastitis. In: *The Bovine Udder and Mastitis*, (eds M. Sandholm, T. Honkanen-Buzalski, L. Kaartinen & S. Pyorala), pp. 149–160. Faculty of Veterinary Medicine, University of Helsinki, Helsinki.

Swan, G.E., Guthrie, A.J., Mulders, M.S.G., Killeen, V.M., Nueton, J.P., Short, C.R. & van den Berg, J.S. (1995) Single and multiple dose pharmacokinetics of gentamicin administered intravenously and intramuscularly in adult conditioned Thoroughbred mares. *Journal of the South African Veterinary Association*, **66**, 151–156.

Toutain, P.L., Lassourd, V., Costes, G., Alvinerie, M., Bret, L., Lefebvre, H.P. & Braun, J.P. (1995) A non-invasive and quantitative method for the study of tissue injury caused by intramuscular injection of drugs in horses. *Journal of Veterinary Pharmacology and Therapeutics*, **18**, 226–235.

Williams, R.T. (1967) Comparative patterns of drug metabolism. *Federation Proceedings*, **26**, 1029–1039.

Wilson, R.C., Duran, S.H., Horton, C.R., Jr & Wright, L.C. (1989) Bioavailability of gentamicin in dogs after intramuscular or subcutaneous injections. *American Journal of Veterinary Research*, **50**, 1748–1750.

Zhanel, G.G. (1993) Once daily aminoglycoside dosing: the result of research on anti-microbial pharmacodynamics. *American Journal of Pharmaceutical Education*, **56**, 156–167.

Ziv, G. (1980) Drug selection and use in mastitis: systemic vs local drug therapy. *Journal of the American Veterinary Medical Association*, **176**, 1109–1115.

Chapter 7
The Bioavailability and Disposition of Antimicrobial Agents in Neonatal Animals

Introduction

Differences between neonatal and adult animals in the intensity and duration of the effects produced by a drug when given at usual (adult) dosage can generally be attributed to increased biovailability and altered disposition (wider distribution and slower elimination) during the neonatal period. The altered pharmacokinetic behaviour of drugs in the neonate affects the plasma drug concentration profile and the concentrations attained at drug receptor sites or, in the case of antimicrobial agents, at sites of infection.

The neonatal period, which is generally considered to be the time span from birth to 1 month of age, varies between species. It appears to be 1–2 weeks in foals, about 8 weeks in calves, lambs and piglets, and 10–12 weeks in puppies. Some characteristic features of the neonatal period include increased drug absorption from the gastrointestinal tract, lower binding to plasma proteins (particularly albumin), lower ratio of body-fat to fluids (affects distribution of lipophilic drugs), larger extracellular fluid volume (affects distribution of hydrophilic drugs), increased permeability of the blood–brain barrier, production of acidic urine and slower elimination (longer half-life) of most drugs (Baggot & Short, 1984). Variations in the rate of maturation of the physiological variables that influence drug bioavailability and disposition account for the species differences in the duration of the neonatal period. In all species, however, profound adaptive changes in the physiological variables occur during the first 24 h of postnatal life. This coincides with the time that the pharmacokinetic behaviour of drugs is most 'unusual'. It could be hypothesized that the initial rapid development is at least partly due to the cessation of a hormonal suppressive influence. Even though absorption (depending on the route of drug administration), distribution, metabolism and excretion collectively influence the dose–effect relationship, the development of these processes can be considered separately for descriptive purposes.

Absorption

Colostral antibodies (macromolecules) are readily absorbed from the gastro-intestinal tract during the first 24 h after birth. This infers that the intestinal epithelium is more permeable during the first 24–36 h of postnatal life. The relatively less acidic pH in the stomach and the nature of the ingesta (mainly milk) influence the extent of drug absorption (systemic availability). Anti-microbial agents, such as penicillins, that are poorly absorbed and likely to cause digestive disturbances in older foals (>4 months of age) and adult horses can be administered to neonatal and young foals for the treatment of some systemic bacterial infections. Oral administration of amoxicillin trihydrate (30 mg/kg), as a 5% oral suspension, to 5–10-day old foals produced serum amoxicillin concentrations above 1 μg/mL for 6 h (Love *et al.*, 1981). The systemic availability of amoxycillin is 30–50% in neonatal foals compared with 5–15% in adult horses (Baggot *et al.*, 1988). Pivampicillin, a pro-drug of ampi-cillin, has systemic availability of 40–53% in foals between 11 days and 4 months of age (Ensink *et al.*, 1994). Although oral administration of amino-benzyl penicillins (ampicillin and amoxycillin) increases their half-life approximately twofold, there is no need to adjust the usual dosage interval (6–8 h). Penicillin V, the phenoxymethyl analogue of penicillin G (benzylpe-nicillin), cannot be recommended (due to low systemic availability and the production of digestive disturbances) for the treatment of bacterial infections in horses of any age (Baggot *et al.*, 1990).

The systemic availability of cefadroxil (5% oral suspension) decreases progressively from 68% in 1-month-old foals to 14.5% in foals 5 months of age (Duffee *et al.*, 1977). The half-life of this first-generation cephalosporin remains unchanged over the 1–5 month age range.

Erythromycin estolate in conjunction with rifampin (both drugs administered orally) can be recommended for the treatment of *Rhodococcus equi* pneumonia in foals. Early diagnosis of the infection and prompt initiation of therapy considerably increase the effectiveness of treatment. Apart from this specific indication, macrolide antibiotics (including erythromycin) and lincosamides (lincomycin and clindamycin) are contra-indicated in horses. Antimicrobial agents in these classes can cause severe disturbance of the balance between commensal bacterial flora in the colon of the horse.

As the rumen takes 4–8 weeks, depending on dietary composition, to develop and become functional, the bioavailability (rate and extent of absorption) of drugs administered orally to pre-ruminant calves resembles that in monogastric species rather than in cattle. Antimicrobial agents that are partly inactivated by ruminal microorganisms or that undergo exten-sive first-pass hepatic metabolism would be expected to have higher sys-temic availability (extent of absorption) in neonatal (pre-ruminant) animals. The systemic availability of orally administered trimethoprim, for example, is far higher in newborn kids than in older kids and adult goats (Nielsen & Rasmussen, 1976).

Distribution

Body composition may largely account for species variations or age-related differences in the extent and pattern of drug distribution. The decreasing extracellular fluid volume, as a percentage of body weight, during the neonatal period reduces the apparent volume of distribution of drugs that are highly ionized or relatively polar (e.g. penicillins, aminoglycosides, non-steroidal anti-inflammatory drugs (NSAIDs)). The increasing ratio of body-fat to fluids contributes to the increasing apparent volume of distribution of lipophilic drugs (e.g. macrolides, fluoroquinolones, trimethoprim) during the neonatal period. The volume of distribution differences are most pronounced between newborn (< 24 h of age) and adult animals.

Drugs reversibly bind in varying degrees to plasma proteins; the extent of protein binding is characteristic of the drug. As only the unbound fraction can diffuse into tissues, extensive (> 80%) binding of a drug to plasma proteins influences the total (bound plus unbound) concentration in the plasma, the extent of distribution and the availability of the drug for elimination (metabolism and excretion). Examples of antimicrobial agents that bind extensively to plasma proteins include cloxacillin, nafcillin, cefazolin, cefoperazone, ceftriaxone, sulphadimethoxine, doxycycline, erythromycin, clindamycin, rifampin and ketoconazole. Acidic drugs (penicillins, cephalosporins, sulphonamides) bind to plasma albumin, while some basic drugs (trimethoprim, macrolides and lincosamides) bind to α_1-acid glycoprotein. In the case of extensively bound drugs, a small change in the concentration of drug binding protein can significantly affect the amount of drug in the systemic circulation that is immediately available for extravascular distribution and elimination. Relative hypoalbuminaemia is a characteristic of neonatal animals, apart from foals; it is most pronounced in newborn piglets. The lower concentration of plasma albumin causes lower binding of acidic drugs and contributes to increased extravascular distribution. The combination of lower protein binding of extensively bound penicillins and cephalosporins and the larger extracellular fluid volume account for the larger apparent volume of distribution of these drugs in neonatal animals. Whereas the concentration of plasma albumin increases during the first 2 weeks of postnatal life, that of α_1-acid glycoprotein decreases in piglets and calves, but gradually increases in foals (Son *et al.*, 1996). This implies that protein binding of organic bases (such as lincomycin, clindamycin, erythromycin and trimethoprim) decreases as neonatal piglets and calves mature (Kinoshita *et al.*, 1995; Tagawa *et al.*, 1994).

Because disposition refers to the simultaneous effects of distribution and elimination, it is necessary to consider both components of the process when interpreting changes that occur during the neonatal period. Comparison of the disposition kinetics of enrofloxacin (2.5 mg/kg administered intravenously) in 1-day-old and 1-week-old calves shows that the volume of distribution ($V_{d(ss)}$) is smaller and the systemic clearance (Cl_B) of the drug is lower in the 1-day-old calves, while the half-life does not differ significantly between the age groups

(Kaartinen *et al.*, 1997) (Table 7.1). The changes in the disposition kinetics of enroflaxacin that occur during the first week of postnatal life in calves could be attributed to differences in plasma protein binding of enrofloxacin and in the body fat-to-fluids ratio because the drug is lipid-soluble. Enrofloxacin is converted by *N*-dealkylation, a hepatic microsomal oxidative reaction, to ciprofloxacin; both agents are antimicrobially active. The rate of formation of the active metabolite (ciprofloxacin) is five times slower and the peak plasma concentration is significantly lower in the 1-day-old than in the 1-week-old calves. Nonetheless, the sum of enrofloxacin and ciprofloxacin concentrations in plasma exceeds 0.10 µg/mL for 30 h and 24 h in 1-day-old and 1-week-old calves, respectively. The minimum inhibitory concentration for the majority of susceptible *Escherichia coli* strains (MIC_{90}) isolated from calves is 0.25 µg/mL. As fluoroquinolones have concentration-dependent bactericidal activity and induce a post-antibiotic effect (although of variable duration) (Craig, 1993), a 24-h dosage interval may be appropriate for enrofloxacin administration to neonatal calves.

Table 7.1 Disposition kinetics of enrofloxacin and formation of ciprofloxcin in newborn and one-week-old Finnish Ayrshire calves. A single dose (2.5 mg/kg) of enrofloxacin was administered by intravenous injection to the calves ($n = 4$ in each age group). Results are expressed as mean $\pm$ SEM and (range).

Pharmacokinetic parameter	Age of calves		Statistical significance
	1 day	1 week	
Enrofloxacin			
$V_{d\ (ss\ )}$ (L/kg)	1.81 $\pm$ 0.10 (1.54–2.01)	2.28 $\pm$ 0.14 (1.88–2.52)	$P = 0.035$
Cl_B (L/h·kg)	0.19 $\pm$ 0.03 (0.14–0.28)	0.39 $\pm$ 0.06 (0.31–0.56)	$P = 0.021$
$t_{1/2}$ (h)	6.61 $\pm$ 1.12 (4.28–9.36)	4.87 $\pm$ 0.68 (3.13–6.43)	NS
Ciprofloxacin			
t_{max} (h)	15.0 $\pm$ 3.0 (12–24)	2.8 $\pm$ 0.8 (1–4)	$P = 0.007$
C_{max} (mg/L)	0.087 $\pm$ 0.017 (0.07–0.14)	0.142 $\pm$ 0.005 (0.13–0.15)	$P = 0.023$

The blood–brain barrier restricts the passage of poorly diffusible drugs (such as aminoglycosides, penicillins, first- and second-generation cephalosporins) from the systemic circulation into the central nervous system. The failure of many antimicrobial agents to attain effective concentrations in cerebrospinal fluid is a well recognized problem in the treatment of bacterial meningitis, especially when caused by Enterobacteriaceae. Passage across the blood–brain barrier is limited to free (unbound) drug in the plasma that is sufficiently lipid-soluble to passively diffuse through both the capillary endothelium and the astrocytic sheath. As this morphological barrier is only partially developed at birth, drugs of moderate lipid solubility and certain endogenous substances (such as bilirubin) that cannot normally enter the extracellular fluid of the brain gain access during the early neonatal period. With regard to the treatment of bacterial meningitis, the parenteral preparation of trimethoprim–sulphadiazine (24 mg/kg, administered by slow intravenous injection at 12-h dosage intervals) could be effective. Greater therapeutic success is likely to be achieved in foals by administering intravenously either cefotaxime (at 8-h dosage intervals) or ceftriaxone (at 12-h dosage intervals, due to its longer half-life). The dose range for both of these third-generation cephalosporins is 15–25 mg/kg body weight. Aminoglycoside antibiotics, due to their polar nature, do not attain effective concentrations in the cerebrospinal fluid.

Metabolism

Metabolism (biotransformation) converts most lipid-soluble drugs into polar metabolites that are far less widely distributed than the parent drug and are readily excreted in the urine, although some drug metabolites (in particular glucuronide conjugates) are also excreted in bile. While the liver is the principal organ of drug metabolism, other organs (lungs and kidneys) and tissues (intestinal mucosa and blood) are capable of metabolizing drugs at least by some pathways. Antimicrobial agents that are mainly eliminated by hepatic metabolism include most sulphonamides, trimethoprim, fluoroquinolones, chloramphenicol, clindamycin, metronidazole, rifampin, ceftiofur (unique among the cephalosporins in this regard), and ketoconazole (but not fluconazole, which is eliminated by renal excretion). Enrofloxacin, difloxacin, ceftiofur and rifampin are initially converted to active metabolites that possess antimicrobial activity at least equal to that of the parent drugs. Pivampicillin, a prodrug, is activated by hydrolysis to ampicillin during absorption from the small intestine.

Most drug metabolic pathways are deficient in newborn animals and their activity progressively develops during the neonatal period. In the majority of species (ruminant animals, pigs, dogs and (presumably) cats), the hepatic microsomal-associated metabolic pathways (various oxidative reactions and glucuronide conjugation) develop rapidly during the first 3–4 weeks after birth, and at 8–12 weeks of age have activity *approaching* that of adult animals (Short & Davis, 1970; Nielsen & Rasmussen, 1976; Reiche, *et al.*, 1980; Reiche, 1983). There is indirect evidence which suggests that glucuronide synthesis develops very rapidly in foals during the first week after birth (Adamson *et al.*, 1991). For extensively metabolized drugs a long dosage interval, relative to that used in adult animals, should be applied during the first 3 days of postnatal life and can gradually be decreased, depending on the animal species, as the neonate matures.

The half-life of trimethoprim, which is mainly metabolized by hepatic microsomal oxidation, is four to five times longer in newborn kids than in adult goats (Nielsen & Rasmussen, 1976). A period of about 8 weeks appears to be required for the half-life of trimethoprim in kids to decrease to the value found in adult goats. This roughly coincides with the development of hepatic microsomal oxidative activity.

Ceftiofur is a third-generation cephalosporin with activity against Gram-positive and Gram-negative aerobes, and some anaerobic bacteria. Conversion of ceftiofur to desfuroylceftiofur is catalysed by an esterase, which is most active in the kidneys followed by the liver (Olson *et al.*, 1998). Desfuroylceftiofur has antibacterial activity similar to that of the parent drug. The active metabolite rapidly becomes reversibly bound to proteins in the plasma and tissues, while the unbound fraction forms conjugates with glutathione and cysteine. The high performance liquid chromatographic (HPLC) assay method measures the combined plasma concentration of ceftiofur and desfuroylceftiofur conjugates as a single derivative (desfurolyceftiofur acetamide), which is expressed as micrograms of ceftiofur free acid equivalents per millilitre (Jaglan *et al.*, 1990). In a study of the influence of age on the disposition of ceftiofur, administered intravenously as ceftiofur sodium at a dose of 2.2 mg ceftiofur free acid equivalents per kg body weight, in Holstein bull calves, it was shown that the volume of distribution ($V_{d(ss)}$) decreases and systemic clearance (Cl_B) increases during the first 3 months after birth (Brown *et al.*, 1996). The progressive decreases in the volume of distribution of the derivative measured (ceftiofur and desfuroylceftiofur conjugates), which is water-soluble, could be attributed to the age-related decrease in extracellular fluid volume. The lower clearance in the 1-week-old and 1-month-old calves than in older calves is due to maturation of the elimination processes for ceftiofur. Because the decreases in volume of distribution are proportionally less than the increases in clearance in calves 1 month of age and older, the half-life decreases more or less in accordance with the increased clearance (Table 7.2). Half-life is a hybrid (composite) pharmacokinetic parameter that depends upon the relationship between the volume of distribution (area method) and the systemic clearance (Cl_B) of a drug:

$$t_{1/2} = \frac{0.693 \cdot V_{d(area)}}{Cl_B}$$

A useful application of half-life is in the selection of the dosage interval.

NSAIDs are weak organic acids that are ionized in the plasma, undergo extensive binding to plasma albumin and are mainly eliminated by hepatic metabolism. The disposition of phenylbutazone, ketoprofen and flunixin shows a consistent pattern of differences between newborn (<1-day-old) foals and adult horses (Wilcke *et al.*, 1993, 1998; Crisman *et al.*, 1996). The volume of distribution is larger, the systemic clearance is lower and the half-life of these

Table 7.2 Comparison of pharmacokinetic values derived from plasma concentrations of ceftiofur and metabolites (measured as desfuroylceftiofur acetamide by HPLC) after intravenous injection of ceftiofur sodium at a dose of 2.2 mg ceftiofur free acid equivalents per kilogram in Holstein bull calves of various ages.

Age	$V_{d(ss)}$ (mL/Kg)	Cl_B (mL/h·kg)	$t_{1/2}$ (h)
1 week	345 ± 62	17.8 ± 3.2	16.1 ± 1.5
1 month	335 ± 92	16.7 ± 3.1	17.2 ± 3.1
3 months	284 ± 49	30.3 ± 4.6	8.2 ± 2.8
6 months	258 ± 72	39.8 ± 14.9	5.95 ± 1.2

drugs is longer in newborn foals (Table 7.3). These differences are due to the larger extracellular fluid volume and lower activity of hepatic microsomal-associated metabolic pathways in neonatal foals.

As adult cats have a relative deficiency in hepatic microsomal glucuronyl transferase activity, glucuronide conjugates of drugs and endogenous substances (such as bilirubin and steroidal substances) are slowly synthesized in

Table 7.3 Comparison of the disposition kinetics of non-steroidal anti-inflammatory drugs in newborn foals and adult horses; values are expressed as median and range.

Pharmacokinetic parameter	Newborn foal	Adult horse
Flunixin[a]		
$V_{d\,(ss)}$ (mL/kg)	220 (165–239)	150
Cl_B (mL/h·kg)	17.0 (9.6–23.3)	92–580
$t_{1/2}$ (h)	8.5 (6.6–12.9)	1.5–4.2
$MRT_{i.v.}$ (h)	12.5 (8.9–20.0)	
Ketoprofen[b]		
$V_{d\,(ss)}$ (mL/kg)	339 (317–417)	153
Cl_B (mL/h·kg)	56.1 (49.4–85.5)	185–289
$t_{1/2}$ (h)	4.6 (3.0–5.5)	1.02–1.06
$MRT_{i.v.}$ (h)	6.0 (4.1–7.4)	
Phenylbutazone[c]		
$V_{d\,(ss)}$ (mL/kg)	274 (190–401)	152
Cl_B (mL/h·kg)	18 (13–38)	36
$t_{1/2}$ (h)	7.4 (6.4–22.1)[d]	3.5–6.0
$MRT_{i.v.}$ (h)	32 (22–41)	

[a] Crisman *et al.* (1996).
[b] Wilcke *et al.* (1998).
[c] Wilcke *et al.* (1993).
[d] Half-life was greatly prolonged in two foals that were less than 12 h of age at the time of dosing.

cats. Further decreased activity of this metabolic pathway would render neonatal kittens particularly susceptible to toxicity with drugs that undergo glucuronide conjugation (e.g. chloramphenicol, salicylate).

Excretion

Renal excretion is the principal elimination process for drugs that are predominantly ionized at physiological pH (such as penicillins and cephalosporins), polar drugs (aminoglycosides), and for molecules with variable solubility in lipid (tetracyclines, apart from doxycycline and minocycline). Exceptions among β-lactam antibiotics include nafcillin, cefoperazone and ceftriaxone, which are excreted in bile, while cephalothin and cefotaxime undergo deacetylation before excretion in urine. Even though fluoroquinolones, trimethoprim and sulphonamides are mainly eliminated by hepatic metabolism, a fraction of the systemically available dose is excreted unchanged in urine.

Renal excretion mechanisms (glomerular filtration and active, carrier-mediated tubular secretion) are incompletely developed at birth in mammalian species. During the early neonatal period glomerular filtration and tubular secretion mature independently at rates that are species-related. The glomerular filtration rate (GFR), based on inulin clearance, attains adult values within 2 days in calves, 2–4 days in lambs, kids and piglets, and may take at least 14 days to mature in puppies. Proximal tubular secretion, based on clearance of *para*-aminohippurate, matures within 2 weeks after birth in the ruminant species and pigs, but may take up to 6 weeks in dogs. In a recently published study of the maturation of renal function in full term pony foals during the first 10 days of postnatal life, it was shown that the GFR and effective renal plasma flow (indicates tubular secretion) remain relatively constant throughout the neonatal period (Holdstock *et al.*, 1998). This implies that the neonatal foal, like the calf, has relatively mature renal function shortly after birth. In newborn animals, the capacity of renal function is adequate to meet physiological requirements. However, when lipid-soluble drugs are administered to neonatal animals, the combined effect of slow hepatic metabolism and inefficient renal excretion considerably decreases the rate of elimination of the parent drugs and their polar metabolites. Urinary pH is acidic in neonates of all species; this would favour tubular reabsorption and extend the half-life of drugs that are weak organic acids and of sufficient lipid solubility to be reabsorbed by passive diffusion (e.g. most sulphonamides).

Following parenteral administration, the distribution of gentamicin is virtually restricted to extracellular fluid, and elimination takes place solely by glomerular filtration. The pattern of age-related changes in the disposition of gentamicin is similar in foals (Cummings *et al.*, 1990) and in calves (Clarke *et al.*, 1985). Values of the systemic clearance of gentamicin in 1- and 5-day-old foals and calves compared with mares and cows, respectively, indicate that glomerular filtration is mature in equine and bovine neonates (Table 7.4). The longer half-life of gentamicin, at least up to 15 days of age, but particularly in 1-day-old foals and calves, is due to the larger apparent volume of distribution of the drug. Although the disposition of gentamicin differs significantly between newborn (4–12 h of age at the time of dosing) and 6-week-old piglets (Giroux *et al.*, 1995), age-related changes in disposition of the drug follow a similar pattern to that in foals and calves. As the volume of distribution decreases during the neonatal period, the half-life of gentamicin becomes shorter. The average half-life of gentamicin is 5.2 h in newborn piglets, and 3.8 h, 3.5 h and 2.7 h in 4–6- and 10-week-old piglets, respectively.

Table 7.4 Age-related changes in the disposition of gentamicin in foals and calves.

Age (days)	$V_{d(ss)}$ (mL/Kg)	Cl_B (mL/min·kg)	$t_{1/2}$ (min)
Foals			
1	307 ± 30	1.75 ± 0.47	127 ± 23
5	350 ± 66	2.98 ± 1.48	90 ± 32
10	344 ± 95	2.60 ± 0.96	101 ± 33
15	325 ± 48	2.40 ± 0.87	106 ± 33
Mares	156 ± 22	1.69 ± 0.65	65 ± 55
Calves			
1	376 ± 41	1.92 ± 0.43	149 ± 38
5	385 ± 44	2.44 ± 0.34	119 ± 20
10	323 ± 20	2.02 ± 0.27	118 ± 13
15	311 ± 29	2.10 ± 0.32	111 ± 8.5
Cows	129 ± 17	1.29 ± 0.26	76 ± 11

Renal excretion mechanisms appear to mature within the first 2 weeks after birth in foals, calves, lambs, kids and piglets, while their maturation in puppies may take 4–6 weeks. In a study of the pharmacokinetics of amikacin in critically ill full-term foals ranging in age from 2 to 12 days, the systemic clearance of the aminoglycoside was lower (indicating impaired renal function) and the half-life was considerably prolonged in uraemic compared with non-uraemic foals (Adland-Davenport *et al.*, 1990).

Oxytetracycline is eliminated by glomerular filtration but, because it distributes more widely in tissues and undergoes enterohepatic circulation, its half-life is much longer than that of aminoglycoside antibiotics and varies between species (from 3.4 h in goats to 9.6 h in horses). The apparent volume of distribution and the half-life of oxytetracycline decrease with age of calves between 3 and 14 weeks old and further in adult cattle (Nouws *et al.*, 1983). The changes in disposition of the drug could be attributed to the decrease in total body water volume and the progressive development of the rumen. Even though the volume of distribution of oxytetracycline is larger in 4–5-day-old foals than in adult horses, the half-life of the drug does not appear to be extended in neonatal foals (Papich *et al.*, 1995). The half-life of ceftriaxone, a third-generation cephalosporin that distributes widely in body fluids (including penetration of the blood–brain barrier) and is eliminated by biliary rather than renal excretion, is twofold longer in 2–12-day-old foals (Ringger *et al.*, 1998) than in adult horses (Ringger *et al.*, 1996). The longer half-life could be due to the larger volume of extracellular fluid in the neonatal foals.

Drug selection and administration

In selecting an antimicrobial agent for use in a neonatal animal, consideration should be given to the immune status of the neonate (especially newborn) and the likely degree of development of the physiological variables that influence the distribution and elimination of drugs: the latter factor is age-dependent and varies between species. It is preferable to select an antimicrobial agent or combination that produces a bactericidal effect and, depending on bacterial susceptibility, has a wide margin of safety. Drugs to consider include penicillins, cephalosporins, amoxycillin or ticarcillin combined with clavulanic acid, trimethoprim–sulphonamide combinations and enrofloxacin (in calves and piglets). Because of their potential to produce nephrotoxic and ototoxic effects and to accumulate upon repeated dosage, an aminoglycoside (gentamicin or amikacin) should be used only when specifically indicated.

The variability associated with drug absorption from the gastrointestinal tract can be overcome by using a parenteral preparation (dosage form). It should preferably be administered either by intravenous infusion or slow intravenous injection to avoid circulatory overload. Intraosseous administration is a useful alternative to intravenous injection of some antimicrobial agents (e.g. sodium ampicillin or amoxycillin, cefotaxime, ceftriaxone, gentamicin or amikacin sulphate) in neonatal foals (Fig. 7.1) (Golenz *et al.*, 1994) and puppies (Lavy *et al.*, 1995). This particularly applies when the neonate is in a state of septic shock and/or dehydration. Total plasma protein concentration is an inaccurate index of hydration status unless monitored (repeatedly measured) and interpreted in conjunction with packed cell volume (PCV).

Age-related species variations in development of the various elimination processes (hepatic metabolic pathways and renal excretion mechanisms) make the prediction of dosage intervals unreliable. However, longer dosage intervals should be applied in neonatal animals (especially during the first 3 days after birth) than in adult animals of the same species. Because of wide individual variation in the plasma concentration profiles obtained following gentamicin administration, at least in neonatal foals, and the relatively narrow margin of safety of the drug, maintenance dosage should be based on measurement of peak and trough plasma gentamicin concentrations.

Drug absorption from intramuscular sites largely depends on regional blood flow, which can vary with formulation (aqueous solution or suspension, salt

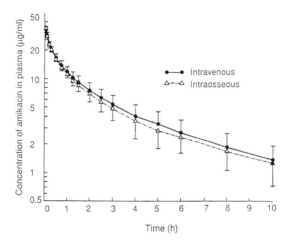

Fig. 7.1   Concentrations (mean ± SD) of amikacin in plasma after i.v. and i.o. administration of amikacin sulphate (7 mg/kg body weight) to six foals at 3–5 days of age.

form and concentration of the drug) of the parenteral dosage form (drug preparation) and the presence of disease states (such as dehydration). The sum of these variables not only influences the plasma concentration profile that will be obtained, but may affect the response to therapy. In kittens, puppies and piglets, there is the added risk of causing tissue damage at the intramuscular injection site. Following the intramuscular injection of 10% aqueous suspension of amoxycillin trihydrate at a dose of 7 mg/kg body weight, a relationship between the body weight (or age) of calves and the serum amoxicillin concentration profile was found (Fig. 7.2) (Marshall & Palmer, 1980). The lower the body weight of calves, the higher the serum amoxicillin concentrations obtained. Even though the serum concentration profiles for amoxycillin (10% aqueous suspension of amoxycillin trihydrate injected intramuscularly at a dose of 7 mg/kg, except in cats 10–12 mg/kg) differ in shape between species, the inverse relationship between body weight and serum amoxycillin concentrations obtained appears to apply (Fig. 7.3). The trend shown is that the physically smaller animals (cats, dogs and piglets) have an early high peak concentration followed by a rapid decline, while larger animals (calves and

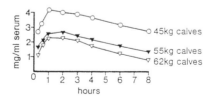

Fig. 7.2   Effect of age and weight on the bioavailability of amoxycillin in calves after intramuscular injection of amoxycillin trihydrate aqueous suspension (100 mg/mL) at a dose of 7 mg/kg body weight.

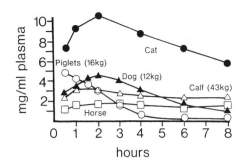

Fig. 7.3 Effect of species and weight on the bioavailability of amoxycillin after intramuscular injection of amoxycillin trihydrate aqueous suspension (100 mg/mL) at the same dose (7 mg/kg) in the various species except cats (10–12 mg/kg).

horses) have a lower and relatively constant serum concentration of amoxycillin throughout the 8 h period of sampling. It is not known whether other drug preparations administered intramuscularly show this relationship.

In mild-to-moderate infections, oral drug administration may be used for maintenance therapy with aminobenzyl penicillins (ampicillin or amoxycillin in dogs and cats; pivampicillin in foals), cefadroxil, trimethoprim–sulphonamide combinations, and enrofloxacin (in calves and piglets). Fluconazole suppresses oral and oesophageal candidiasis in immunosuppressed foals and may be effective in the treatment of systemic candidiasis.

The systemic availability of orally administered antimicrobials is higher in neonates and elimination, particularly when hepatic metabolism is involved, takes place more slowly. At 1 week of age the foal appears to have a relatively greater ability to eliminate drugs than neonates of other animal species.

The success of antimicrobial therapy depends upon the prompt initiation of treatment according to a well-informed empirical approach, followed by specific therapy based on precise identification of the causative pathogenic microorganism and knowledge of its susceptibility; supportive measures should be provided. Selection of the antimicrobial agent of choice and the optimum dosage rate for treatment of infections caused by microorganisms of unpredictable susceptibility (*Escherichia coli. Klebsiella, Proteus* and *Salmonella* spp. and coagulase-positive staphylococci) requires knowledge of quantitative susceptibility, determined by the broth dilution method which measures minimum inhibitory concentration (MIC), of the bacterial pathogen. In the treatment of severe systemic infections caused by *Pseudomonas aeruginosa*, the concurrent use of gentamicin and ticarcillin could be justified on the basis of the generally synergistic action of the combination against *Pseudomonas* sp.

The physiological features of the neonatal period that influence the bioavailability and disposition of drugs should be considered when selecting the route of administration and the dosage interval. An appreciation of species differences in the rate at which age-related physiological variables mature, and knowledge of the elimination processes for the drug selected serve as guidelines for dosage estimation in neonatal animals.

References

Adamson, P.J.W., Wilson, W.D., Baggot, J.D., Hietala, S.K. & Mihalyi, J.E. (1991) Influence of age on the disposition kinetics of chloramphenicol in equine neonates. *American Journal of Veterinary Research*, **52**, 426–431.

Adland-Davenport, P., Brown, M.P., Robinson, J.D. & Derendorf, H.C. (1990) Pharmacokinetics of amikacin in critically ill neonatal foals treated for presumed or confirmed sepsis. *Equine Veterinary Journal*, **22**, 18–22.

Baggot, J.D. & Short, C.R. (1984) Drug disposition in neonatal animals, with particular reference to the foal. *Equine Veterinary Journal*, **16**, 364–367.

Baggot, J.D., Love, D.N., Stewart, J. & Raus, J. (1988) Bioavailability and disposition kinetics of amoxycillin in neonatal foals. *Equine Veterinary Journal*, **20**, 125–127.

Baggot, J.D., Love, D.N., Love, R.J., Raus, J. & Rose, R.J. (1990) Oral dosage of penicillin V in adult horses and foals. *Equine Veterinary Journal*, **22**, 290–291.

Brown, S.A., Chester, S.T. & Robb, E.J. (1996) Effects of age on the pharmacokinetics of single dose ceftiofur sodium administered intramuscularly or intravenously to cattle. *Journal of Veterinary Pharmacology and Therapeutics*, **19**, 32–38.

Clarke, C.R., Short, C.R., Hsu, R.-C. & Baggot, J.D. (1985) Pharmacokinetics of gentamicin in the calf: Developmental changes. *American Journal of Veterinary Research*, **46**, 2461–2466.

Craig, W. (1993) Pharmacodynamics of antimicrobial agents as a basis for determination of dosage regimens. *European Journal of Clinical Microbial Infectious Disease*, **1**, 6–8.

Crisman, M.V., Wilcke, J.R. & Sams, R.A. (1996) Pharmacokinetics of flunixin meglumine in healthy foals less than twenty-four hours old. *American Journal of Veterinary Research*, **57**, 1759–1761.

Cummings, L.E., Guthrie, A.J., Harkins, J.D. & Short, C.R. (1990) Pharmacokinetics of gentamicin in newborn to 30-day-old foals. *American Journal of Veterinary Research*, **51**, 1988–1992.

Duffee, N.E., Stang, B.E. & Schaeffer, D.J. (1977) The pharmacokinetics of cefadroxil over a range of oral doses and animal ages in the foal. *Journal of Veterinary Pharmacology and Therapeutics*, **20**, 427–433.

Ensink, J.M., Barneveld, A., Klein, W.R., van Miert, A.S.J.P.A.M. & Vulto, A.G. (1994) Oral bioavailability of pivampicillin in foals at different ages. *Veterinary Quarterly*, **16**, 5113–5116.

Giroux, D., Sirois, G. & Martineau, G.-P. (1995) Gentamicin pharmacokinetics in newborn and 42-day-old male piglets. *Journal of Veterinary Pharmacology and Therapeutics*, **18**, 407–412.

Golenz, M.R., Wilson, W.D., Carlson, G.P., Craychee, T.J., Mihalyi, J.E. & Knox, L. (1994) Effect of route of administration and age on the pharmacokinetics of amikacin administered by the intravenous and intraosseous routes to 3- and 5-day-old foals. *Equine Veterinary Journal*, **26**, 367–373.

Holdstock, N.B., Ousey, J.C. & Rossdale, P.D. (1998) Glomerular filtration rate, effective renal plasma flow, blood pressure and pulse rate in the equine neonate during the first 10 days *post partum*. *Equine Veterinary Journal*, **30**, 335–343.

Jaglan, P.S., Cox, B.L., Arnold, T.S., Kubicek, M.F., Stewart, D.J. & Gilbertson, J.J. (1990) Liquid chromatographic determination of desfuroylceftiofur metabolite of ceftiofur as residue in cattle plasma *Journal of the Association of Official Analytical Chemists*, **73**, 26–30.

Kaartinen, L., Pyorala, S., Moilanen, M. & Raisanen, S. (1997) Pharmacokinetics of enrofloxacin in newborn and one-week-old calves. *Journal of Veterinary Pharmacology and Therapeutics*, **20**, 479–482.

Kinoshita, T., Son, D.-S., Shimoda, M. & Kokue, E. (1995) Impact of age-related alteration of plasma α_1-acid glycoprotein concentration on erythromycin pharmacokinetics in pigs. *American Journal of Veterinary Research*, **56**, 362–365.

Lavy, E., Goldstein, R., Shem-Tov, M., Glickman, A., Ziv, G. & Bark, H. (1995) Disposition kinetics of ampicillin administered intravenously and intraosseously to canine puppies. *Journal of Veterinary Pharmacology and Therapeutics*, **18**, 379–381.

Love, D.N., Rose, R.J., Martin, I.C.A. & Baily, M. (1981) Serum levels of amoxycillin following its oral administration to Thoroughbred foals. *Equine Veterinary Journal*, **13**, 53–55.

Marshall, A.B. & Palmer, G.H. (1980) Injection sites and drug bioavailability. In: *Trends in Veterinary Pharmacology and Toxicology*, (eds A.S.J.P.A.M. van Miert, J. Frens & F.W. van der Kreek), pp. 54–60. Elsevier, Amsterdam.

Nielsen, P. & Rasmussen, F. (1976) Influence of age on half-life of trimethoprim and sulphadoxine in goats. *Acta Pharmacologica et Toxicologica*, **38**, 113–119.

Nouws, J.F.M., van Ginneken, C.A.M. & Ziv, G. (1983) Age-dependant pharmacokinetics of oxytetracycline in ruminants. *Journal of Veterinary Pharmacology and Therapeutics*, **6**, 59–66.

Olson, S.C., Beconi-Barker, M.G., Smith, E.B., Martin, R.A., Vidmar, T.J. & Adams, L.D. (1998) *In vitro* metabolism of ceftiofur in bovine tissues. *Journal of Veterinary Pharmacology and Therapeutics*, **21**, 112–120.

Papich, M.G., Wright, A.K., Petrie, L. & Korsrud, G.O. (1995) Pharmacokinetics of oxytetracycline administered intravenously to 4 to 5-day-old foals. *Journal of Veterinary Pharmacology and Therapeutics*, **18**, 375–378.

Reiche, R. (1983) Drug disposition in the newborn. In: *Veterinary Pharmacology and Toxicology*, (eds Y. Ruckebusch, P.-L. Toutain and G.D. Koritz), pp. 49–55. MTP Press, Lancaster, U.K.

Reiche, R., Mulling, M. & Frey, H.-H. (1980) Pharmacokinetics of chloramphenicol in calves during the first weeks of life. *Journal of Veterinary Pharmacology and Therapeutics*, **3**, 95–106.

Ringger, N.C., Pearson, E.G., Gronwall, R.R. & Kohlepp, S.J. (1996) Pharmacokinetics of ceftriaxone in healthy horses. *Equine Veterinary Journal*, **28**, 476–479.

Ringger, N.C., Brown, M.P., Kohlepp, S.J., Gronwall, R.R. & Merritt, K. (1998) Pharmacokinetics of ceftriaxone in neonatal foals. *Equine Veterinary Journal*, **30**, 163–165.

Short, C.R. & Davis, L.E. (1970) Perinatal development of drug-metabolizing enzyme activity in swine. *Journal of Pharmacology and Experimental Therapeutics*, **174**, 185–196.

Son, D-S., Hariya, S., Shimoda, M. & Kokue, E. (1996) Contribution of α_1-acid glycoprotein to plasma protein binding of some basic antimicrobials in pigs. *Journal of Veterinary Pharmacology and Therapeutics*, **19**, 176–183.

Tagawa, Y., Kokue, E., Shimoda, M. & Son, D. (1994) α_1-Acid glycoprotein-binding as a factor in age-related changes in the pharmacokinetics of trimethoprim in piglets. *Veterinary Quarterly*, **16**, 13–17.

Wilcke, J.R., Crisman, M.V., Sams, R.A. & Gerken, D.F. (1993) Pharmacokinetics of phenylbutazone in neonatal foals. *American Journal of Veterinary Research*, **54**, 2064–2067.

Wilcke, J.R., Crisman, M.V., Scarratt, W.K. & Sams, R.A. (1998) Pharmacokinetics of ketoprofen in healthy foals less than twenty-four hours old. *American Journal of Veterinary Research*, **59**, 290–292.

Appendix
Pharmacokinetic Terms: Symbols and Units

With regard to the symbols used for pharmacokinetic terms, discrepancies between pharmacokinetic computer programs as well as between papers in the literature are quite common. Consistency in the use of symbols would reduce errors that could arise with the interpretation of values reported for various terms. The units in which pharmacokinetic terms are expressed are a feature of how the terms are defined and influence the numerical values obtained. Careful consideration of the units associated with a term can often serve to clarify the precise meaning of the term or concept as defined. The insertion of units associated with the numerical values of individual terms in equations is particularly useful in ensuring that the equation is correctly applied and in verifying the units in which the parameter calculated should be expressed. Because pharmacokinetic parameters are quantitative terms, it is important that the units in which they are expressed are correctly presented. In the human literature, which is largely concerned with a single species, clearance and apparent volume of distribution are expressed in units of mL/min and mL (or L), respectively. In the veterinary literature and for comparative purposes, these pharmacokinetic parameters as well as dose level and infusion rate are expressed on a unit body weight (per kg) basis. The unit of body weight is in the denominator of the terms in which it occurs, e.g. dose level (mg/kg), infusion rate (μg/min·kg), clearance (mL/min·kg), apparent volume of distribution (mL/kg).

Terms and units

Unit of drug concentration: μg/mL or ng/mL

C_p	plasma drug concentration at any time t
A, B	coefficients of biexponential equation describing disposition curve
$C_{p(0)}$	estimated initial (zero-time) drug concentration in plasma; sum of the coefficients associated with phases of the disposition curve

$C_{p(12\,h)}$	plasma drug concentration at 12 hours (or any specified time) after administration of the drug
$C_{p(last)}$	the last measured plasma drug concentration, with reference to the time of collection of the last of a series of blood samples for drug assay.
$C_{p,ss}$	plasma drug concentration at steady-state during a constant rate intravenous infusion
$C_{p,ss(max)}$	maximum desirable plasma drug concentration at steady-state on administering a fixed dose at constant dosage intervals
$C_{p,ass(min)}$	minimum effective plasma drug concentration at steady-state on administering a fixed dose at constant dosage intervals
$C_{p(avg)}$	(desired) average plasma concentration of drug during a dosage interval at steady-state (multiple dosing)
C_{max}	maximum (peak) concentration of drug in blood plasma (applied to extravascular drug administration)
C_{min}	minimum observed (or could infer lowest effective) concentration of drug in blood plasma

Unit of time: minutes (min) or hours (h)

$t_{1/2}$	half-life, which may be qualified by the process to which it refers. For example, $t_{1/2(\beta)}$ refers to the elimination half-life of a drug when the disposition curve following intravenous administration of the dose can be adequately described by a biexponential equation.
$t_{1/2(a)}$	absorption half-life
$t_{1/2(d)}$	apparent half-life following oral or extravascular administration of a drug; d represents disposition
MRT	mean residence time, which may be qualified by the route of administration
MAT	mean absorption time
t_{max}	(observed) time after drug administration at which peak plasma concentration occurs
τ (tau)	dosage interval (h)

Rate constants: min^{-1} or h^{-1} (reciprocal time)

α, β	exponents of biexponential equation describing the disposition curve; α and β are the first-order rate constants associated with the distribution and elimination phases, respectively, of the disposition curve. When the curve is best described by a triexponential equation, γ (gamma) is the first-order rate constant associated with the linear terminal elimination phase

k_{12} and k_{21} first-order rate constants associated with transfer of unbound drug between the central (1) and peripheral (2) compartments, respectively, of the two-compartment pharmacokinetic model

k_{el} first-order rate constant for elimination of drug from the central compartment of the pharmacokinetic model

k_a apparent first-order absorption rate constant

k_d apparent first-order disposition (mainly elimination) rate constant when drug is administered orally or by any other extra-vascular route.

Volume terms: mL/kg or L/kg

$V_{d(area)}$ apparent volume of distribution based on area under the curve (AUC)

$V_{d(ss)}$ apparent volume of distribution at steady-state

V_c apparent volume of central compartment of pharmacokinetic model

For comparative purposes, clearance is expressed in units of mL/min·kg or mL/h·kg

The centred dot · represents × (multiplied by)

Cl_B body (systemic) clearance

Cl_R renal clearance

Cl_H hepatic clearance

Q_{organ} blood flow to the specific organ (mL/min); expressed on a unit body weight basis (mL/min·kg)

R_0 rate of intravenous infusion; µg/min·kg (µg/min × kg)

Area under the curve (AUC) is expressed in units of µg·h/mL (µg × h/mL)

AUC   total area under the plasma drug concentration–time curve (from time zero to infinity). Whenever the determination of AUC is partial (incomplete), the time period over which it is determined should be specified; for example, AUC_{0-12h} refers to area under the curve from time zero to 12 h after drug administration

AUMC   total area under the first moment curve is expressed in units of $\mu g \cdot h^2 / mL$ ($\mu g \times h^2 / mL$)

Fraction terms: value ≤ 1, usually expressed as per cent (%)

F fraction of the administered dose which reaches the systemic circulation unchanged (systemic availability of a drug)

f_{el} fraction of dose eliminated during a dosage interval

f_r fraction of dose remaining at the end of a dosage interval

f_{ex} fraction of dose excreted unchanged in the urine

f_b	fraction of drug bound to plasma proteins
E	extraction ratio (no units)
E_H	hepatic extraction ratio

Weight (Mass)

D	dose (amount) of drug to be administered, which may be qualified by the route of administration; mg/kg or µg/kg
W	body weight of animal; kg

Equations

Bioexponential equation

$$C_p = Ae^{-\alpha t} + Be^{-\beta t}$$

Triexponential equation

$$C_p = Ae^{-\alpha t} + Be^{-\beta t} + \Gamma e^{-\gamma t}$$

The coefficients (A, B, Γ) associated with the polyexponential equation describing the disposition curve could be replaced by C_1, C_2, C_3 and the exponents (α, β, γ) be replaced by $\lambda_1, \lambda_2, \lambda_3$.

Index

absorption
  neonatal animals, 253
  topical preparations, 179–81
acepromazine, 4
acetaminophen *see* paracetamol
acetazolamide, 23
acetylation, 14, 16, 18–19
acetylcysteine, 20
acetylsalicylic acid *see* aspirin
acquired resistance, 215–17
action of drugs, 1–2
acyclovir, 157
adrenaline
  biotransformation processes, 13, 20
  physiological antagonism, 158
aflatoxin, 20
albendazole, 21, 163
  bioavailability, 70
  controlled-release bolus, 73
  drug interactions, 120
  effect of fasting on liver function, 111–12
  stereoisomerism, 170–2
albumin, plasma protein binding, 92,
    99–102, 103–4
allopurinol, 23, 120
amidases, 14
amikacin, 161, 224–5, 260
aminoglycosides, 217, 224
  clearance, 44, 115
  clinical effectiveness, 229
  duration of therapy, 244
  extent of distribution, 39, 92
  mechanism of action, 214, 229
  neonatal animals, 256
  resistance, 215, 216, 225
  selective tissue binding, 92
  selectivity and toxicity, 160, 161, 225–6
  variables that influence clinical
    response, 245
aminophylline, 8, 46, 147
amitraz, 162
  topical preparations, 184, 186, 188, 190,
    194–5
amoxycillin, 197, 224

bioavailability, 64, 65, 67, 78–9, 80
bovine mastitis therapy, 248
combinations, 243
neonatal animals, 253, 262–3
resistance, 215, 216
amphetamine
  biotransformation processes, 10
  elimination, 33
  plasma protein binding, 99
  renal clearance, 117
amphotericin, 159, 161, 214
ampicillin, 223, 224
  bioavailability, 64, 77, 79, 81–2
  bovine mastitis therapy, 247, 248
  changes in drug disposition
    febrile state, 96, 97
    renal disease, 113
  clearance, 126
  combinations, 243
  interspecies scaling, 124
  resistance, 215
anaesthetic agents, species variation in
    drug disposition, 2–6
antagonism, 141, 151–3
  chemical, 157–8
  pharmacological, 151–3
  physiological, 158
  selective inhibition of enzymes, 153–7
anthelmintics, selectivity and toxicity,
    162–4
antifungal agents, 202
  topical preparations, 199–202
antimicrobials
  active metabolites, 227
  classification, 210–12
  distribution and elimination, 217–27
  effects on intestinal microorganisms,
    159–60, 213, 222–3
  mechanisms of action, 213–14
  neonatal animals, 253
  plasma concentrations and clinical
    effectiveness, 228–30
  potential pharmacokinetic interactions,
    227–8

resistance, 214–17
  acquired, 215–17
  cross-resistance, 217
  inherent, 215
  transferable, 217
selectivity and toxicity, 159–62
therapy, 230–5
  administration and dosage, 235–41
  bacterial culture and susceptibility
    testing, 233–4
  bovine mastitis, 246–9
  combinations, 241–4
  duration, 244–5
  initial (empirical), 230–2
  maintenance therapy, 234–5
topical preparations, 196–9
variables influencing clinical response,
  245–6
antipyrine
  changes in drug disposition
    effect of fasting on hepatic function,
      109–10
    febrile state, 98
    hepatic disease, 107–8
  elimination, 32, 126–7
apramycin, 124
ascorbic acid, 20
aspirin (acetylsalicylic acid; salicylate)
  bioavailability, 58, 62, 70
  biotransformation processes, 14
  clearance, 43
  elimination, 30, 34
  plasma protein binding, 99–100
  renal clearance, 117
  selective inhibition of enzymes, 155
  species variation in dosage
    requirements, 8
atenolol, 141
  clinical selectivity, 150
  stereoisomerism, 166
atropine, 23, 156
  clinical selectivity, 150–1
avermectins, 78, 163, 185, 189, 190
azathioprine, 120
azithromycin, 221

bacampicillin, 64
bacitracin, 197, 198, 214
baquiloprim, 160
benzimidazole, 22
  bioavailability, 58, 70, 71
  effect of fasting on hepatic function,
    110–12
  species variation in dosage
    requirements, 9
benzocaine, 198

benzyl alcohol, 8
benzyl benzoate, 8, 184, 191
benzyl peroxide, 183
benzylpenicillin, 26
biliary excretion, 15, 25, 28–9
bioavailability, 55–85
  bioequivalence, 82–5
  effect of food, 64–7
  estimation, 56–60
  factors influencing, 60–1
  first-pass effect, 61–4
  intramuscular injection, 74–82
  modified-release dosage forms, 71–4
  rectal, 67–8
  ruminant species, 68–71
bioequivalence, 82–5
biotransformation processes, 10–25
  acetylation, 14, 16, 18–19
  changes in rate of, 22–4
  cutaneous, 183–4
  drug interactions and, 119–21
  first-pass effect, 61–4
  glucorinide synthesis, 16, 17–18, 23, 33,
    114, 184, 220
    neonatal animals, 256–9
  glutathione conjugation, 16, 20, 23
  glycine conjugation, 16, 18
  hydrolysis, 14–16, 18, 24
  hydroxylation, 11–12, 34
  intestinal microorganisms and, 24–5
  metabolic activation, 21–2
  methylation, 16, 20
  microsomal oxidative reactions, 10–13,
    22–3, 62, 64, 114, 119
  neonatal animals, 256–9
  non-microsomal oxidative reactions,
    13–14
  stereoisomerism and, 166
birds
  antimicrobial treatment, 222–3
  biotransformation, 18
  clearance, 43, 45, 124
  elimination, 33, 45
  intramuscular injection, 81
bispyridinium oxime HI-6, 23, 124, 156
bovine mastitis therapy, 246–9
bumetanide, 75–6
bupivacaine, 172
butorphanol tartrate, 32

caffeine
  biotransformation processes, 13
  elimination, 29, 32
calcium disodium edetate, chemical
    antagonism, 157–8
captopril, 142–3

carbamazepine, 22
  dosages, 147
  drug interactions, 120
  elimination, 30
carbaril, 184, 194
carbenicillin, 124, 243
cardiac disease *see* heart disease
cardiac glycosides, 28
carprofen, 28
  selective inhibition of enzymes, 155, 156
  stereoisomerism, 168–9
cats
  antifungal agents, 200, 201, 202
  antimicrobial treatment, 197, 198
  biotransformation, 18, 19, 20, 22, 220
  cardiac drugs, 141, 142
  changes in drug disposition, renal
      clearance, 117
  clearance, 45
  dosage requirements, 6, 7, 8
  drug toxicity
    anthelmintics, 162
    antimicrobials, 160, 161
  ectoparasiticides, 192–6
  elimination, 29, 32, 33, 220
  intramuscular injection, 80, 81
  intravenous anaesthetic agents, 3, 6
  neonatal animals, 258–9
  skin, 178, 182
    topical preparations, 184, 192–6, 200,
        203
  stereoisomerism of drugs and, 168
cattle
  antifungal agents, 200, 202
  antimicrobial agents, bovine mastitis,
      246–9
  bioavailability of drugs, 68–71
    estimation, 58
    intramuscular injection, 78, 79, 80
    modified-release dosage forms, 73–4
  biotransformation, 22
  changes in drug disposition
    drug interactions, 121–2
    effect of fasting on hepatic function,
        111–12
    febrile state, 97–8, 99
    renal clearance, 117
  dosages for, 6, 7, 8, 9, 238
  ectoparasiticides, 186
  elimination, 29, 32, 33, 45, 221, 223
  excretion, 28
  intravenous anaesthetic agents, 6
  mastitis therapy, 246–9
  neonatal animals, 252, 259–60
  skin, 178, 180
    topical preparations, 186, 200

  stereoisomerism of drugs and, 167, 168
cefadroxil, 64, 65, 197, 223, 253
cefazolin, 77, 223
cefixime, 64
cefoperazone, 99, 218, 223, 224, 247
ceftiofur, 21–2
  elimination, 30, 33
  intramuscular injection, 77–8
  neonatal animals, 257
ceftizoxime, 124
ceftriaxone, 99, 103, 218, 223, 224
cefuroxime, 64, 247
cephadrine, 77
cephalexin, 61, 64, 197, 223
cephalosporins, 217, 223
  bioavailability, 64
  elimination, 33
  mechanisms of action, 214, 228
  plasma protein binding, 100
  resistance, 215, 216
  selectivity and toxicity, 160
cephapirin, 124
chelation, 118, 157
chemical antagonism, 157–8
chirality (stereoisomerism), 155–6, 164–73
chloral hydrate, 13
chloramphenicol, 23, 64, 159, 217–18
  bioavailability, 61, 69
  biotransformation processes, 10, 24, 64
  drug interactions, 120
  effect of fasting on hepatic function, 110
  elimination, 32, 33, 220
  mechanism of action, 214
  selective enzyme inhibition, 157
chlordiazepoxide, 77
chlorhexidine gluconate, 199, 200
chlortetracycline, 67, 124, 198
cholestyramine resin, 118
cholinesterase, 7, 23
cimetidine, 23, 116, 201
  drug interactions, 120, 121
  selective enzyme inhibition, 157
ciprofloxacin, 22, 62, 227
  clearance, 43–4, 46
  elimination, 36, 220, 221
  neonatal animals, 255
cisapride, 68
clarithromycin, 64, 221
clavulanate, 76, 224, 243
clavulanic acid, 197
clearance
  renal, 114–17
  systemic, 9, 42–6, 93
clenbuterol, 150
clindamycin, 77, 162, 218, 221
clinical selectivity *see* selectivity

clonazepam, 30, 60
clonidine, 205
clorsulon, 9, 163, 164
closantel, 163–4
　bioavailability, 70
　elimination, 30
　species variation in dosage
　　requirements, 9
clotrimazole, 199, 200
cloxacillin, 103, 218, 223, 247, 248
colistimethate, 161, 162
combination therapies
　antimicrobials, 241–4
　chemotherapy, 158
concentration profile, 1, 2
　clinical effectiveness of antimicrobials
　　and, 228–30
　steady-state plasma concentration,
　　137–40
controlled-release ruminal boluses, 9, 71,
　73–4
corticosteroids
　bovine mastitis therapy, 248
　topical preparations, 202–4
crocodiles, dosage requirements, 7
cross-resistance, 217
culture, bacterial, 233–4
cutaneous biotransformation, 183–4
cyanogenetic glycosides, 24, 69
cypermethrin, 164, 172
　topical preparations, 181, 186, 188, 189,
　　190–1
cyromazine, 189–90
cytarabine, 157
cythioate, 185–6
cytochrome P450 enzymes, 11–13, 14, 22,
　23, 119, 183

deer
　bioavailability of drugs
　　intramuscular injection, 79
　　modified-release dosage forms, 73
　dosage requirements, 6
deltamethrin, 186, 189, 190
desfuroylceftiofur, 21, 22, 227
desmethyldiazepam, 103
detomidine, 32, 151
dexamethasone, 22, 23
dextropropoxyphene, 172
diaminopyrimidines, 160, 217, 218
diazepam, 67, 77
　bioavailability, 61, 68
　biotransformation processes, 10, 62
　changes in drug disposition
　　displacement, 103
　　drug interactions, 120

　plasma protein binding, 101, 102,
　　103
　elimination, 30, 32
　extent of distribution, 39, 92
　interspecies scaling, 124
dichlorodiphenyl-trichloroethane (DDT),
　22, 119
dichlorvos, 184, 192, 194
dicloxacillin, 77, 103
dieldrin, 22, 119
diemthylsulphoxide, 180–1
diet *see* nutrition
diethylcarbamazine, 163
diethyltoluamide, 194
difloxacin, 221
digitalis glycosides, 69
digitoxin, 102, 103
digoxin, 77
　bioavailability, 61, 64
　biotransformation processes, 24
　changes in drug disposition
　　displacement, 103, 119
　　drug interactions, 118
　　renal clearance, 115
　　renal disease, 113, 114
　dosages, 141–2, 146
　elimination, 34, 146
　extent of distribution, 39, 92
diltiazem, 72
dimeticone, 71
dimpylate, 184, 188, 189, 194
diphenhydramine, 152, 158
diphenoxylate, 14
diprenorphine, 6
disease states
　biotransformation processes and, 23–4
　changes in drug disposition and, 93–4,
　　245
　　febrile state, 94–9
disopyramide, 99
disposition of drugs, changes in, 92–129
　displacement, 102–4, 118–19
　drug interactions, 117–22
　effects of fasting on hepatic function,
　　109–12
　febrile state, 94–9
　hepatic disease, 101, 104–9
　interspecies scaling, 122–9
　plasma protein binding, 99–102, 118
　renal clearance, 114–17
　renal disease, 101–2, 112–14
distribution of drugs, 9, 38–41, 92
　antimicrobials, 217–27
　interspecies scaling, 129
　neonatal animals, 254–6
disulfiram, 23

dobutamine
  clinical selectivity, 150
  dosages, 143–4, 148
  stereoisomerism, 172
dogs
  antifungal agents, 200, 201, 202
  antimicrobial treatment, 197, 198
  bioavailability of drugs
    estimation, 58
    first-pass effect, 62
    intramuscular injection, 75, 76, 77, 80,
      81
    modified-release dosage forms, 71,
      72–3
    rectal, 67–8
  biotransformation, 18, 19
  changes in drug disposition
    drug interactions, 119, 120, 121, 122
    febrile state, 94, 95, 98
    hepatic disease, 107, 108
    plasma protein binding, 101, 102
    renal clearance, 115, 117
    renal disease, 113
  clearance, 43, 44, 45
  distribution extent, 40
  dosages, 6–7, 8, 146, 147
    cardiac drugs, 140, 141–2, 144
    clinical selectivity, 150
  drug toxicity
    anthelmintics, 162
    antimicrobials, 161
  duration of therapy, 245
  ectoparasiticides, 192–6
  elimination, 29, 30, 32, 33, 45, 220, 221,
    223, 224
  intravenous anaesthetic agents, 3–4, 6
  neonatal animals, 252
  skin, 178, 182, 200
    irritation, 76
    topical preparations, 192–6, 200, 202,
      203
  stereoisomerism of drugs and, 168, 169,
    170, 171
donkeys
  clearance, 45
  elimination, 30, 33, 35, 223
doramectin, 78, 186, 189, 190
dosages of drugs
  antimicrobial therapy, 235–41
  cardiac drugs, 140–4
  concentration profile, 1, 2, 137–40,
    144–9
  modified-release dosage forms, 9, 71–4
  neonatal animals, 261–4
  pharmacological effect and, 1
  rates, 46–7

regimen, 136–49
  calculation, 2, 40–1
  fluctuations in steady-state plasma
    concentration, 144–9
  species variation in dosage
    requirements, 6–9
doxapram, 158
doxycycline
  bioavailability, 64
  distribution, 39, 223
  elimination, 34, 223
  protein binding, 218
  soluble salt, 60
dromedaries
  bioavailability of drugs, 79
  elimination, 29

ectoparasiticides, topical preparations,
  185–96
elimination of drugs
  antimicrobials, 217–27
  biotransformation, 10–25, 61–4, 119–21
  clearance, 9, 42–6, 93, 114–17
  excretion, 10, 15, 25–9, 33–4, 259–61
  interspecies scaling, 122–9
  plasma protein binding and, 100
  processes, 10–29
  rate of, 29–37
enalapril, 21, 143
enilconazole, 199, 200
enrofloxacin, 197
  bioavailability, 67
  biotransformation processes, 62
  changes in drug disposition
    drug interactions, 120
    febrile state, 96, 97, 98–9
  clearance, 43, 126
  elimination, 33, 36, 220, 221
  interactions, 227, 228
  neonatal animals, 255
enterohepatic circulation, 24, 25, 28, 29, 34,
  118
erythromycin, 23, 64, 159, 162, 221, 222,
  226
  biliary excretion, 28
  bioavailability, 64, 65
  combinations, 243
  elimination, 221
  interspecies scaling, 124
  neonatal animals, 253
  protein binding, 218
  stomach acids and, 61
ethanol
  biotransformation processes, 13, 23
  elimination, 34
etorphine, 6

excretion, 10, 25–9
  by kidneys, 15, 25–8, 33–4
  by liver, 15, 25, 28–9
  neonatal animals, 259–61

febantel, 21, 70, 163, 171
fenbendazole, 21, 163
  bioavailability, 61, 70
  controlled-release bolus, 73
  species variation in dosage
      requirements, 9
  stereoisomerism, 170–1
fenitrothion, 194
fenoprofen, 168
fenoxycarb, 190
fentanyl, 102, 205–6
fenthion, 194
fenvalerate, 194
ferrets, 45
fever, changes in drug disposition and,
      94–9
fipronil, 194
first-pass effect, 61–4
fish
  biotransformation, 18
  clearance, 43, 44, 45, 46
  distribution extent, 40
  dosages for, 241
  drug toxicity
      anthelmintics, 162, 164
      pyrethroids, 189
  ectoparasiticides, 192
  elimination, 33, 35–6, 220, 223, 241
  half-life of drugs, 35–6
flip-flop phenomenon, 58, 77
florfenicol, 36, 216
fluazuron, 186
fluconazole, 199, 200, 201, 214, 263
flucytosine, 22, 157, 159, 161
flumethrin, 188, 189
flunixin
  bioavailability, 77
  bovine mastitis therapy, 248
  elimination, 30, 32
  extent of distribution, 41
  selective inhibition of enzymes, 155
fluocinolone acetonide, 180
fluoroquinolones, 217
  bioavailability, 61, 64
  biotransformation processes, 64
  clinical effectiveness, 229
  distribution, 39, 219
  elimination, 221
  mechanism of action, 214, 229
  resistance, 216
  selectivity and toxicity, 160–1

variables that influence clinical
      response, 245
fluorouracil, 157
fungal infections, 199–202
furosemide
  changes in drug disposition
      displacement, 103, 118
      drug interactions, 122
      renal disease, 113
  dosages, 143–4, 148
  extent of distribution, 39
fusidic acid, 198

gall bladder, 28
gentamicin
  bioavailability, 75
  changes in drug disposition
      drug interactions, 122
      febrile state, 94
      renal clearance, 115
  clearance, 44–6, 115, 123–4, 126
  combinations, 243
  elimination, 33, 224, 259–60
  interspecies scaling, 123–4
  neonatal animals, 259–60
  nephrotoxicity, 161
giraffes, dosage requirements, 6
glucocorticoids, selective inhibition of
      enzymes, 155
glucorinide synthesis, 16, 17–18, 23, 33,
      114, 184, 220
  neonatal animals, 256–9
glucoronyl transferase, 8, 18
ß-glucoside conjugation, 18
glutathione conjugation, 16, 20, 23
glyceryl trinitrate, 64
glycine conjugation, 16, 18
goats, 187
  bioavailability of drugs, 68–71
      intramuscular injection, 79, 81
  changes in drug disposition
      effect of fasting on hepatic function,
          110
      febrile state, 97, 98, 99
      renal clearance, 117
  clearance, 43, 44
  dosage requirements, 9
  elimination, 29, 30, 32, 33, 45, 223
  intravenous anaesthetic agents, 3, 4
  neonatal animals, 257
  skin, 178
  stereoisomerism of drugs and, 171
griseofulvin, 60, 64, 184, 199, 202
guinea pigs
  clearance, 45
  skin, 182

half-life of drugs, 9, 29–37, 93
  applications of, 36–7, 93
  fish, 35–6
  mammals and birds, 29–35
halothane, renal clearance and, 115–16
haloxon, 192
heart disease, 24
  cardiac drugs, 140–4
  changes in drug disposition and, 101
heparin, chemical antagonism, 157
hepatic *see* liver
hetacillin, 64
hexobarbital, 166
hexobarbitone, 32
histamine, 13, 20
horses
  antifungal agents, 200, 201, 202
  antimicrobial treatment, 159, 197, 198,
    199, 213, 222
  bioavailability of drugs
    effect of food, 64–5, 67
    estimation, 58
    intramuscular injection, 75–6, 77, 78,
      80–1
    modified-release dosage forms, 72
    rectal, 67, 68
  cardiac drugs, 140, 141, 142, 144
  changes in drug disposition
    drug interactions, 122
    effect of fasting on hepatic function,
      109–10
    renal clearance, 115, 117
  clearance, 43, 44, 45
  distribution extent, 40
  dosages for, 8, 238, 241
  drug toxicity
    anthelmintics, 162
    antimicrobials, 159
  ectoparasiticides, 190–2
  elimination, 29, 30, 32, 33, 35, 220, 221,
    224
  excretion, 28
  intravenous anaesthetic agents, 6
  neonatal animals, 252, 256, 257–8,
    259–60, 261
  skin, 178, 197, 200
    irritation, 76, 162
    topical preparations, 190–2, 198, 199,
      200, 201, 203
  stereoisomerism of drugs and, 167, 168
  sweat, 180
humans
  changes in drug disposition
    drug interactions, 119
    effect of fasting on hepatic function,
      109

    febrile state, 94
    hepatic disease, 107, 108
    plasma protein binding, 99
    renal clearance, 117
  clearance, 127
  elimination, 29, 30, 32, 35, 223, 224
  excretion, 27
  intravenous anaesthetic agents, 3, 4, 6
  skin, 178, 180, 182, 199
  stereoisomerism of drugs and, 168, 169,
    170, 171
  sweat, 180
hydrocortisone, 180
hydrolysis, 14–16, 18, 24
hydroxylation, 11–12, 34
hypoxanthine, 23

ibuprofen
  displacement, 103
  elimination, 30
  selective inhibition of enzymes, 156
imidazoles, 23, 199, 200
imidocarb, 98
indomethacin
  biliary excretion, 28
  bioavailability, 75
  selective inhibition of enzymes, 155
inherent resistance, 215
interactions of drugs
  antimicrobials, 227–8
  biotransformation processes and,
    119–21
  synergism, 158–9
  see also antagonism; combination
    therapies
intestinal microorganisms
  biotransformation processes and, 24–5
  effects of antimicrobials, 159–60, 213,
    222–3
intraconazole, 200
intramuscular injection
  bioavailability of drugs and, 74–82
  skin irritation, 76, 162
intravenous anaesthetic agents, 2–6
  species variation in drug disposition,
    2–6
ion trapping effect, 92
ionophore antibiotics, 159
ipratropium, 150
isoniazid, 19
isoproterenol, 13
itraconazole, 103, 160, 199
ivermectin, 163, 191–2
  bioavailability, 71, 78, 189
  controlled-release bolus, 73
  extent of distribution, 92

idiosyncratic toxicity of, 6–7
injection, 78, 189, 195
species variation in dosage
    requirements, 9
topical preparations, 186, 189

kanamycin, 161
ketamine
    clearance, 43
    drug interactions, 121–2
    species variation in drug disposition, 4,
        6
    stereoisomerism, 169
ketoconazole, 23, 199, 200, 201
    bioavailability, 64
    changes in drug disposition,
        displacement, 103, 118
    mechanism of action, 214
    selective enzyme inhibition, 157
ketoprofen
    bioavailability, rectal, 68
    changes in drug disposition,
        displacement, 103
    extent of distribution, 41
    selective inhibition of enzymes, 155
    stereoisomerism, 167, 168
kidneys
    changes in drug disposition
        renal clearance, 114–17
        renal disease, 101–2, 112–14
    excretion through, 15, 25–8, 33–4
        neonatal animals, 259–61
    functional units, 25–6
    nephrotoxicity of drugs, 161–2
koalas, 109

levamisole, 162, 163
    bioavailability, 71
    stereoisomerism, 172, 173
    topical preparations, 180, 181
levopropoxyphene, 172
life span, 128
lignocaine, 99
    biotransformation processes, 10, 14, 24
    changes in drug disposition
        drug interactions, 120, 121
        effect of fasting on hepatic function,
            109
        hepatic disease, 107
        plasma protein binding, 102
    dosages, 140
lincomycin, 67, 197, 221
lincosamides, 99, 217
    distribution, 39, 219, 221
    effect on intestinal microorganisms, 159,
        222

elimination, 221
mechanism of action, 214
neonatal animals, 253
protein binding, 218
resistance, 217
selectivity and toxicity, 160
liver
    biotransformation processes in, 10
        microsomal oxidative reactions,
            10–13, 22–3, 62, 64, 114, 119
    changes in drug disposition
        drug interactions, 121
        effects of fasting on hepatic function,
            109–12
        hepatic disease, 101, 104–9
    damage to, 24
    excretion through, 15, 25, 28–9
llamas, 45

macrolides, 23, 99, 217
    distribution, 39, 92, 219, 221
    effect on intestinal microorganisms, 159,
        222
    elimination, 221
    endectocides, 162, 163
    mechanism of action, 214
    protein binding, 218
    resistance, 217
maintenance therapy, 234–5
marbofloxacin, 77, 221
mean residence time, 9, 47–9
meclofenamate, 155
meclofenamic acid, 58, 77
meloxicam, 155
meperidine *see* pethidine
mercaptopurine, 120, 157
metabolic activation, 21–2
metabolism *see* biotransformation
    processes
methaemoglobinaemia, 8
methimazole, 13, 119, 120
methoprene, 190
methotrexate, 116, 122, 124
methscopolamine, 61
methylation, 16, 20
methylthionium chloride, 69
methylxanthines
    biotransformation processes, 13
    elimination, 29
    see also caffeine; theophylline
metoclopramide, 61, 118
metronidazole, 23, 64, 217
    bioavailability, 65
    biotransformation processes, 64
    changes in drug disposition, drug
        interactions, 120

dosages, 8, 47, 238
  extent of distribution, 39
  mechanism of action, 214
  resistance, 215
  topical preparations, 184
miconazole, 199, 200, 214
microorganisms, intestinal *see* intestinal
    microorganisms
microsomal oxidative reactions, 10–13,
    22–3, 62, 64, 114, 119
milbemycins, 78, 163, 185, 195
minocycline, 34, 223
modified-release dosage forms,
    bioavailability of drugs and, 71–4
monensin, 71, 159
monkeys
  elimination, 30, 32
  skin, 182, 183
  stereoisomerism of drugs and, 168
monofluoroacetate, 22, 156
monofluorocitrate, 22, 156
morantel, 9, 73, 163
morphine
  biliary excretion, 28
  biotransformation processes, 24
  changes in drug disposition, renal
      disease, 113
  dosages, 6, 8
    sustained-release dosage forms, 72
moxidectin, 78, 186, 195–6

nabumetone, 155
nafcillin, 223, 224
naproxen, 146
  displacement, 103, 118
  dosages, 146
  elimination, 30
  plasma protein binding, 99, 103
  selective inhibition of enzymes, 155, 156
  stereoisomerism, 166, 167
natamycin, 199, 201–2, 214
neomycin, 161, 162, 197–8
neonatal animals, 252–64
  absorption, 253
  distribution, 254–6
  drug selection and administration,
      261–4
  excretion, 259–61
  metabolism, 256–9
neostigmine, 23
nerve gases, 23, 156
netobimin, 21, 70, 120, 163, 171
nimesulide, 155
nitrite poisoning, 69
nitrofurantoin, 64
nitrofurazone, 198

nitroglycerin, 64, 205
nitroimidazoles, 10
nitroxynil, 10, 24, 69, 163, 164
non-microsomal oxidative reactions,
    13–14
non-steroidal anti-inflammatory drugs
    (NSAIDs)
  bovine mastitis therapy, 248
  neonatal animals, 257–8
  selective inhibition of enzymes, 153,
      155–6
  stereoisomerism, 167–8
noradrenaline, 20
norfloxacin, 30, 33, 61, 221, 227
nutrition
  biotransformation processes and, 16
  effect of food on bioavailability of
      drugs, 64–7
  effects of fasting on hepatic function,
      109–12
nystatin, 199, 201

obidoxime, 23
organophosphates, 23, 156, 162
  topical preparations, 182, 188–9
ornithine, 18
oxazepam, 102, 103
oxfendazole
  bioavailability, 70
  controlled-release bolus, 73–4
  species variation in dosage
      requirements, 9
oxidative reactions, 10–14
oxprenolol, 102
oxyclozanide, 70, 163
oxyphenbutazone, 118
oxytetracycline, 197, 199, 226
  bioavailability, 59, 67, 79, 80
  bovine mastitis therapy, 247
  changes in drug disposition, febrile
      state, 96, 97
  clearance, 46, 126
  dosage, 237–8, 240–1
  elimination, 34, 35–6, 223, 241, 260–1
  interspecies scaling, 124
  neonatal animals, 260–1
  soluble salt, 60
  topical preparations, 198
oxytocin, 249

paracetamol
  biotransformation processes, 20
  effect of fasting on hepatic function,
      109
  toxicity, 8, 20, 22
parathion, 22, 181

penicillins, 26, 197, 198, 217, 223
  bioavailability, 64, 65, 67
    intramuscular injection, 80–1
  changes in drug disposition
    drug interactions, 118, 122
    febrile state, 95, 96–7
    renal clearance, 116
  combinations, 243
  dosages, 238, 241
  effect on intestinal microorganisms, 159
  elimination, 33
  mechanisms of action, 214, 228–9
  neonatal animals, 253, 263
  plasma protein binding, 100, 223–4
  resistance, 215, 216
  selectivity and toxicity, 159, 160
  stomach acids and, 61
pentobarbital, 3, 102
permethrin, 164
  topical preparations, 181, 186, 190, 191,
    192, 194
pethidine, 99
  biotransformation processes, 24
  elimination, 32
  extent of distribution, 92
phenacetin, 20
phenobarbital, 22, 60, 68
phenobarbitone, 62, 119, 146
  dosages, 146
  drug interactions, 119
  elimination, 30, 33
  renal clearance, 117
phenoxybenzamine, 153
phenylbutazone, 22, 28, 116, 119
  bioavailability, 58, 61, 67
  biotransformation processes, 62
  changes in drug disposition
    displacement, 103, 118
    drug interactions, 120, 122
    plasma protein binding, 102, 103
  clearance, 43
  elimination, 29, 30, 34
  extent of distribution, 39, 41
  selective inhibition of enzymes, 155
phenytoin, 22, 67, 77, 119
  clearance, 43
  displacement, 118, 119
  drug interactions, 119, 120
  elimination, 30
  soluble salt, 60
  sustained-release dosage forms, 72
phosmet, 186, 194
physiological antagonism, 158
physostigmine, 23
pigs
  antimicrobials, 197, 198

bioavailability of drugs
  effect of food, 67
  intramuscular injection, 78, 79, 80, 81
changes in drug disposition
  febrile state, 96–7, 98–9
  plasma protein binding, 102
clearance, 43, 44
dosages for, 238
ectoparasiticides, 190
elimination, 32, 33, 35, 223
intravenous anaesthetic agents, 6
neonatal animals, 252, 260
skin, 178, 182
  topical preparations, 190, 198
piperazine, 163
piperonyl butoxide, 159, 190, 191, 192
piroxicam, 155
pivampicillin, 21
  bioavailability, 62, 64, 65
  neonatal animals, 253
plasma
  concentration profile
    clinical effectiveness of antimicrobials
      and, 228–30
    fluctuations in steady-state plasma
      concentration, 144–9
  drug concentration profile, 1, 2
    steady-state plasma concentration,
      137–40
  plasma protein binding, 92, 99–102, 218,
    223–4
    drug displacement and, 102–4, 118–19
poloxalene, 71
polychlorinated biphenyls (PCBs), 22, 119
polyethylene glycol, 198
polymyxins, 161, 162, 197, 198, 214
povidone-iodine, 199
pralidoxime, 23, 156
praziquantel, 163
prednisolone, 124
primidone, 62
probenecid, 122, 224
  inhibition of tubular secretion by, 26,
    116, 122
procainamide, 116
  biotransformation processes, 14, 19
  dosages, 140
    sustained-release dosage forms, 72
  elimination, 33
procaine, 14, 118, 197, 226, 238
prodrugs
  effect of foods, 64
  metabolic activation, 21–2, 24
prontosil, 10
propantheline, 61, 150
propetamphos, 188, 189

propofol, 4, 43
propoxur, 184, 194
propoxyphene, 114
propranolol, 99
  antagonism, 152
  bioavailability, 61
  biotransformation processes, 10, 24,
    183–4
  changes in drug disposition
    drug interactions, 120, 121
    hepatic disease, 107
    plasma protein binding, 102
    renal disease, 114
  clinical selectivity, 150
  dosages, 140–1
    sustained-release dosage forms, 72
  extent of distribution, 92
  soluble salt, 60
  stereoisomerism, 166, 170, 172, 184
propylene glycol, 77, 180, 198
protamine, 157
pseudocholinesterase, 7, 14
pyrantel, 163
pyrethrins, 159, 164, 172, 192–3
pyrimethamine, 65, 160, 214

quinidine, 77, 99
  dosages, 140, 142
    sustained-release dosage forms, 72
  drug interactions, 119
  plasma protein binding, 101, 102
  soluble salt, 60
quinine, 96

rabbits
  atropine resistance, 151
  changes in drug disposition
    febrile state, 98
    hepatic disease, 106
  clearance, 45
  elimination, 223
  skin, 182
rafoxanide, 70, 163–4
rats
  dosage requirements, 7
  skin, 182
  stereoisomerism of drugs and, 168, 171
rectal bioavailability of drugs, 67–8
renal *see* kidneys
reptiles
  bioavailability of drugs, 81
  clearance, 124
  dosages for, 241
  elimination, 33, 241
resistance
  antimicrobials, 214–17

    acquired, 215–17
    cross-resistance, 217
    inherent, 215
    transferable, 217
rifampin, 22, 64, 119, 217
  bioavailability, 65
  biotransformation processes, 64
  combinations, 243
  drug interactions, 119
  elimination, 34
  extent of distribution, 39
  mechanism of action, 214
  resistance, 215, 216, 217
  synergism, 159
rofecoxib, 155

salicylanilides, 163
salicylate *see* aspirin
sarin, 23, 156
selamectin, 196, 204
selectivity
  antimicrobials and anthelmintics,
    159–64
  selective tissue binding, 92
  significance of antagonism, 141, 151–3
    chemical, 157–8
    pharmacological, 151–3
    physiological, 158
    selective inhibition of enzymes, 153–7
sheep
  bioavailability of drugs, 68–71
    intramuscular injection, 75, 77–8
    modified-release dosage forms, 73
  changes in drug disposition
    drug interactions, 120
    febrile state, 99
  clearance, 43
  distribution extent, 40
  dosage requirements, 9
  elimination, 29, 30, 33, 35, 37, 223, 224
  excretion, 28
  footrot, 197
  intravenous anaesthetic agents, 3, 6
  neonatal animals, 252
  skin, 180
    topical preparations, 187–9
  stereoisomerism of drugs and, 167, 171
skin, 178–9
  irritation through intramuscular
    injection, 76, 162
  sweat, 180
  see also topical preparations
slow-release ruminal boluses, 71, 73
sodium nitrite, 69
sodium thiosulphate, 69
soman, 23, 156

sotalol, 140–1
spiramycin, 67
spironolactone, 60, 152
steady-state plasma concentration, 137–40
    fluctuations in, 144–9
stereoisomerism, 155–6, 164–73
steroids, topical preparations, 202–4
streptomycin, 161
succinylcholine, 7, 14, 121
sulbactam, 224
sulindac, 28, 155
sulphadiazine, 197
    bioavailability, 67
    bovine mastitis therapy, 247
    changes in drug disposition, renal
        clearance, 117
    clearance, 44, 117
    elimination, 33, 35, 220–1, 241
    neonatal animals, 256
    topical preparations, 198
sulphadimethoxine
    biotransformation processes, 19
    elimination, 33
    febrile state and, 96, 97
    protein binding, 218
sulphadimidine, 46, 96, 97
sulphamethazine, 30, 70
sulphamethoxazole, 96, 97
sulphasalazine, 24
sulphate conjugation, 16
sulphathiazole, 15
sulphisoxazole, 19
sulphobromophthalein (BSP), 28, 109
sulphonamides, 217
    bioavailability, 64
    biotransformation processes, 64
    changes in drug disposition
        febrile state, 96
        plasma protein binding, 99, 100
    clearance, 44
    combinations, 243
    elimination, 32, 34
    extent of distribution, 39
    mechanism of action, 214
    resistance, 216–17
    selectivity and toxicity, 160
    synergism, 158
susceptibility testing, 233–4
sustained-release dosage forms, 71–3
suxibuzone, 61
sweat, 180
synergism, 158–9
systemic clearance, 9, 42–6, 93

tabun, 23
teflubenzuron, 192

terrapins, 7
tetracyclines, 217
    biliary excretion, 28
    bioavailability, 64, 67
    changes in drug disposition
        drug interactions, 118
        plasma protein binding, 99
        renal disease, 113
    distribution, 39, 219, 223
    effect on intestinal microorganisms, 159
    elimination, 34, 223
    interspecies scaling, 124
    mechanism of action, 214
    resistance, 215, 216, 217
    selectivity and toxicity, 160
theophylline, 8, 23, 46
    biotransformation processes, 13
    changes in drug disposition
        drug interactions, 120
        plasma protein binding, 101
    clearance, 46, 126–7
    dosages, 147
        sustained-release dosage forms, 72
    elimination, 29, 32
    interactions, 227–8
thiamylal, 3–4, 5
thiopental, 3–4, 5, 99
thiopentone, 3, 5
tiamulin, 222
ticarcillin, 76, 216, 243
timolol, 150
tinidazone, 220
tobramycin, 161
tolfenamic acid, 155
tolnaftate, 199, 202
topical preparations, 178–206
    absorption process, 179–81
    antibacterial agents, 196–9
    antifungal agents, 199–202
    corticosteroids, 202–4
    cutaneous biotransformation, 183–4
    ectoparasiticides, 185–96
    species variations, 181–3
    susceptibility of cats, 184
    transdermal therapeutic systems, 204–6
tortoises, 7
toxicity, 148
    chemical antagonism in treatment of,
        157–8
    nephrotoxicity, 161–2
    selective inhibition of enzymes, 156–7
transdermal therapeutic systems, 204–6
transferable resistance, 217
triamterene, 102
triazoles, 200
triclabendazole, 21, 61, 70, 163

trimethoprim, 99, 159, 160, 197
  bioavailability, 64, 65, 67, 69
  biotransformation processes, 24, 64
  bovine mastitis therapy, 247
  changes in drug disposition
    febrile state, 96, 97, 98
    renal clearance, 117
  clearance, 44
  combinations, 243
  distribution, 39, 219
  dosages, 241
  elimination, 30, 33, 35
  neonatal animals, 253, 256, 257
  selectivity and toxicity, 160
  synergism, 158
turtles, 7

urinary pH, 27–8, 34, 116–17

valproate, 30, 103, 105, 118
valproic acid, 72–3, 99, 147
vancomycin, 214
verapamil
  stereoisomerism, 166, 169–70, 173
  sustained-release dosage forms, 72
VX nerve gas, 156

warfarin, 103, 106, 118, 119

xylazine, 32
  clinical selectivity, 151
  drug interactions, 121–2
  extent of distribution, 39, 40, 92
  species variation in dosage
    requirements, 6

young *see* neonatal animals